T0127651

A Systematic Review of Key Issues in Public Health

Stefania Boccia • Paolo Villari • Walter Ricciardi
Editors

A Systematic Review of Key Issues in Public Health

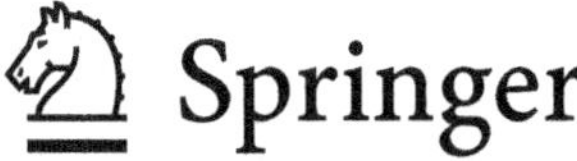

Editors
Stefania Boccia
Università Cattolica del Sacro Cuore
Institute of Hygiene Faculty of Medicine
Rome
Italy

Walter Ricciardi
Institute of Hygiene, Faculty of Medicine
Università Cattolica del Sacro Cuore
Rome
Italy

Paolo Villari
Public Health and Infectious Diseases
Sapienza University of Rome
Rome
Italy

ISBN 978-3-319-37482-6 ISBN 978-3-319-13620-2 (eBook)
DOI 10.1007/978-3-319-13620-2

Springer Cham Heidelberg New York Dordrecht London

Softcover reprint of the hardcover 1st edition 2015

Printed on acid-free paper

Springer is part of Springer Science+Business Media (www.springer.com)

Preface

Anyone watching the television news or reading a newspaper today, in 2014, could be forgiven for lapsing into despair. Europe has yet to emerge from the longest economic recession in over 500 years and its leading political institutions show no sign of even understanding its main cause, their collective failure to tackle the reckless, and in some cases criminal behaviour of the corporate financial institutions. In several parts of the globe, such as Central Africa and the Middle East, conflicts are wreaking carnage among innocent bystanders on a massive scale, often involving unspeakable atrocities, in some cases by states using sophisticated modern weapons to attack densely populated areas. Countries that once aspired to lofty principles of democracy and freedom have been exposed as being engaged in kidnapping (now sanitised by the term "rendition") and torture. In many places, including parts of Western Europe, anyone who is in any way different, by virtue of their skin colour or the outward signs of their religious belief, risks persecution or worse, with explicitly racist parties achieving significant electoral success for the first time since the 1930s. Politicians, who now including a vanishingly small number of individuals with any scientific training, let alone understanding, are incapable of responding to the profound damage we are doing to our environments, remaining in denial and the evidence of harm accumulates. Media commentators offer not hope for a better future but gloom and doom, representing older people who would once have been valued for their accumulated wisdom as a burden that can no longer be afforded.

Yet, as has so often been the case in the past, times of crisis bring out the best in some people, who have the vision to see into the future, to make the connections, and to propose workable solutions. The challenges listed above have two main things in common. They all have profound implications for population health and they are all what are termed "wicked" problems, characterised by incomplete information and complex interdependencies and thus resistant to easy solutions. They require joined up thinking on a large-scale, drawing on a broad range of disciplinary perspectives, from epidemiology and statistics to sociology and political science. As the editors of this excellent volume note, the skills required are those of a participant in the decathlon. The decathlete may not have the speed off the blocks of Usain Bolt or the endurance of Mo Farah, but they instead have the combination of talents in a broad range of areas that are required to find possible solutions to these wicked problems.

This book is in many ways a manual for the public health decathlete, although the editors have gone much further by including 15, not 10, items. These items cover many of the contemporary challenges confronting population health. Seven chapters review the changing burden of disease and injury, providing many examples of the tremendous successes of the public health community. The most celebrated have been those in the struggle against communicable disease, with the authors noting achievements in transforming acquired immune deficiency syndrome (AIDS) into a condition that those infected die with rather than from. However, there are others, less well-recognised, such as the 50 % decline in mortality from cardiovascular disease in North Western Europe in the past four decades. Yet, as the authors of all of these chapters note, progress is not inevitable. Communicable diseases that once seemed to be coming under control are reappearing, such as tuberculosis, but now in a much more alarming drug-resistant form. Indeed, antimicrobial resistance is now recognised as a global threat, potentially posing an existential threat to humanity, just like climate change. Failure by governments to act against the vectors of non-communicable disease, and especially the major corporations that profit from sales of unhealthy products, for example by placing considerations of health above those of trade liberalisation, has permitted the spread of obesogenic and alcogenic environments, with profound consequences for our future health.

Other chapters in this volume explore topics that, while not exactly new, have achieved much greater importance in recent decades. These include the topic on urban health. Even though it has long been known that those who moved to the cities that emerged during the industrial revolution became less healthy than those who stayed in the countryside, the growth of megacities has created health challenges on an entirely different scale. They also include public mental health, long put in a distant second place by public health professionals, echoing the way in which those with mental illness were themselves confined in faraway places, behind high walls where they could be kept out of sight. 150 years on, Gregor Mendel would be astonished at the progress that has been made since his experiments with cross pollination of peas. Genomics brings many opportunities for our understanding of the aetiology of disease and, by enabling improved therapeutic targeting, potentially some advances in treatment. Yet, by creating yet another way to separate groups within the population, it also poses threats to collective actions based on solidarity. It is an issue that is poorly understood by many commentators, as is ageing, also addressed in this volume. The fact that populations are ageing should surely be celebrated as a success, yet too often it is seen as a threat. As the authors note, the challenge is to achieve active ageing, adding life to years and not simply years to life.

As the authors of these individual chapters show, the challenge of understanding and responding to these issues must be based on concerted interdisciplinary activities, drawing together those with a range of skills and expertise. However, the whole is greater than the sum of the individual parts, so two concluding chapters look at the ways of bringing these issues together, highlighting the need to embed health in all policies (including those where it is too often absent, such as fiscal, defence, and criminal justice policies) and to undertake assessments of the health impacts of all policies. Reflecting on the situation today, had someone assessed, and taken seriously, the health impact of the austerity policies still being pursued in many countries, many of those who found life no longer worth living might still be alive today.

The need for active, engaged, informed, and highly skilled public health professionals is greater now than ever, if we are to raise awareness of the health consequences of the many challenges we now face and are to offer workable solutions. This excellent book, written by some of Europe's leading experts on public health, will help to achieve this goal.

Professor of European Public Health Martin McKee
London School of Hygiene and Tropical Medicine

Contents

1 **Introduction and Global Burden of Disease** 1
Andrea Silenzi, Maria Rosaria Gualano and Walter Ricciardi

2 **Health Trends of Communicable Diseases** 5
Alessio Santoro, Benedetto Simone and Aura Timen

3 **Global Burden and Health Trends of Non-Communicable Diseases** 19
Silvio Capizzi, Chiara de Waure and Stefania Boccia

4 **Cardiovascular Disease (CVD)** 33
Elvira D´Andrea, Iveta Nagyova and Paolo Villari

5 **Epidemiology of Cancer and Principles of Prevention** 65
Stefania Boccia, Carlo La Vecchia and Paolo Boffetta

6 **Obesity and Diabetes** 89
Anna Maria Ferriero and Maria Lucia Specchia

7 **Respiratory Diseases and Health Disorders Related to Indoor and Outdoor Air Pollution** 109
Francesco Di Nardo and Patrizia Laurenti

8 **Public Health Gerontology and Active Aging** 129
Andrea Poscia, Francesco Landi and Agnese Collamati

9 **Some Ethical Reflections in Public Health** 153
Maria Luisa Di Pietro

10 **Injury Prevention and Safety Promotion** 169
Johan Lund, Paolo Di Giannantonio and Alice Mannocci

11 Migrant and Ethnic Minority Health ... 189
M.L. Essink-Bot, C.O Agyemang, K Stronks and A Krasnik

12 Public Mental Health ... 205
Chiara Cadeddu, Carolina Ianuale and Jutta Lindert

13 Urban Public Health ... 223
Umberto Moscato and Andrea Poscia

14 Genomics and Public Health ... 249
Stefania Boccia and Ron Zimmern

15 Health Impact Assessment: HIA ... 263
Roberto Falvo, Marcia Regina Cubas and Gabriel Gulis

16 Health in All Policies ... 277
Agnese Lazzari, Chiara de Waure and Natasha Azzopardi-Muscat

Index ... 287

Contributors

C.O Agyemang Department of Public Health, Academic Medical Center—University of Amsterdam, Amsterdam, The Netherlands

Natasha Azzopardi Muscat Department of Health Services Management, Faculty of Health Sciences, University of Malta, Msida, Malta

Benedetto Simone Institute of Public Health, Section of Hygiene, Università Cattolica del Sacro Cuore, L. go F. Vito 1, Rome, Italy

Paolo Boffetta Mount Sinai School of Medicine Tisch Cancer Institute, New York, NY, USA

Chiara Cadeddu Institute of Public Health, Section of Hygiene, Università Cattolica del Sacro Cuore, Rome, Italy

Silvio Capizzi Institute of Public Health, Section of Hygiene, Università Cattolica del Sacro Cuore, L. go F. Vito 1, Rome, Italy

Agnese Collamati Institute of Gerontology, Università Cattolica del Sacro Cuore, L.go F. Vito 1, Rome, Italy

Elvira D'Andrea Department of Public Health and Infectious Diseases, Sapienza University of Rome, ple Aldo Moro 5, Rome, Italy

Chiara de Waure Institute of Public Health, Section of Hygiene, Università Cattolica del Sacro Cuore, Rome, Italy

Paolo Di Giannantonio Institute of Public Health, Section of Hygiene, Università Cattolica del Sacro Cuore, Rome, Italy

Francesco Di Nardo Institute of Public Health, Section of Hygiene, Università Cattolica del Sacro Cuore, Rome, Italy

M.L. Essink-Bot Department of Public Health, Academic Medical Center—University of Amsterdam, Amsterdam, The Netherlands

Roberto Falvo Section of Hygiene, Institute of Public Health, Università Cattolica del Sacro Cuore, Rome, Italy

Anna Maria Ferriero Section of Hygiene, Institute of Public Health, Università Cattolica del Sacro Cuore, Rome, Italy

Gualano Department of Public Health Sciences, University of Turin, Turin, Italy

Gabriel Gulis Unit for Health Promotion Research, University of Southern Denmark, Esbjerg, Denmark

Carolina Ianuale Institute of Public Health, Section of Hygiene, Università Cattolica del Sacro Cuore, Rome, Italy

A Krasnik Faculty of Health Sciences Department of Public Health CSS, Danish Research Centre for Migration Ethnicity and Health (MESU) University of Copenhagen, Copenhagen, Denmark

Carlo La Vecchia Department of Clinical Sciences and Community Health, Universitá degli Studi di Milano, Milan, Italy

Francesco Landi Institute of Gerontology, Catholic University of Sacred Heart, Rome, Italy

Patrizia Laurenti Institute of Public Health, Section of Hygiene, Università Cattolica del Sacro Cuore, Rome, Italy

Agnese Lazzari Institute of Public Health, Section of Hygiene, Università Cattolica del Sacro Cuore, Rome, Italy

Jutta Lindert Protestant University of Ludwigsburg, Ludwigsburg, Germany University of Leipzig, Leipzig, Germany

Harvard School of Public Health, Boston, USA

Maria Luisa Di Pietro Institute of Public Health, Section of Hygiene, Università Cattolica del Sacro Cuore, Rome, Italy

Johan Lund Institute of Health and Society, Section for Social Medicine, University of Oslo, Oslo, Norway

Alice Mannocci Department of Public Health and Infectious Diseases, Sapienza University of Rome, Rome, Italy

Umberto Moscato Institute of Public Health, Section of Hygiene, Università Cattolica del Sacro Cuore, L.go F. Vito 1, Rome, Italy

Iveta Nagyova Department of Public Health, PJ Safarik University, Kosice, Tr SNP 1, Slovakia

Andrea Poscia Institute of Public Health, Section of Hygiene, Università Cattolica del Sacro Cuore, Rome, Italy

Marcia Regina Cubas Pós-Graduação em Tecnologia em Saúde, Pontifícia Universidade Católica do Paraná, Curitiba, PR, Brazil

Walter Ricciardi Institute of Public Health, Section of Hygiene, Università Cattolica del Sacro Cuore, Rome, Italy

Alessio Santoro Institute of Public Health, Section of Hygiene, Università Cattolica del Sacro Cuore, Rome, Italy

Andrea Silenzi Institute of Public Health, Section of Hygiene, Università Cattolica del Sacro Cuore, Rome, Italy

Maria Lucia Specchia Section of Hygiene, Institute of Public Health, Università Cattolica del Sacro Cuore, Rome, Italy

K Stronks Department of Public Health, Academic Medical Center—University of Amsterdam, Amsterdam, The Netherlands

Aura Timen Centre for Infectious Disease Control, National Institute of Public Health and the Environment, Bilthoven, The Netherlands

Paolo Villari Department of Public Health and Infectious Diseases, Sapienza University of Rome, ple Aldo Moro 5, Rome, Italy

Ron Zimmern PHG Foundation, Cambridge, UK

Chapter 1
Introduction and Global Burden of Disease

Andrea Silenzi, Maria Rosaria Gualano and Walter Ricciardi

In 1920, when two young undergraduates of Yale University visited Charles-Edward Amory Winslow in his laboratory and asked him whether to take up a career in public health, he answered: "it is essential that worker in this domain of applied science should see clearly the goal toward which he is aiming, however far ahead of the immediate possibilities of the moment it may appear to be".

This advice, after about a 100 years, is valid now more than ever. Every worker involved in the protean field of public health has to face multifactorial problems that, actually, represent extremely interesting challenges and incentives to practice the "science and art of preventing disease, prolonging life and promoting health through the organized efforts of society" [1].

If we want to compare the public health professional with an athlete and his sport, certainly the discipline that is more likely to be used as a paradigm would be the decathlon. In fact, if the decathlon is a "combined event in athletics consisting of ten track and field events", public health incorporates a real interdisciplinary approach based on epidemiology, biostatistics and health planning [2]. Environmental health, community health, behavioural health, health economics, public policy, insurance medicine and occupational medicine are other important and apparently different subfields, linked by the mainstream of prevention.

A. Silenzi (✉) · W. Ricciardi
Institute of Public Health, Section of Hygiene, Università Cattolica del Sacro Cuore, L.go F. Vito 1, 00168 Rome, Italy
e-mail: andrea.silenzi@rm.unicatt.it

M. R. Gualano
Department of Public Health Sciences University of Turin P.zza Polonia 94, 10126 Turin, Italy
e-mail: mar.guala@gmail.com

W. Ricciardi
e-mail: wricciardi@rm.unicatt.it

S. Boccia et al. (eds.), *A Systematic Review of Key Issues in Public Health*,
DOI 10.1007/978-3-319-13620-2_1

It is intuitive and also supported by evidences that tackling causes of diseases can prevent much premature death and suffering.

In fact, the removal of upstream causes is often more cost-effective than the removal of proximal medical causes since upstream causes bring about a plethora of downstream sufferings: this is one of the goals of public health.

Similarly, another goal of this discipline is to take care of health and wellbeing of people, both in the individual dimension and in the community. This means, primarily, promoting a longer life with a better quality of living, free from disease and disability.

Several key principles are inherent in the public health approach: the importance of analysing the problem (any disease but also a new policy, a new model of health care delivery, etc.) with an epidemiologic method, proposing a solution and, finally, assessing the impact of interventions; the need for flexibility and urgency in response to ongoing monitoring and operational research; the need to intervene against health inequalities, no matter how difficult it is to access occurrences of the problem or how minor the perceived problem is in a particular community [3].

Indubitably, the epidemiological transition that signed the last century, witnessed by a sudden and stark increase in population growth rates (brought about by medical innovation in disease or sickness therapy and treatment), accounts for the replacement of infectious diseases by non-communicable diseases over time. This was due to better treatments and new technologies used in medical practice and widespread sanitation, but even more to a growing public health approach all over the world. In fact, during the twentieth century, heart diseases, cancer and other chronic conditions assumed more dominant roles and new concerns also came to medical attention (e.g. the terrifying consequences of thermonuclear war, the effects of environmental pollution and climate change) [4]. At the moment, optimism about prospects for the health of future generations persists but remains tempered by the concern about the "pathologies of civilization". An obesity epidemic, feared at the beginning of the 1900s, has become a reality and the management of an increasing community of elderly people represents the most challenging duty to face nowadays. Our previously steady increase in life expectancy has stalled, as reported in different national statistical and epidemiological reports, and may even be reversed [5].

Currently, the protean dynamism of the burden of disease poses challenges: how do we define disease meaningfully, and how do we measure our burden of disease and set health policy priorities? Although repeated assessment of burden of disease would allow comparisons between populations and over time, since mortality and morbidity are multifactorial, any changes in terms of incidence and prevalence are difficult to attribute to actions taken by the health sector in terms of planning and management.

A given health system might achieve the best possible population health, given its budget, but burden of disease could increase because of changes in other causes of disease (e.g. changing food supply or climatic conditions). Similarly, a system might provide substandard care while burden of disease falls. Even in high-income countries, the correlation between quality of care and mortality is low [6].

Public health shapes the context within people and communities can be safe and healthy and, by its very nature, it requires support by citizens, its beneficiaries [7]. For this reason, some authors suggest that the best way to improve population health is to think less about the organization and more about the solutions and high-value interventions, starting from the citizens' perspectives [8].

We need to know that, due to budget limits, a decision to invest in a particular set of interventions means that we are implicitly deciding not to invest in others. And "even if an effective intervention is delivered at high quality without waste, it may still represent low value if greater value could be achieved by using that resources to treat another group of patient" [9].

Often there is only a tenuous link between research questions and the decision on problems faced by policymakers aiming to maximise health, and only by prioritising high-value interventions, we will make the most of available resources.

The mission of public health is to maximise population health, changing culture, orienting and influencing decision-making, taking into account and promoting equity and social values.

The important issues are those we can do something about, those for which we have effective interventions because "the world changes when the boldest thinking is directed at the toughest problems".

Public health is innovation and

> [...] it simply requires thinking in new ways about the barriers that prevent progress [because] innovation is not a single solution. It is a process. It is a frame of mind, a way of constantly looking at problems from new angles so that you can see more and more powerful solutions, try them out, and keep improving on them. [10]

The topics addressed with this book are relevant more than ever at this time, because the financial crisis across Western countries has increased the awareness of maximizing health benefits with the lowest possible expenditure.

In this book, a comprehensive review of different key issues in public health will illustrate some of the challenges they pose worldwide and a systematic report of the best practice example in terms of cost-effectiveness of certain health policy intervention might help policymakers to engage more meaningful and successful decisions.

References

1. Winslow CEA (1920) The untilled fields of public health. Science 51(1306):23–33
2. "Decathlon" Wikipedia. Available at http://en.wikipedia.org/wiki/Decathlon. Accessed 28 March 2014
3. Guest C, Ricciardi W, Kawachi I, Lang I (2013) Oxford handbook of public health practice, 3rd edn. Oxford University Press, Oxford
4. Jones DS, Podolsky SH, Greene JA (2012) The burden of disease and the changing task of medicine. N Engl J Med 366:2333–2338
5. The National Observatory on Health Status in the Italian Regions (2012). Osservasalute Report. Prex, Milan, Italy

6. Roberts I, Jackson R (2013) Beyond disease burden: towards solution-oriented population health. Lancet 381(9884):2219–2221
7. Institute of Medicine (1988) The future of public health. National Academies Press, Washington, DC
8. Gray JAM (2007) How to get better value healthcare. Offox, Oxford
9. Gray JAM (2013) The shift to personalised and population medicine. Lancet 382(9888):200–201
10. Gates M (2013) Reinvent a better world: a series. "Impatient Optimists Blog" by Bill and Melinda Gates Fundation. Avaible at http://www.impatientoptimists.org/Posts/2013/08/The-Key-to-Reinventing-a-Better-World. Accessed 28 March 2014

Chapter 2
Health Trends of Communicable Diseases

Alessio Santoro, Benedetto Simone and Aura Timen

Introduction

Although the burden of communicable diseases has been steadily decreasing in past decades in industrialised countries, it is still considerable worldwide. Lower respiratory infections, diarrhoeal disease and HIV/acquired immunodeficiency syndrome (AIDS) are still among the top major killers in 2011 (Fig. 2.1, the ten leading causes of death in the world in 2011 according to the World Health Organization), and communicable diseases in general are responsible for considerable morbidity in all parts of the world [1].

There is, however, a marked difference in terms of burden of disease, morbidity and mortality between industrialized low-income countries.

In industrialized countries, chronic diseases such as cardiovascular diseases, cancer and diabetes have the highest burden. In low-income countries, infectious diseases still represent the biggest issue. Lower respiratory infections, HIV/AIDS,

A. Santoro (✉) · B. Simone
Institute of Public Health, Section of Hygiene, Università Cattolica del Sacro Cuore,
L.go F. Vito 1, 00168 Rome, Italy
e-mail: alessio.santoro@live.it

B. Simone
e-mail: benedetto.simone@yahoo.it

A. Timen
Centre for Infectious Disease Control, National Institute of Public Health and the Environment,
P.O. box 1, 3720 BA Bilthoven, The Netherlands
e-mail: aura.timen@rivm.nl

S. Boccia et al. (eds.), *A Systematic Review of Key Issues in Public Health*,
DOI 10.1007/978-3-319-13620-2_2

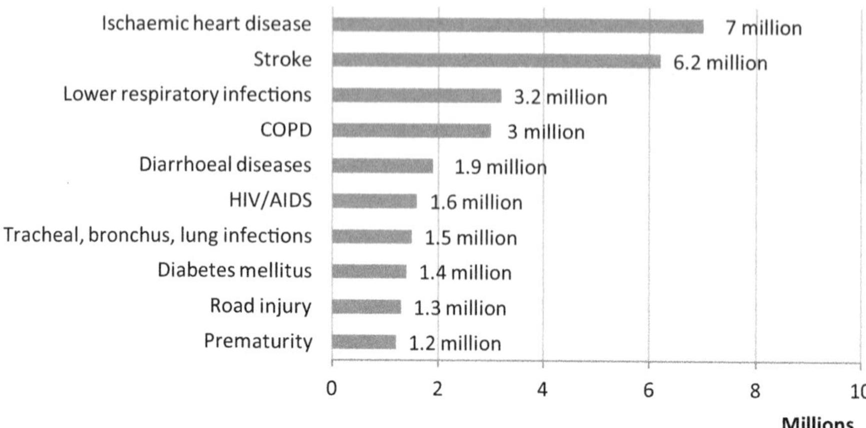

Fig. 2.1 The ten leading causes of death in the world in 2011 according to the World Health Organization [1]. *COPD* chronic obstructive pulmonary disease

diarrhoeal diseases, malaria and tuberculosis (TB) collectively account for around one third of all deaths.

Despite these differences, there is a wide range of emerging and re-emerging infectious diseases with varying potentials for spread in the world. Multidrug-resistant (MDR) TB and vancomycin-resistant *Staphylococcus aureus* are examples of emerging infections that do not immediately involve large numbers of persons but that will ultimately have a serious impact on public health throughout the world [1].

This chapter considers a selected number of infectious diseases, or of groups of diseases, which, for their burden, are of particular importance in low-income or in industrialized countries.

Tuberculosis

Mycobacterium tuberculosis is an aerogenic transmitted agent which represents the most frequent cause of TB. *Mycobacterium tuberculosis* can stay latent for years; symptoms, which can be both pulmonary and extra-pulmonary, occur when, under favourable conditions, the agent multiplies. Correct treatment of active cases is crucial to prevent the occurrence of MDR TB and extensively drug-resistant (XDR) TB. The Bacille Calmette–Guérin (BCG) vaccine is a live, weakened vaccine; hence, every sort of immunosuppression, as well as pregnancy, represents absolute contraindications. BCG vaccine protects against severe forms of TB, particularly non-pulmonary localizations. WHO recommends BCG vaccination in all newborns in high-incidence TB countries. In Europe, vaccination is recommended in all people with an increased risk of contracting TB: among them, children with parents coming from high-incidence countries and who travel regularly to their home countries [2].

Table 2.1 Economic impact of tuberculosis (TB) in European countries according to the European Centre for Disease Prevention and Control [5]

In the old EU-15 countries (+Cyprus, Malta and Slovenia), the costs per case were:	In the remaining new EU countries, the costs per case were:
€ 10,282 for drug-susceptible TB	€ 3,427 for drug-susceptible TB
€ 57,213 for multidrug-resistant (MDR) TB	€ 24,166 for M/XDR-TB
€ 170,744 for extensively drug-resistant (XDR) TB	–

Twenty-two high-burden countries account for over 80 % of the world's TB cases; in those countries, both incidence and mortality for TB are downscaling. These findings are consistent with the global data which reveal that incidence and mortality are falling down in all WHO Regions. However, within the global scenario, huge variations can be underlined: the Millennium Development Goals (MDGs) of halving the 1990 levels by 2015 are not on track to be achieved in the African and European Regions [2].

Although enormous progress has been done, despite regional variations, the global burden of TB is still relevant; data referring to 2011 revealed 8.7 million new cases of TB (13 % coinfected with HIV) and 1.4 million people deaths due to such disease. TB prevalence is higher in Asia and Africa. In Asia, India and China together account for almost 40 % of the worldwide TB cases while the African Region registered the 24 % of all the global cases, and the highest rates of cases and deaths per capita [2]. In the WHO European Region, the estimated TB prevalence is more than 500,000 cases; most recent data reported 44,000 victims, the vast majority in Eastern Europe and Central Asia [3, 4].

Unfortunately, steps further in responding to M/XDR-TB are still slow. India, China, the Russian Federation and South Africa have almost 60 % of the worldwide cases of M/XDR-TB. However, with over half of the world's countries with the highest percentage of M/XDR-TB cases, the WHO European Region is a gravity centre for such disease, particularly Eastern European and Central Asian countries [3, 4].

In 2004, WHO recommended the implementation of collaborative TB/HIV activities on a global scale; progress on this issue has proceeded. Around 80 % of TB cases among people living with HIV were located in Africa. In 2011, in the WHO European Region, 6 % of TB patients were coinfected with HIV [2].

With regard to TB costs, most recent data, referring to 2011, strengthened the awareness of the gigantic economic impact of TB in the WHO European Region. Table 2.1 reports the economic impact of TB [5].

Other relevant data reported that:

- The 70,340 susceptible TB cases, the 1.488 MDR-TB and the 136 XDR-TB cases notified in 2011 cost € 536.890.315 in 2012.
- The 103,104 disability adjusted life years (DALYs) caused by these cases, when stated in monetary terms, amounted to € 5.361.408.000 in 2012.

In 2006, the Global Plan to Stop TB 2006–2015 reiterated WHO pledges in halting, and beginning to reverse, the TB epidemic by 2015 and in halving TB prevalence and death rates by 2015 compared with 1990 levels. The "directly observed treatment, short course (DOTS) strategy" of the global plan points out main issues to be strengthened. They are:

- Political commitment (through long-term strategic plans) and financing (through national governments)
- Case detection through quality-assured bacteriology (by using sputum smear microscopy and then culture/drug susceptibility testing)
- Standardized treatment, with supervision and patient support (through the most effective, standardized, short-course regimens to facilitate adherence)
- Effective drug supply and management system (through a reliable system of procurement and distribution of all essential anti-TB drugs to all health facilities)
- Monitoring/evaluation of system, and measure of the impact [6]

In Cambodia, the adherence to the Stop TB Plan resulted in a downscale of the TB prevalence in 2011 by 45 % compared to 2002 through the decentralization of TB control services from provincial/district hospitals to health centres [7].

At the European level, Switzerland implemented a strategic plan to fight against TB; it represents a benchmark with regard to the strict collaboration between a national government and WHO EURO. This nationwide plan aims at specifically focusing the fight against TB towards the reduction of inequalities, the access to screening and diagnosis, the strengthening of the treatment according to DOTS guidance, the improvement of the epidemiologic surveillance network, the upgrade of communication/information campaigns and the setting of new international collaborations [8].

With regard to MDR/XDR TB, in the high-prevalence Eastern European and Central Asian countries, stakeholders and decision-makers are recommended to address targeted evidence-based interventions policies. Main efforts have to be focused on:

- Identifying and addressing risk factors contributing to the spread of drug-resistant TB
- Strengthening the health system response in providing accessible, affordable and acceptable services
- Working in regional, national and international partnerships on TB prevention, control and care
- Monitoring the trends of M/XDR-TB and measuring the impact of interventions [9, 10]

HIV/AIDS

The pathogenetic mechanism of the HIV consists in attacking the immune system. The long incubation period ends with a lifelong severe disease culminating in AIDS. AIDS is defined by the presence of one or more "opportunistic" illnesses. Sexual contacts with an infected person and sharing needles/syringes with someone who is infected represent the most common modalities of transmission. Less commonly, HIV can be contracted through transfusions of infected blood. Finally, newborns of HIV-infected women may become infected before or during birth, or through breast feeding. Since the mid-1990s, the quality of life of HIV patients has been deeply scaled up through effective combination therapies. These drugs delayed the onset of AIDS and the related death; however, the occurrence of side effects raises concerns [11].

In 2011, the global prevalence of HIV accounted for 34 million people; 69 % of them lived in Sub-Saharan Africa. Around five million people are living with HIV in South, South-East and East Asia combined. Other high-prevalence regions include the Caribbean, Eastern Europe and Central Asia [11].

Worldwide, HIV incidence is in downturn. In 2011, 2.5 million people acquired HIV infection; this number was 20 % lower than in 2001. Sharpest declines in the incidence have been recorded in the Caribbean (42 %) and Sub-Saharan Africa (25 %). However, variation among regions gives rise to concerns; since 2001, a 35 % increase of HIV incidence has been reported in the Middle East and North Africa. The number of newly infected people in Eastern Europe and Central Asia has been scaling up since 2001, as well [11].

As for HIV mortality rates, the number of people dying from AIDS-related causes has been reducing since the mid-2000s, because of the improved antiretroviral therapy [12, 13]. In 2011, the Joint United Nations Programme on HIV and AIDS (UNAIDS) estimated that 1.7 million people died from AIDS-related causes worldwide, thus recording a 24 % decline compared with 2005 statistics. However, huge variations between regions have been reported, as well. Although Sub-Saharan Africa still accounts for 70 % of all AIDS-related deaths, a 32 % downturn was underlined in this region, in 2011. Consistent findings have been reported in the Caribbean, (reduction achieved was 48 %), in Oceania (41 %) and in Latin America (10 %). According to data referring to incidence rates, increased AIDS-related mortality has been highlighted in Eastern Europe/Central Asia (21 %) and in the Middle East/North Africa (17 %) [11].

The steady scaling up of HIV incidence in the WHO European Region raises many concerns and underpinned further investigations to point out high-risk groups. The highest number of HIV cases in Europe was reported among men who have sex with men (MSM, 38 %), individuals infected by heterosexual contact (24 %) and injecting drug use (4 %). Noteworthy, transmission patterns are widely different across Europe: MSM route of transmission accounted for a disproportionate amount cases in the UK and in the Netherlands, heterosexual contacts in Western/Central Europe and injection drug users in Eastern Europe [14, 15].

Although evidence of cost-effective interventions is not clear and straightforward neither for Western countries nor for developing ones, some analysis outlined interesting results. In developing countries, mass media campaigns and interventions for sex workers, preventative measures to interrupt mother-to-child transmission, voluntary counselling and school-based education have been shown to be cost-effective [16].

In Europe, interesting findings have been reported with regard to structural interventions (as mass media campaigns and large-scale condom distributions), and individually focused interventions to change risk behaviour, respectively in low- and high-prevalence populations [17]. However, with regard to behavioural interventions in high-prevalence settings, a UK study pointed out the effectiveness of group- and community-level interventions but unclear findings were recorded in terms of individual-level interventions [18].

Globally, others evaluations reported the cost-effectiveness of:

- Community empowerment approach to HIV prevention and treatment across sex workers, with projected impact beyond the sex worker community
- Needle/syringe programmes among drug users' groups
- Behavioural interventions for MSM to reduce the rate of unprotected anal intercourse (27 % downturn vs. no HIV-preventive interventions) [19, 20, 21].

In Europe, most successful HIV control programmes emerge from the awareness that HIV transmission is higher among injecting drug users; in turn, people who inject drugs are at greater risk of contracting TB. Hence, in order to foster people to seek and maintain treatment, the city of Porto has brought services for opioid substitution therapy (OST), HIV and TB together, focusing services on people's needs instead than on diseases. The WHO assessment of the Porto's model showed that integrating services for HIV, TB and drug-dependence treatments improve the accessibility and quality of care for people who inject drugs [22].

Crucial tools to drive decisions of stakeholders and policymakers should rely on scientific evidence and on the burden of disease. As for the latter, statistics show that in Europe high-risk groups are MSM (36 and 22 % in Western and Central Europe, respectively), injecting drug users (33 % in Eastern Europe) and male and transgender sex workers [19, 23]. Policymakers and HIV programme implementers should target their policies to high-prevalence groups, in order to streamline efforts. According to most recent evidence-based recommendations, stakeholders and policymakers should take into account that most successful HIV campaigns should be addressed to social change as decriminalization of sex workers, de-stigmatisation of sex between men and of drug use. In this framework, policies should be focused on HIV testing and distribution of condoms (at individual level), and on policy efforts to decriminalize MSM behaviour and anti-homophobia programmes (at community level) [23].

Other Sexually Transmitted Infections

Sexually transmitted infections (STIs) are a heterogeneous group of infections which recognize a common transmission pathway. They include:

- Chlamydia, caused by the *Chlamydia trachomatis* bacteria
- Gonorrhoea, caused by *Neisseria gonorrhoeae* bacteria

- Syphilis caused by *Treponema pallidum* bacteria (syphilis may also be transmitted from mother to child, thus resulting in congenital syphilis)
- Blood-borne viruses which could be sexually transmitted, as well (HIV, hepatitis B and hepatitis C viruses are the most common ones) [24]

STIs are contracted through vaginal, oral and anal sexual intercourse.

STIs raise public health concerns because of the profound consequences of these infections on sexual and reproductive health. During pregnancy, syphilis leads to foetal/neonatal deaths, prematurity, low birth weight or congenital disease. As for gonorrhoea and chlamydia, they represent an important cause of infertility. Noteworthy, contracting an STI increases the chances of acquiring HIV infection by threefold or more.

In recent years, HIV addressed all the public health efforts and the strong association between STIs and HIV acquisition has been underestimated [24].

Worldwide, an estimated 499 million new cases of curable STIs (as gonorrhoea, chlamydia and syphilis) occurred in 2008; these findings suggested no improvement compared to the 448 million cases occurring in 2005. However, wide variations in the incidence of STIs are reported among different regions; the burden of STIs mainly occurs in low-income countries [24].

In the European Union (EU), chlamydia is the most frequently reported STI; more than 340,000 new cases have been reported in 2010. However, the true incidence of chlamydia is likely to be higher than the officially reported one; underreporting and asymptomatic disease are common when referring to chlamydia infection. On the other hand, the scaling up of the reported cases of chlamydia infection (incidence rates have more than doubled over the past 10 years) represents a straightforward attempt of Member States to tackle the problem of STIs by improving the diagnosis of the infection. In Europe, three quarters of all new cases of chlamydia were contracted by young people (particularly women). Furthermore, almost 95 % of cases are reported from six Western/Northern Europe countries reflecting the considerable variation in screening, diagnostic and surveillance programmes across EU countries [15].

With regard to gonorrhoea, more than 25 % of cases are reported among MSM. Furthermore, almost 40 % of the overall incidence occurs in people below 25 years of age. Main public health concerns on gonorrhoea arose after 2009; indeed, the European Gonococcal Antimicrobial Surveillance Programme (EuroGASP) reported decreased susceptibility to cefixime. As ceftriaxone, cefixime represents the recommended therapy for gonorrhoea across Europe; decreased susceptibility to this orally administered antibiotic may have major health and economic implications in the case of parenterally administered ceftriaxone becomes the only viable option [25].

As for syphilis, in 2010 the overall incidence rate was around 4.4 per 100,000 people within the EU. Around 83 % of all cases were reported among people older than 25 years of age. The highest incidence occurred in MSM. However, the 2010 incidence of 4.4 represents a huge achievement compared to the 8.4 per 100,000 people, recorded in 2000 [15].

Table 2.2 Implementation steps for control of chlamydia infections according to the European Centre for Disease Prevention and Control [27]

Level A	Primary prevention: health promotion, sex education, school programmes and condom distribution
Level B	Case management: Level A+chlamydia diagnostic and clinical services, and patient/partner management services, supported by clear evidence-based guidance
Level C	Opportunistic testing: Level B+testing with the aim of case finding of asymptomatic cases
Level D	Screening programme: Level C+as it is difficult to identify asymptomatic cases, a more systematic screening programme
Level C/D	The evidence for the impact of Level C/D programmes is limited; therefore, whether implemented, they need to be evaluated to guide future policies

HIV discussion has been developed separately, in a dedicated section.

As for the cost-effectiveness of STIs interventions, further investigation is required. However, evidence-based cost-saving interventions include: widespread condom provision, school education programmes, safe sex training for high-risk groups, wide choice of contraceptive services and high-quality rapid access to STI services [26].

According to the crucial burden of chlamydia infection in Europe, we decided to focus our further discussion around this disease. The economic impact of chlamydia infection has been deeply investigated; in the UK, the cost of chlamydia complications has been estimated to a minimum of € 110 million, annually [26]. Each year, in the USA, direct costs of chlamydia and its complications range between € 1 and 3 billion.

To tackle the burden of chlamydia in Europe, in 2009, the European Centre for Disease Control in Stockholm (ECDC) released a guidance to develop an effective chlamydia national control programme which, as a prerequisite, requires the involvement of national authorities, key stakeholders and policymakers. Implementations steps are reported in Table 2.2 [27].

In 2008, the ECDC evaluated in depth the availability of national chlamydia control programmes across EU Member States. Results of the assessment showed a wide variability among countries; main findings are reported in Table 2.3 [28].

Table 2.3 Availability of national chlamydia control programmes across EU Member States. (Source: Review of chlamydia control activities in EU countries. ECDC Technical Report, 2008)

No organized activities *No guidelines for effective diagnosis and management of diagnosed chlamydia cases*	Case management *Guidelines covering minimum of diagnostic tests and antibiotic treatment, for at least one group of health care professionals*	Case finding *Case management + either guidelines covering partner notification or guidelines including offer of chlamydia testing for sexual contacts of people with chlamydia*	Opportunistic testing *Case finding + either guidelines stating that at least one specified group of asymptomatic people is offered chlamydia tests or guidelines include a list of asymptomatic people to whom chlamydia testing should be offered*	Organized screening *Opportunistic testing + organised chlamydia screening available to a substantial part of the population within the public health system*
Bulgaria	Austria	Belgium	Denmark	The Netherlands
Finland	Czech Republic	France	Estonia	The UK
Greece	Germany	Hungary	Latvia	–
Ireland	Italy	–	Sweden	–
Luxembourg	Lithuania	–	–	–
Malta	–	–	–	–
Portugal	–	–	–	–
Romania	–	–	–	–
Slovenia	–	–	–	–
Spain	–	–	–	–

At the EU level, the reduction of countries reporting no organised activity should be set as the minimal target [27, 29]

Influenza

Seasonal influenza viruses are classified into three groups according to the specific variety of the haemagglutinin (or "H" protein) and the neuraminidase (or "N" protein). Specific combinations of these two proteins label A, B and C seasonal influenza viruses; furthermore, type A influenza viruses are further divided into subtypes [30].

In temperate climates, seasonal influenza tends to spread in winter months, following a person-to-person transmission pattern. The continuous evolution of seasonal influenza viruses explains why people can contract the disease multiple times, throughout life [30].

The currently circulating seasonal influenza A virus subtypes are the influenza A(H1N1) and A(H3N2). Influenza A(H1N1) virus is the same virus that caused pandemic influenza in 2009, which is currently circulating seasonally. In addition, there are two type B viruses that are circulating as seasonal influenza viruses, as well. A and B influenza viruses are included in the seasonal influenza vaccine, which represents the most effective way to prevent the disease and its potential severe outcomes. Influenza C virus is excluded from the vaccine, according to the lower burden of disease [30].

A pandemic influenza occurs when an influenza virus, which was not previously circulating among humans and to which most people do not have immunity, emerges and transmits among humans; whether this happens, these viruses may result in large influenza outbreaks outside seasonal patterns. Pandemic influenza outbreaks can occur when humans are infected with influenza viruses that are routinely circulating in animals, such as avian influenza virus and swine influenza virus. Indeed, animal viruses neither easily transmit to humans nor, if it happens, transmit among them. Occasionally, some animal viruses infect humans but human infections of zoonotic influenza do not spread far among humans. If such a virus acquires the capacity to spread easily among people, either through adaptation or through acquisition of certain genes from human viruses, a pandemic could start. Currently, there are no pandemic viruses circulating in the world [30].

The burden of seasonal influenza varies, globally, in different regions. The 2012–2013 influenza season was characterized by crucial differences, reported below:

- Influenza A(H3N2) was the most common virus in North America and in temperate Asia
- A(H1N1)pdm09 (pandemic 2009) affected Europe, North Africa and the Middle East
- Influenza type B was reported in North America and Europe, by the end of the season [31]

With regard to costs of influenza, results of a 2007 study, referring to 2003 data, highlighted the huge economic brunt of the burden of influenza in the USA, accounting for US$ 87.1 billion across all age groups [32].

As reported above, vaccination is the most effective modality to prevent the occurrence of influenza and of its potential severe outcomes. Two types of influenza vaccines are available: trivalent inactivated influenza vaccine (TIV) and live attenuated influenza vaccine (LAIV). Both TIV and LAIV contain three strains of influenza viruses and are administered annually.

The selection of strains to be included in the vaccine is taken according to the information gathered from the Global Influenza Surveillance Network (GISN), a partnership which encompasses 5 WHO Collaborating Centres, 136 National Influenza Centres in 106 countries and several laboratories. Apart from the crucial role of obtaining reliable virus information to update influenza vaccines, other GISN functions are to:

- Monitor the burden of human influenza
- Detect and obtain isolates of pandemic potential viruses [33]

The influenza vaccine is made up of strains of influenza A(H3N2) viruses, A(H1N1) and B. Each year, one or more virus strains might be changed according to results provided by GISN in order to reflect the most recent circulating influenza A(H3N2),

A(H1N1) and B viruses. In the large majority of countries, TIV remains the cornerstone of influenza vaccination [33].

Although influenza vaccination rates are scaling up globally, particularly in Central/Eastern Europe and in Latin America, no country has fully implemented WHO vaccine recommendations, so far. Consistent findings also encompass industrialized countries where significant proportions of the groups at risk of complications from influenza are not vaccinated. In high-risk groups, influenza is a serious public health problem, potentially leading to severe illness and death. For these reasons, WHO specifically recommends vaccination to the following categories:

- Pregnant women (even to extend protection to infants under 6 months who are not eligible for immunization)
- Children 6–59 months of age (particularly in children 6–23 months)
- Elderly individuals who are above a nationally defined age limit (often >65 years)
- Persons > 6 months with specific chronic diseases (pulmonary, cardiovascular, metabolic, renal dysfunction, immunosuppression as AIDS and transplant recipients)
- Health care workers (even to protect vulnerable patients) [34]

Hence, policymakers and stakeholders should address their efforts towards the implementation and the strengthening of influenza vaccination programmes, taking into account the potential health impacts of influenza in high-risk groups as well as its huge economic brunt.

Malaria

Malaria is caused by the parasite *Plasmodium,* which is borne by mosquitoes of the species *Anopheles*. In the human body, the parasites multiply in the liver, and then infect red blood cells [35].

Symptoms of malaria include fever, headache and vomiting, and usually appear between 10 and 15 days after contact with the mosquito. If not treated, malaria is potentially lethal as it can disrupt the blood supply to vital organs. In many parts of the world, the parasites have developed resistance to a number of malaria medicines [36].

It is estimated that in 2010 alone, malaria caused 216 million clinical episodes and 655,000 deaths. An estimated 91 % of deaths in 2010 were in the African Region, followed by 6 % in the South-East Asian Region and 3 % in the Eastern Mediterranean Region (3 %). About 86 % of deaths globally were in children. A total of 3.3 billion people (half the world's population) live in areas at risk of malaria transmission in 106 countries and territories [35, 36].

Malaria imposes substantial costs to both individuals and governments. Direct costs for malaria have been estimated to be at least US$ 12 billion per year worldwide [35, 36].

Key interventions to control malaria include: prompt and effective treatment with artemisinin-based combination therapies, use of insecticidal nets by people at risk, and indoor residual spraying with insecticide to control the vector mosquitoes. Success in malaria control, however, requires strong, sustained political and budgetary commitment at national and international levels.

Zambia and Ethiopia, which achieved substantial progress in malaria control, are examples of strong political support behind malaria control programmes. The Zambian government has supported the establishment and implementation of a 6-year strategy and has taken the lead on coordinating all partners. The Ethiopian government has established joint steering committees at the national and regional levels to strengthen accountability by removing taxes and tariffs on malaria preventive tools and by promoting demand through communication efforts [36].

Diarrhoeal Diseases

Diarrhoea is defined as the passage of three or more loose or liquid stools per day (or more frequent passage than is normal for the individual). It is generally the symptom of an infection in the intestinal tract, which can be caused by several of bacterial, viral and parasitic organisms. Infection is spread through contaminated food or drinking water, or from person to person as a result of poor hygiene [37].

Globally, most cases in children are caused by rotavirus. In adults, norovirus and *Campylobacter* are the most common. Less common causes include other bacteria (or their toxins) and parasites. Transmission can occur due to consumption of improperly prepared foods or contaminated water or via close contact with individuals who are infectious [38].

Diarrhoeal diseases amount to an estimated 4.1 % of the total disability-adjusted life years (DALY) global burden of disease, and are responsible for 1.8 million deaths every year. An estimated 88 % of that burden is attributable to unsafe supply of water, sanitation and hygiene [39]. Children in the developing world are the most affected by diarrhoeal disease: It is estimated that diarrhoeal diseases account for one in nine child deaths worldwide, making diarrhoea the second leading cause of death among children under the age of 5 after pneumonia [40].

Two recent advances in managing diarrhoeal disease—(1) oral rehydration salts (ORS) containing lower concentrations of glucose and salt, and zinc supplementation as part of the treatment; and (2) rotavirus vaccine—can drastically reduce the number of child deaths. These new methods, used in addition to prevention and treatment with appropriate fluids, breastfeeding, continued feeding and selective use of antibiotics, have been shown to reduce the duration and severity of diarrhoeal episodes and lower their incidence [41].

Diarrhoea prevention focused on safe water and improved hygiene and sanitation, however, remains the most successful and cost-effective intervention in diarrhoeal diseases control: every US$ 1 invested yields an average return of US$ 25.50 [42].

References

1. The top 10 causes of death. Fact sheet N°310 (Updated July 2013) World Health Organization, Global burden of disease. http://www.who.int/mediacentre/factsheets/fs310/en/index.html. Accessed 28 Jan 2015
2. WHO (2012) Global Tuberculosis Report 2012. World Health Organization, Geneva
3. WHO-EURO (2013) TB is everywhere, and its treatment and care must be so, too. World Health Organization Regional Office for Europe, Copenhagen
4. ECDC/WHO-EURO (2013) Tuberculosis surveillance and monitoring in Europe. ECDC, Stockholm
5. Diel R, Vandeputte J, de Vries G, Stillo J, Wanlin M, Nienhaus A (2014) Costs of tuberculosis disease in the EU—a systematic analysis and cost calculation. Eur Respir J 43(2):554-65
6. WHO (2006) The stop TB strategy, building on and enhancing DOTS to meet the TB-related millennium development goals. World Health Organization, Geneva
7. CENAT (2007) Strategic plan for tuberculosis laboratories for TB control in Cambodia 2007–2010. Ministry of Health
8. DFI (2012) Stratégie nationale de lutte contre la tuberculose 2012–2017. Confederation Suisse
9. WHO-EURO (2011) Consolidated action plan to prevent and combat multidrug- and extensively drug-resistant tuberculosis in the WHO European Region 2011–2015. World Health Organization Regional Office for Europe, Baku
10. Dara M, Kluge H (2011) Roadmap to prevent and combat drug-resistant tuberculosis, the consolidated action plan to prevent and combat multidrug- and extensively drug-resistant tuberculosis in the WHO European Region, 2011–2015. World Health Organization Regional Office for Europe, Copenhagen
11. UNAIDS (2013). UNAIDS report on the global AIDS epidemic 2013. UNAIDS.
12. Ortblad KF, Lozano R, Murray CJ (2013) The burden of HIV: insights from the Global Burden of Disease Study 2010. AIDS 27(13):2003–2017
13. Lozano R, Ortblad KF, Lopez AD, Murray CJ (2013). Mortality from HIV in the Global Burden of Disease study—authors reply. Lancet 381(9871):991–992
14. ECDC/WHO-EURO (2008) HIV/AIDS surveillance in Europe 2007. ECDC/WHO Europe, Stockholm
15. ECDC (2012) Annual epidemiological report—reporting on 2010 surveillance data and 2011 epidemic intelligence data. ECDC, Stockholm
16. Hogan DR, Baltussen R, Hayashi C, Lauer JA, Salomon JA (2005) Cost effectiveness analysis of strategies to combat HIV/AIDS in developing countries. BMJ 331(7530):1431–1437
17. Cohen DA, Wu SY, Farley TA (2004) Comparing the cost-effectiveness of HIV prevention interventions. J Acquir Immune Defic Syndr 37(3):1404–1414
18. Kegeles SM, Hart GJ (1998) Recent HIV-prevention interventions for gay men: individual, small-group and community-based studies. AIDS 12(Suppl A):S209–S215
19. Beyrer C (2011) The global HIV epidemics among men who have sex with men. World Bank, Washington, D.C
20. Kerrigan D, Wirtz A, Baral S, Decker M, Murray L, Poteat T, Pretorius C, Sherman S, Sweat M, Semini I, N'Jie N'D, Stanciole A, Butler J, Osornprasop S, Oelrichs R, Beyrer C (2013) The global HIV epidemics among sex workers. World Bank, Washington, D.C
21. Dutta A, Wirtz A, Stanciole A, Oelrichs A, Semini A, Baral S, et al (2013) The global HIV epidemics among people who inject drugs. World Bank, Washington, D.C
22. Grenfell P, Carvalho A, Martins A, Cosme D, Barros H, Rhodes T (2012) Accessibility and integration of HIV, TB and harm reduction services for people who inject drugs in Portugal. World Health Organization Regional Office for Europe, Copenhagen
23. Platt L (2013) HIV epidemics in the European region: vulnerability and response. World Bank, Washington, D.C
24. WHO (2013) Sexually transmitted infections (STIs). World Health Organization, Geneva

25. ECDC (2009) Gonococcal antimicrobial susceptibility surveillance in Europe. ECDC, Stockholm
26. Adams EJ, Turner KM, Edmunds WJ (2007) The cost effectiveness of opportunistic chlamydia screening in England. Sex Transm Infect 83(4):267–274; discussion 74–5
27. ECDC (2009) Chlamydia control in Europe. ECDC, Stockholm
28. ECDC (2008) Review of chlamydia control activities in EU countries. ECDC, Stockholm
29. Richens J, Fairclough L, Khotenashvili L (2011) Scaling up sexually transmitted infection prevention and control in the WHO European region, 2012. World Health Organization Regional Office for Europe, Ljubliana
30. WHO (2013) Influenza virus infections in humans. World Health Organization, Geneva
31. WHO (2013). Review of the 2012–2013 winter influenza season, northern hemisphere. World Health Organization, Geneva
32. Molinari NA, Ortega-Sanchez IR, Messonnier ML, Thompson WW, Wortley PM, Weintraub E, et al (2007) The annual impact of seasonal influenza in the US: measuring disease burden and costs. Vaccine 25(27):5086–5096
33. WHO (2013). Recommended composition of influenza virus vaccines for use in the 2013–2014 northern hemisphere influenza season. World Health Organization, Geneva
34. SAGE (2012) Working group. Background paper on influenza vaccines and immunization. World Health Organization, Geneva
35. World Malaria Report 2011, World Health Organization. http://www.who.int/malaria/world_malaria_report_2011/en/index.html. Accessed 28 Jan 2015
36. The Global Malaria action Plan for a Malaria Free World. http://www.rollbackmalaria.org/gmap/. Accessed 28 Jan 2015
37. Diarrhoea: why children are still dying and what can be done. World Health Organization 2009. http://www.who.int/maternal_child_adolescent/documents/9789241598415/en/. Accessed 28 Jan 2015
38. Tate JE, Burton AH, Boschi-Pinto C, Steele AD, Duque J, Parashar UD (2012) 2008 estimate of worldwide rotavirus-associated mortality in children younger than 5 years before the introduction of universal rotavirus vaccination programmes: a systematic review and meta-analysis. Lancet Infect Dis 12(2):136–141
39. Cairncross S, Hunt C, Boisson S, Bostoen K, Curtis V, Fung IC, Schmidt WP (2010). Water, sanitation and hygiene for the prevention of diarrhoea. Int J Epidemiol 39(Suppl 1):i193–i205
40. Aiello AE, Coulborn RM, Perez V, Larson EL (2008) Effect of hand hygiene on infectious disease risk in the community setting: a meta-analysis. Am J Public Health 98(8):1372–1381
41. Clasen TF, Roberts IG, Rabie T, Schmidt WP, Cairncross S.(2006) Interventions to improve water quality for preventing diarrhoea. Cochrane Database Syst Rev 2006(3):CD004794. doi:10.1002/14651858.CD004794.pub2
42. Evaluation of the Costs and Benefits of Water and Sanitation Improvements at the Global Level, WHO 2004. http://www.who.int/water_sanitation_health/wsh0404.pdf. Accessed 28 Jan 2015

Chapter 3
Global Burden and Health Trends of Non-Communicable Diseases

Silvio Capizzi, Chiara de Waure and Stefania Boccia

The non-communicable disease (NCD) epidemic, which is expected to increase in the future, has a serious negative impact on development in human, social and economic realms. NCDs reduce productivity and contribute to poverty. NCDs already pose a substantial economic burden: The macroeconomic simulations suggest a cumulative output loss of US$ 47 trillion over the next two decades. Cardiovascular disease is the dominant contributor to the global economic burden of NCDs.

The majority of NCDs can be prevented through population-wide and individual interventions that reduce major risk factors. Best practices related to reducing risks and preventing diseases exist in many countries with different income levels. Interventions that combine a range of evidence-based approaches show better results.

Definition of NCDs

NCDs are defined as diseases of long duration and, generally, slow progression, and they are the major cause of adult mortality and morbidity worldwide [1]. Four main diseases are generally considered to be dominant in NCDs' mortality and morbidity: cardiovascular diseases, diabetes, cancer and chronic respiratory diseases (see Table 3.1) [2].

S. Capizzi (✉) · C. de Waure · S. Boccia
Institute of Public Health, Section of Hygiene, Università Cattolica del Sacro Cuore, L. go F. Vito 1, 00168 Rome, Italy
e-mail: silviocapizzi@virgilio.it

C. de Waure
e-mail: chiara.dewaure@rm.unicatt.it

S. Boccia
e-mail: sboccia@rm.unicatt.it

S. Boccia et al. (eds.), *A Systematic Review of Key Issues in Public Health*,
DOI 10.1007/978-3-319-13620-2_3

Table 3.1 A snapshot of the four major NCDs [2]

Cardiovascular disease (CVD)	A group of diseases involving the heart, blood vessels or the sequelae of poor blood supply due to a diseased vascular supply. Over 82 % of CVD mortality burden is caused by ischaemic or coronary heart disease (IHD), stroke (both haemorrhagic and ischaemic), hypertensive heart disease or congestive heart failure (CHF). Over the past decade, CVD has become the single largest cause of death worldwide, representing nearly 30 % of all deaths and about 50 % of NCDs deaths. In 2008, CVD caused an estimated 17 million deaths and led to 151 million disability adjusted life years (DALYs) (representing 10 % of all DALYs in that year). Behavioural risk factors such as physical inactivity, tobacco use and unhealthy diet explain nearly 80 % of the CVD burden
Cancer	A rapid growth and division of abnormal cells in a part of the body. These cells outlive normal cells and have the ability to metastasize, or invade parts of the body and spread to other organs. There are more than 100 types of cancers, and different risk factors contribute to the development of cancers in different sites. Cancer is the second largest cause of death worldwide, representing about 13 % of all deaths (7.6 million). Recent literature estimated the number of new cancer cases in 2009 alone at 12.9 million, and this number is projected to rise to nearly 17 million by 2020
Diabetes	A metabolic disorder in which the body is unable to appropriately regulate the level of sugar, specifically glucose, in the blood, either by poor sensitivity to the protein insulin or due to an inadequate production of insulin by the pancreas. Type 2 diabetes accounts for 90–95 % of all cases. Diabetes itself is not a high-mortality condition (1.3 million deaths globally), but it is a major risk factor for other causes of death and has a high attributable disability. Diabetes is also a major risk factor for CVD, kidney disease and blindness
Chronic respiratory diseases	Chronic diseases of the airways and other structures of the lung. Some of the most common are asthma, chronic obstructive pulmonary disease (COPD), respiratory allergies, occupational lung diseases and pulmonary hypertension, which together account for 7% of all deaths worldwide (4.2 million). COPD refers to a group of progressive lung diseases that make it difficult to breathe—including chronic bronchitis and emphysema (assessed by pulmonary function and x-ray evidence). Affecting more than 210 million people worldwide, COPD accounts for 3–8 % of total deaths in high-income countries and 4–9 % of total deaths in low- and middle-income countries

Global Burden and Health Trends: Mortality and Morbidity

NCDs are the leading global cause of death worldwide, being responsible for more deaths than all other causes combined. In fact, more than 60 % of all deaths worldwide currently stem from NCDs [3].

In 2008, the leading causes of all NCD deaths (36 million) were:

- CVD (17 million, or 48 % of NCD deaths);
- Cancer (7.6 million, or 21 % of NCD deaths);
- Respiratory diseases (4.2 million, or 12 % of NCD deaths)
- Diabetes (1.3 million, 4 % of NCD deaths) [4].

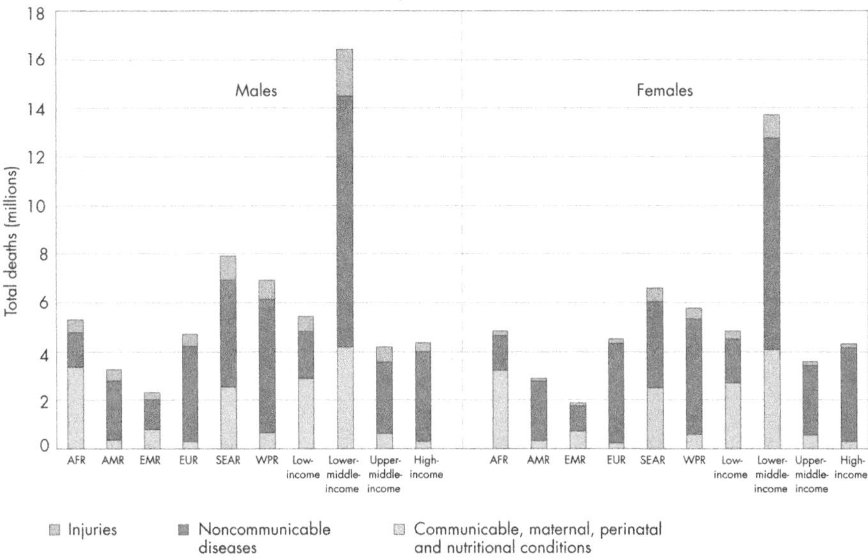

(Note: AFR=African Region, AMR=Region of the Americas, EMR= Eastern Mediterranean Region, EUR= European Region, SEAR=South-East Asia Region, WPR=Western Pacific Region).

Fig. 3.1 Total deaths by broad cause group, by WHO Region, World Bank income group and sex (2008). (Reproduced from WHO 2011) [4]

Population growth and improved longevity are leading to an increased number and proportion of elderly. Because of populations ageing, annual NCD deaths are projected to rise to 52 million in 2030. Contrary to popular opinion, nearly 80 % of NCD deaths occur in low- and middle-income countries [4], up sharply from just under 40 % in 1990 [5]. NCDs are the most frequent causes of death in most countries in the Americas, Eastern Mediterranean, Europe, South-East Asia and the Western Pacific. In the African Region, there are still more deaths from infectious diseases than NCDs (Fig. 3.1) [4]. Even there, however, NCDs are rising rapidly and are projected to exceed communicable, maternal, perinatal and nutritional diseases as the most common causes of death by 2030 [6].

Low- and lower-middle-income countries have the highest proportion of deaths from NCDs under 60 years. Premature deaths under 60 years for high-income countries were 13 and 25 % for upper-middle-income countries. In lower-middle-income countries, the proportion of premature NCD deaths under 60 years rose to 28 %, more than double the proportion in high-income countries. In low-income countries, the proportion of premature NCD deaths under 60 years is 41 %, three times the proportion in high-income countries [7].

With respect to trends, from 1990 to 2010, an important decrease in age-standardized death rates has been observed for major vascular diseases, especially heart disease and strokes, as well as chronic respiratory disease and cancer (respectively, − 21.2, − 41.9 and − 13.8 %). Notwithstanding, an increase in absolute number of deaths from CVD and cancer has been shown. Similarly, the number

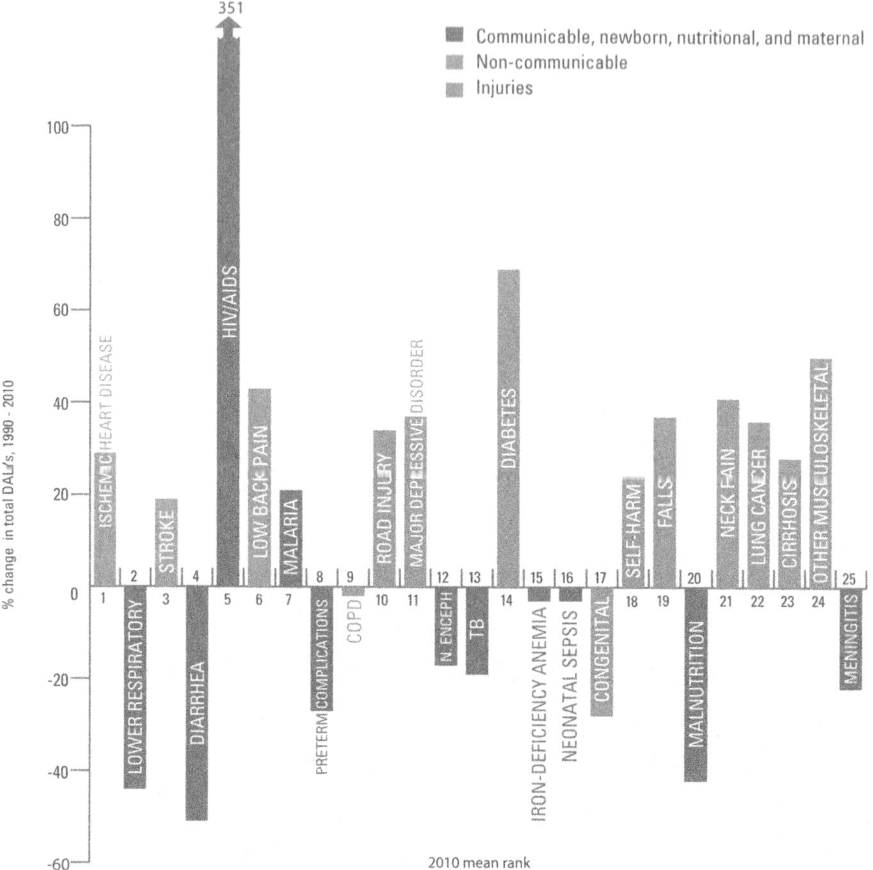

Fig. 3.2 Shifts in leading causes of DALYs from 1990 to 2010. (Reproduced from Institute for Health Metrics and Evaluation 2011)[9]

of deaths due to diabetes has increased as well as age-standardized mortality rates [8]. Generally speaking, death rates from NCDs decreased from 645.9 to 520.4 per 100,000 over 1990–2010 [9].

In addition to information about NCD-related deaths, morbidity data are important for the management of health care systems and for planning and evaluation of health service delivery.

However, reliable data on NCD morbidity are unavailable in many countries. It is anyway well known that ageing, increase in NCDs, shifts toward disabling causes and away from fatal causes and changes in risk factors have led to a shift in the leading causes of DALYs worldwide [9] (Fig. 3.2).

Overall, NCDs account for more than 50 % of DALYs in most counties. This percentage rises to over 80 % in Australia, Japan and the richest countries of Western Europe and North America worldwide [9].

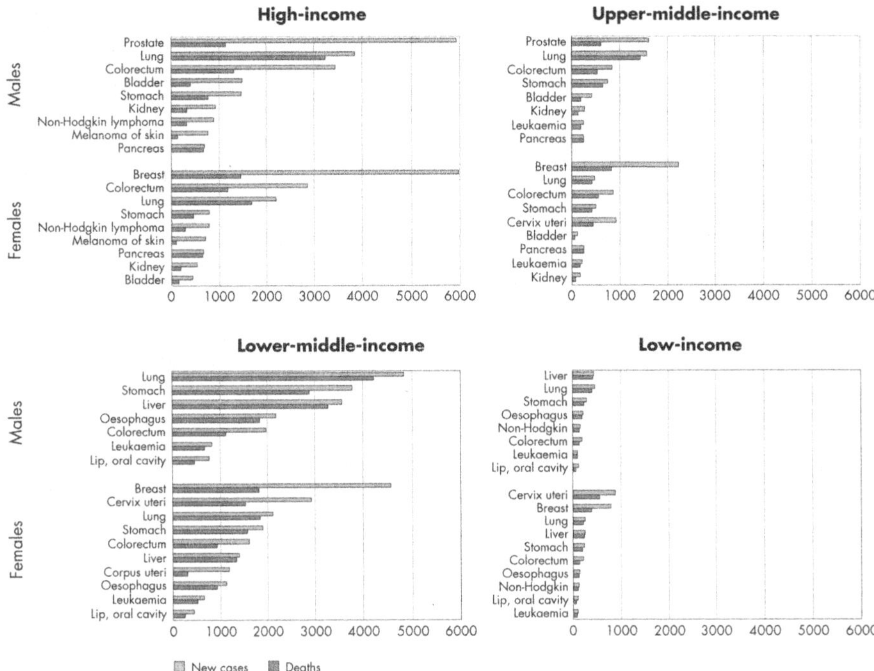

Fig. 3.3 Estimated annual number of new cases and deaths for the ten most common cancers, by World Bank income groups and sex, 2008. (Reproduced from WHO 2011) [4]

The most comprehensive and available morbidity data relate to cancer and diabetes.

Cancer is predicted to be an increasingly important cause of morbidity in the next few decades in all regions of the world. The estimated incidence of 12.7 million new cancer cases in 2008 [10] will rise to 21.4 million by 2030, with nearly two thirds of all cancer occurring in low- and middle-income countries. This estimated percentage increase in cancer incidence by 2030 (compared with 2008) will be greater in low- (82 %) and lower-middle-income countries (70 %) compared with the upper-middle- (58 %) and high-income countries (40 %). Without any changes in underlying risk factors and on the base of anticipated demographic changes only, between 10 and 11 million cancers will be diagnosed annually in 2030 in low- and lower-middle-income countries [11].

Within upper-middle-income and high-income countries, prostate and breast cancers are the most common in males and females, respectively, with lung and colorectal cancers representing the next most common types in both sexes. Within low-income countries, lung and breast cancers remain among the most common but cancers with an infection-related aetiology—cervix, stomach and liver are also frequent. Within the lower-middle-income countries, the three most common types of cancer are lung, stomach and liver cancers in males, and breast, cervix and lung cancer in females (Fig. 3.3) [4].

The global prevalence of diabetes was estimated to be 10 % in adults aged 25+ years. The prevalence of diabetes was highest in the Eastern Mediterranean Region and Americas (11 % for both sexes) and lowest in the WHO European and Western Pacific Regions (9 % for both sexes).

Moreover, the estimated prevalence of diabetes was relatively consistent across countries with low-income ones showing the lowest prevalence (8 % for both sexes), and the upper-middle-income countries showing the highest (10 % for both sexes) [4]. People with diabetes have a twofold increase in the risk of stroke [12]. Diabetes is the leading cause of renal failure in many populations in both developed and developing countries [4]. Lower-limb amputations are at least 10 times more common in people with diabetes than in nondiabetic individuals in developed countries, and more than half of all nontraumatic lower limb amputations are due to diabetes [13].

Furthermore, diabetes is one of the leading causes of visual impairment and blindness in developed countries [14]. People with diabetes require at least two to three times health care resources compared to people who are not affected [15].

Risk Factors

With respect to etiopathogenesis, NCDs are due to a complex of interacting factors and recognize several risk factors.

Behavioural Risk Factors

A large percentage of NCDs are preventable through the reduction of five main behavioural risk factors:

1. *Tobacco:* Almost six million people die from tobacco each year, from both direct use and second-hand smoke [16]. By 2020, this number will increase to 7.5 million, accounting for 10 % of all deaths [17]. Smoking is estimated to cause about 71 % of lung cancer, 42 % of chronic respiratory disease and nearly 10 % of CVD [18]. Smoking prevalence is generally higher in upper-middle-income countries than lower-middle-income ones [4].
2. *Physical inactivity:* Approximately 3.2 million people die each year due to physical inactivity [19]. People who are insufficiently physically active have a 20–30 % increased risk of all-cause mortality. Regular physical activity reduces the risk of CVD, including high blood pressure, diabetes, breast and colon cancer and depression [20]. Insufficient physical activity is higher in high-income countries, but very high levels are now also seen in some middle-income countries especially in women [4].
3. *Alcohol:* Approximately 2.3 million die each year from the harmful use of alcohol. More than half of these deaths occur from NCDs including cancers, CVD

and liver cirrhosis [21]. Adult per capita consumption is higher in high-income countries [4].

4. *Unhealthy diet:* approximately 16.0 million (1 %) DALYs (a measure of the potential life lost due to premature mortality and of years of productive life lost due to disability) and 1.7 million (2.8 %) of deaths worldwide are attributable to low fruit and vegetable consumption. Adequate consumption of fruit and vegetables reduces the risk for CVD, stomach cancer and colorectal cancer [22]. Most populations consume much higher levels of salt than recommended by WHO for disease prevention; high salt consumption is an important determinant of high blood pressure and cardiovascular risk [23, 24]. High consumption of saturated fats and *trans*-fatty acids is linked to heart disease [25]. Unhealthy diet is rising quickly in lower-resource settings. Available data suggest that fat intake has been rising rapidly in lower-middle-income countries since the 1980s [4].
5. *Infections associated to cancer:* At least two million cancer cases per year (18 % of the global cancer burden) are attributable to chronic infections by human papillomavirus, hepatitis B virus, hepatitis C virus and *Helicobacter pylori*. These infections are largely preventable or treatable [4].

Metabolic Risk Factors

1. *Raised blood pressure:* it is a major risk factor for CVD and it is estimated to cause 7.5 million deaths, about 12.8 % of all [22]. The prevalence of raised blood pressure is similar across all income groups, though it is generally lowest in high-income populations [4].
2. *Overweight and obesity:* At least 2.8 million people die each year as a result of being overweight or obese. Raised body mass index (BMI) increases risks of heart disease, strokes, diabetes and certain cancers. Once considered a high-income country problem, overweight and obesity are now on the rise in low- and middle-income countries too, particularly in urban settings. In 2011, more than 40 million children under the age of 5 were overweight (more than 30 million are living in developing countries and 10 million in developed countries) [26].
3. *Raised cholesterol:* Raised cholesterol increases the risks of heart disease and stroke and causes 2.6 million deaths annually. Raised cholesterol is highest in high-income countries [4].

Social Determinants

There is strong evidence of association between social determinants (especially education level, household income and access to health care) and NCDs. In fact, vulnerable and socially disadvantaged people get sicker and die sooner than people belonging to a higher social position, especially because they are at greater risk of being exposed to harmful products, such as tobacco or unhealthy food, and have limited access to health services.

Moreover, since in poorer countries most health care costs must be paid by patients out of pocket, NCDs creates significant strain on household budgets, particularly for lower-income families. In low-resource settings, health care costs for CVD, cancers, diabetes or chronic lung diseases can quickly drain household resources, driving families into poverty. Each year, an estimated 100 million people are pushed into poverty because they have to pay directly for health services [27].

Economic Burden

NCDs have been established as a clear threat not only to human health but also to the economic growth. Claiming more than 60 % of all deaths, these diseases are currently the world's main killers. Eighty percent of these deaths now occur in low- and middle-income countries. Half of those who die of NCDs are in the prime of their productive years, and thus, disability and lives lost are also endangering the market [2].

Globally, NCDs have reduced the quality and quantity of the labour force and human capital [28]. In the USA, men with chronic disease worked 6.1 % fewer hours and women worked 3.9 % fewer hours [29]. A healthy lifestyle in the US working-age population reduced health care costs by 49 % in adults aged 40 or older. Instead, obesity increased individual annual health care costs by 36 %, smoking by 21 % and heavy drinking by 10 % [28].

Over the next 20 years, NCDs will cost more than US$ 47 trillion, representing 75 % of global gross domestic product in 2010, and pushing millions of people below the poverty line [2].

In particular, the global cost of CVD is estimated in 2010 at US$ 863 billion (an average per capita of US$ 125), and it is estimated to rise to US$ 1044 billion in 2030—a 22% increase. Overall, the cost for CVD could be as high as US$ 20 trillion over the 20-year period (an average per capita of nearly US$ 3000). Currently, about US$ 474 billion (55 %) is due to direct health care costs and the remaining 45 % to productivity loss from disability or premature death, or time loss from work because of illness or the need to seek care.

Diabetes costs the global economy nearly US$ 500 billion in 2010, and that figure is projected to rise to at least US$ 745 billion in 2030, with developing countries increasingly taking on a much greater share of the outlays.

The 13.3 million new cases of cancer in 2010 were estimated to cost US$ 290 billion. Medical costs accounted for the greatest share at US$ 154 billion (53 % of the total), while non-medical costs and income losses accounted for US$ 67 billion and US$ 69 billion, respectively. The total costs were expected to rise to US$ 458 billion in the year 2030.

The global cost of illness for COPD will rise from US$ 2.1 trillion in 2010 to US$ 4.8 trillion in 2030. Approximately half of all global costs for COPD will arise in developing countries [2].

By contrast, mounting evidence highlights how millions of deaths can be averted and economic losses reduced by preventive initiatives: population-based measures for reducing tobacco and harmful alcohol use, as well as unhealthy diet and physical inactivity, are estimated to cost US$ 2 billion per year for all low- and middle-income countries, which in fact translates to less than US$ 0.40 per person [2].

Reducing Risks and Preventing Disease: Population-Wide and Individual Interventions Effectiveness and Cost-Effectiveness

Interventions to prevent NCDs on a population-wide basis are not only feasible but also cost-effective [30]. Moreover, low-cost solutions can work anywhere to reduce the major risk factors for NCDs.

While many interventions may be cost-effective, some are considered "best buys"—actions that should be undertaken immediately to produce accelerated results in terms of lives saved, diseases prevented and heavy costs avoided [4].

Best buys include:

- Protecting people from tobacco smoke and banning smoking in public places;
- Warning about the dangers of tobacco use
- Enforcing bans on tobacco advertising, promotion and sponsorship
- Raising taxes on tobacco
- Restricting access to retailed alcohol
- Enforcing bans on alcohol advertising
- Raising taxes on alcohol
- Reduce salt intake and salt content of food
- Replacing transfat in food with polyunsaturated fat
- Promoting public awareness about diet and physical activity

In addition to best buys, there are many other cost-effective and low-cost population-wide interventions that can reduce risk factors for NCDs [4]. These include:

- Nicotine dependence treatment
- Promoting adequate breastfeeding and complementary feeding
- Enforcing drink-driving laws
- Restrictions on marketing of foods and beverages high in salt, fats and sugar, especially to children
- Food taxes and subsidies to promote healthy diets

Also, there is strong evidence for the following interventions:

- Healthy nutrition environments in schools
- Nutrition information and counselling in health care
- National physical activity guidelines
- School-based physical activity programmes for children
- Workplace programmes for physical activity and healthy diets
- Community programmes for physical activity and healthy diets
- Designing workplace and environmental spaces in order to promote physical activity

There are also population-wide interventions that focus on cancer prevention. Vaccination against hepatitis B, a major cause of liver cancer, is a best buy. Vaccination against human papillomavirus (HPV), the main cause of cervical cancer, is also recommended. Protection against environmental or occupational risk factors for cancer, such as aflatoxin, asbestos and contaminants in drinking water, can be included in effective prevention strategies. Screening for breast and cervical cancer can be effective in reducing the cancer burden [4].

Population-wide interventions for NCDs prevention and control can be complemented by efforts to reduce the burden of NCDs on individuals and families. In fact, like population-wide interventions, there are also best buys in individual health care interventions:

- Counselling and multidrug therapy, including glycaemic control for diabetes for people ≥30 years old with a 10-year risk of fatal or nonfatal cardiovascular events ≥30 %
- Aspirin therapy for acute myocardial infarction
- Screening for cervical cancer, once, at age 40, followed by removal of any discovered cancerous lesion
- Early case finding for breast cancer through biennial mammographic screening (50–70 years) and treatment of all stages
- Early detection of colorectal and oral cancer
- Treatment of persistent asthma with inhaled corticosteroids and beta-2 agonists

Financing and strengthening health systems to deliver cost-effective individual interventions through a primary health care approach is a pragmatic first step to achieve the long-term vision of universal care coverage [4].

Identification of the Best Practice

Best practices related to reducing risks and preventing diseases exist in many countries with different income levels.

For example, declines in tobacco use prevalence are apparent in high-income countries that conduct regular population-based surveys of tobacco use (e.g. Australia, Canada, Finland, the Netherlands and the UK) [4].

Moreover, there are some low- and middle-income countries that have also a documented decline:

- Turkey recently became one of the 17 smoke-free countries in the world. It increased tobacco taxes by 77 %, which led to a 62 % price increase on cigarettes. Turkey also adopted and implemented comprehensive tobacco control measures, including pictorial health warnings on tobacco packaging, a comprehensive ban on tobacco advertising, promotion and sponsorship in all media, as well as a comprehensive smoke-free law for all public and work places.
- Egypt increased taxes by 87 % for cigarettes and 100 % for loose tobacco. This will lead to an estimated increase of 44 % in average retail prices and a 21 % reduction in cigarette consumption.
- Ukraine elevated taxes by 127 % on filtered cigarettes, leading to a 73 % increase in retail prices between February 2009 and May 2010 [4, 31, 32].

As regards the promotion of healthy diets, the UK salt reduction programme has involved working with industry to reduce levels of salt in food, raise consumer awareness and improve food labelling. The average intake was 9.5 g/day in 2000–2001, considerably above the recommended national level of no more than 6 g/day for adults. Voluntary salt reduction targets were set, and industry made public commitments to reduce the amount of salt in food products.

Public awareness campaigns about health issues, recommended salt intakes and consumer advice took place between 2004 and 2010. Levels of salt in foods have been reduced in some products by up to 55 %, with significant reductions in those food categories contributing most salt to the diet. Consumer awareness of the 6-g/day maximum recommended intake increased tenfold, and the number of people who say they make a special effort to reduce their intake doubled. By 2008, average intake declined from 9.0 to 8.6 g/day, which is estimated to prevent more than 6,000 premature deaths and save £ 1.5 billion every year, dramatically more than the cost of running the salt reduction programme [23, 33].

Another successful community-based programme—the North Karelia Project—was launched in 1972 in Finland. It addressed diet and smoking through a model which relied on media, health services and community activities in partnership with various organizations and environmental and policy actions [34]. Before the launch of the project, almost all people used butter on their bread and in cooking; afterwards, less than 5 % used butter and 60 % used mainly vegetable oil in cooking. As far as smoking is concerned, prevalence of smokers in men declined from more than 50 % in the early 1970s to around 20 % in 2006. Furthermore, the overall average level of blood cholesterol dropped by over 20 %. This ended up in an 85-% reduction of mortality from 1969–1971 to 2006 with a gain of 7 and 6 years in life expectancy for men and women, respectively [35].

Several countries have explored fiscal measures such as increased taxation on foods that should be consumed in lower quantities and decreased taxation, price subsidies or production incentives for foods that are encouraged. A longitudinal study of food prices and consumption in China found that increases in the prices of unhealthy foods were associated with decreased consumption of those foods

[36]. In the USA, programmes to reduce the price of healthy foods led to a 78 % increase in their consumption [37]. Modelling studies suggest that a combination of tax reduction on healthy foods and tax increases on unhealthy foods may result in a stimulation of the consumption of healthy food, particularly in lower-income populations [38].

Key Elements for Decision Makers

- NCDs are the biggest global killers today. More than 60 % of all deaths are caused by NCDs.
- Nearly 80 % of these deaths occur in low- and middle-income countries, where the highest proportion of deaths under the age of 60 from NCDs occur.
- The prevalence of NCDs, and the resulting number of related deaths, is expected to increase substantially in the future, particularly in low- and middle-income countries.
- The NCD epidemic has a serious negative impact on development in human, social and economic realms. NCDs reduce productivity and contribute to poverty.
- NCDs already pose a substantial economic burden: The macroeconomic simulations suggest a cumulative output loss of US$ 47 trillion over the next two decades.
- Cardiovascular disease is the dominant contributor to the global economic burden of NCDs.
- The majority of NCDs can be averted through population-wide and individual interventions that reduce major risk factors. Interventions that combine a range of evidence-based approaches show better results.

References

1. World Health Organization (2005) Preventing chronic diseases: a vital investment. http://www.who.int/chp/chronic_disease_report/en. Accessed 04 April 2014
2. Bloom DE, Cafiero ET, Jané-Llopis E et al (2011) The global economic burden of non-communicable diseases. http://www3.weforum.org/docs/WEF_Harvard_HE_GlobalEconomicBurdenNonCommunicableDiseases_2011.pdf. Accessed 04 April 2014
3. Alwan A et al (2010) Monitoring and surveillance of chronic non-communicable diseases: progress and capacity in high-burden countries. Lancet 376:1861–1868
4. World Health Organization (2011) Global status report on non-communicable diseases 2010. http://www.who.int/nmh/publications/ncd_report_full_en.pdf. Accessed 04 April 2014
5. Murray CJ, Lopez AD (1997) Mortality by cause for eight regions of the world: Global Burden of Disease Study. Lancet 349(9061):1269–1276
6. World Health Organization (2008) The global burden of disease: 2004 update. Geneva, http://www.who.int/healthinfo/global_burden_disease/2004_report_update/en. Accessed 04 April 2014

7. World Health Organization (2011) Non-communicable diseases country profiles 2011. Geneva: World Health Organization. http://www.who.int/nmh/publications/ncd_profiles2011/en. Accessed 04 April 2014
8. Lozano R, Naghavi M, Foreman K et al (2012) Global and regional mortality from 235 causes of death for 20 age groups in 1990 and 2010: a systematic analysis for the Global Burden of Disease Study 2010. Lancet 380(9859):2095–2128
9. Institute for Health Metrics and Evaluation (2013) The global burden of disease: generating evidence, guiding policy. http://www.healthmetricsandevaluation.org/gbd/publications/policy-report/global-burden-disease-generating-evidence-guiding-policy. Accessed 04 April 2014
10. Ferlay J et al (2010) Estimates of worldwide burden of cancer in 2008: GLOBOCAN 2008. Int J Cancer 127:2893–2917
11. IARC (2012) Estimated cancer incidence, mortality and prevalence worldwide in 2012. http://www.iarc.fr. Accessed 04 April 2014
12. Boden-Albala B et al (2008) Diabetes, fasting glucose levels, and risk of ischemic stroke and vascular events: findings from the Northern Manhattan Study (NOMAS). Diabetes Care 31:1132–1137
13. Icks A et al (2009) Incidence of lower-limb amputations in the diabetic compared to the non-diabetic population. Findings from nationwide insurance data, Germany, 2005-2007. Exp Clin Endocrinol Diabetes 117:500–504
14. Resnikoff S et al (2004) Global data on visual impairment in the year 2002. Bull World Health Organ 82(11):844–851
15. Zhang P et al (2010) Global healthcare expenditure on diabetes for 2010 and 2030. Diabetes Res Clin Pract 87:293–301
16. World Health Organization (2012) Tobacco. Fact sheet N.°339 http://www.who.int/mediacentre/factsheets/fs339/en. Accessed 04 April 2014
17. Mathers CD, Loncar D (2006) Projections of global mortality and burden of disease from 2002 to 2030. PLoS Med 3(11):e442
18. Line H et al (2007) Tobacco smoke, indoor air pollution and tuberculosis: a systematic review and metaanalysis. PLoS Med 4:e20
19. World Health Organization (2011) New physical activity recommendations for reducing disease and prevent deaths. http://www.who.int/chp/media/news/releases/2011_2_physicalactivity/en. Accessed 04 April 2014
20. World Health Organization (2010) Global recommendations on physical activity for health. http://www.who.int/dietphysicalactivity/factsheet_recommendations/en. Accessed 04 April 2014
21. World Health Organization (2011) Alcohol. Fact sheet. http://www.who.int/mediacentre/factsheets/fs349/en. Accessed 04 April 2014
22. World Health Organization (2009) Global health risks: mortality and burden of disease attributable to selected major risks. http://www.who.int/healthinfo/global_burden_disease/GlobalHealthRisks_report_full.pdf. Accessed 04 April 2014
23. Brown IJ et al (2009) Salt intakes around the world: implications for public health. Int J Epidemiol 38:791–813
24. He FJ, MacGregor GA (2009) A comprehensive review on salt and health and current experience of worldwide salt reduction programmes. J Hum Hypertens 23:363–384
25. Murray SC, Miller J (2009) Dietary fat and coronary heart disease: summary of evidence from prospective cohort and randomised controlled trials. Ann Nutr Metab 55:173–201
26. World Health Organization (2013) Obesity and overweight. Fact sheet N.°311. http://www.who.int/mediacentre/factsheets/fs311/en. Accessed 04 April 2014
27. World Health Organization (2013) Non communicable diseases. Fact sheet. http://www.who.int/mediacentre/factsheets/fs355/en. Accessed 04 April 2014
28. Mayer-Foulkes D (2011) A survey of macro damages from non-communicable chronic diseases: another challenge for global governance. Glob Econ J 11(1):1–25

29. Suhrcke M, Stuckler D, Rocco L (2006) Chronic Disease: An economic perspective. Oxford Health Alliance, Oxford
30. Pan American Health Organization (2012) Non-communicable Diseases in the Americas: cost-effective interventions for prevention and control. http://www.paho.org/hq/index.php?option=com_docman&task=doc_view&gid=16220&Itemid. Accessed 04 April 2014
31. World Health Organization (2010) WHO technical manual on tobacco tax administration. http://www.who.int/tobacco/publications/tax_administration/en. Accessed 04 April 2014
32. Center for Disease Control and Prevention (2014) Best practices for comprehensive tobacco control programs—2014. www.cdc.gov/tobacco/stateandcommunity/best_practices/index.htm?source=govdelivery. Accessed 04 April 2014
33. World health Organization (2010) Creating an enabling environment for population-based salt reduction strategies: report of a joint technical meeting held by WHO and the Food Standards Agency, United Kingdom. http://whqlibdoc.who.int/publications/2010/9789241500777_eng.pdf. Accessed 04 April 2014
34. Puska P (2008) The North Karelia Project: 30 years successfully preventing chronic diseases. Diabetes Voices 53:173–201
35. Pekka P, Pirjo P, Ulla U (2002) Influencing public nutrition for noncommunicable disease prevention: from community intervention to national program- experiences from Finland. Public Health Nutr 5:245–251
36. Guo X et al (1999) Food price policy can favorably alter macronutrient intake in China. J Nutr 129:994–1001
37. Suhrcke M et al (2005) Economic consequences of chronic diseases and the economic rationale for public and private intervention. Oxford Health Alliance, London
38. Danish Academy of Technical Sciences (2007) Economic nutrition policy tools—useful in the challenge to combat obesity and poor nutrition? http://www.atv.dk/uploads/1227087410economicnutrition.pdf. Accessed 04 April 2014

Chapter 4
Cardiovascular Disease (CVD)

Elvira D´Andrea, Iveta Nagyova and Paolo Villari

Introduction

Cardiovascular disease (CVD) is the leading cause of death and disability worldwide. The majority of deaths from CVD (almost 80 %) are due to coronary heart disease (CHD; e.g., heart attack) and cerebrovascular disease (e.g., stroke) [1]. These two types of CVD share a common underlying pathological process of the blood vessels known as atherosclerosis. There is strong scientific evidence that behavioral (e.g., tobacco use; physical inactivity; harmful use of alcohol; unhealthy diet—rich in salt, fat, and calories) and metabolic (e.g., hypertension, diabetes, dyslipidemia, overweight and obesity) risk factors play a key role in the etiology of atherosclerosis [2].

CVD is often thought to be a problem of industrialized and wealthy (high-income) nations, but it also has an important impact on developing (low- and middle-income) countries, where they account for over two thirds of deaths. In fact, over the past two decades, deaths from CVD have been declining in high-income countries, while they have increased in low- and middle-income countries [1, 2].

When a country's economy and health system develops, it undergoes a phenomenon called epidemiological transition, referring to the changes in the predominant types of disease and mortality burdening a population. Typically, there is a shift from infectious to chronic diseases [3]. This transition is caused by improvements

E. D´Andrea (✉) · P. Villari
Department of Public Health and Infectious Diseases, Sapienza University of Rome, ple Aldo Moro 5, 00185 Rome, Italy
e-mail: elvira.dandrea@gmail.com

P. Villari
e-mail: paolo.villari@uniroma1.it

I. Nagyova
Department of Public Health, PJ Safarik University, Tr SNP 1, 04011 Kosice, Slovakia
e-mail: iveta.nagyova@upjs.sk

S. Boccia et al. (eds.), *A Systematic Review of Key Issues in Public Health*,
DOI 10.1007/978-3-319-13620-2_4

in health care, leading to a decrease in infant mortality rate; by ageing of the population, with a corresponding increase in rates of chronic diseases that affect older people; and by public health interventions such as vaccinations and the provision of clean water and sanitation, which reduce the incidence of infectious diseases. As life expectancy increases, populations face “new” risks such as smoking and alcohol abuse, physical inactivity, overweight and obesity, etc. The impact of these risks varies at different levels of socioeconomic development, and the major causes of death and disability shift to the chronic and noncommunicable diseases (NCDs).

Increasing exposure to these behavioral risks is not inevitable, and scientific evidence suggests that two thirds of premature deaths due to chronic diseases, including CVD, can be prevented by primary prevention, and another one third by improving health systems to respond more effectively and equitably to health care needs [3]. Therefore, the implementation of preventive interventions through population-wide measures and individual health care interventions can reduce and potentially eliminate the health and socioeconomic burden caused by these diseases and their risk factors. These interventions, which are evidence based and cost-effective, are known as “best buys,” and they provide workable solutions and represent the best economic investment both in high-income and in low- and middle-income nations [4, 5]. Cost-effective prevention strategies and interventions are needed if the growing burden of CVD is to be arrested; this is one of the major health challenges to be overcome in the near future in both developed and developing countries.

This chapter describes the current burden, CVD trends over time, and strategies for prevention of CVD globally, with a particular focus on Europe. It lays out the major risk factors associated with CHD and stroke throughout the course of life. It aims to review and discuss the scientific evidence on the effectiveness and cost-effectiveness of primary and secondary prevention policies. Finally, a reasoned analysis has been performed to identify best practices for CVD prevention strategies and to provide guidance on what drivers play a key role in the decision-making process required to actually implement and improve these prevention strategies.

To provide an overview of the current literature, we conducted a systematic search of current epidemiological (descriptive and analytic), public health (primary and secondary prevention strategies), and health economic literature on CVD, as well as documentation on regulatory and policy issues. For the descriptive and analytical epidemiology of CVD and for primary and secondary prevention strategies, institutional websites of authoritative scientific societies, international organizations, and referenced universities were surveyed and the relevant reports, textbooks, and position papers on the topic were collected. For the effectiveness and cost-effectiveness of primary and secondary prevention policies, a search was performed on several electronic databases (Cochrane Database, PubMed–Medline, NHS Economic Evaluation Database, and SCOPUS), using keywords related to CVD and cost-effectiveness of the primary and secondary CVD policies to retrieve reviews and systematic reviews. In addition, key references from relevant articles were selected.

Cardiovascular Disease: Definitions and Classifications

CVD encompasses a group of medical conditions caused by disorders of the heart and blood vessels. There are different types of CVD that can be classified into two groups based on whether or not the disease results from atherosclerosis. The first group, which involves atherosclerosis, comprises CHD, i.e., disease of the blood vessels supplying the heart muscle (e.g., heart attack); cerebrovascular disease, i.e., disease of the blood vessels supplying the brain (e.g., stroke); diseases of the aorta and arteries, including hypertension; and peripheral vascular disease (PVD), i.e., disease of the blood vessels supplying the arms and legs. The second group includes congenital heart disease, i.e., malformations of heart structure existing at birth; rheumatic heart disease, i.e., damage to the heart muscle and heart valves from rheumatic fever caused by streptococcal bacteria; deep vein thrombosis and pulmonary embolism, i.e., blood clots that occur in the leg veins and can dislodge and move to the heart and lungs; and cardiomyopathies and arrhythmias [4, 6].

Among all types of CVD, heart attack and stroke are responsible for almost 80 % of deaths [1, 4]. These disorders are usually acute events and are mainly caused by a blockage that prevents blood from flowing to the heart or brain. The most common reason for such a blockage is a buildup of fatty deposits on the inner walls of the blood vessels that supply the heart or the brain; this process is known as atherosclerosis [4].

Atherosclerosis is a multifactorial, multistep pathological process that involves chronic inflammation in medium- and large-sized blood vessels. When blood vessel endothelium is exposed to raised levels of low-density lipoprotein (LDL) cholesterol and other substances, it becomes permeable to cells of the immune system, such as monocytes and lymphocytes. The migration of these cells into the deep layers of the endothelium causes the breakdown of various substances and the attraction of LDL cholesterol particles to the site. These LDL particles are engulfed by monocytes, which then differentiate into macrophages (foam cells). From deeper layers of the vessel lining (the media), smooth muscle cells migrate to the site and combine with collagen fibers to form a fibrous cap. At the same time, the macrophages die, so that a necrotic core develops under the fibrous cap. These lesions, known as atheromatous plaques, enlarge as cells and lipids accumulate in them, and they begin to protrude into the vessel lumen. Later, the fibrous cap thins and a fissure on the endothelial surface of the plaque occurs. With the rupture of the plaque, lipid fragments and cellular debris are released into the vessel lumen. These particles are exposed to thrombogenic agents on the endothelial surface, resulting in the formation of a thrombus, or blood clot. If the thrombus is large enough to block circulation of coronary or cerebral blood vessels, this results in a heart attack or stroke [4, 6]. Atherosclerosis with thrombus formation has been recognized as a major cause of cardiovascular death. It begins early in childhood and progresses in adult life when it can potentially manifest as CHD, stroke, and/or PVD [4, 6].

CHD, also called coronary artery disease or ischemic heart disease, is responsible for over 40 % of the global burden due to CVD [1]. Disease develops when an atherosclerotic plaque builds up in the arteries that supply the heart, i.e., the coronary arteries. Through these arteries, the heart muscle (myocardium) acquires the oxygen and other nutrients it needs to continue pumping blood. When the blood flow to the heart is decreased, different symptoms start to appear. These usually occur during exercise or activity because the heart muscle's increased demand for nutrients and oxygen is not being met by the blocked coronary blood vessel. The most common symptom is chest pain (angina pectoris) due to ischemia. Other common symptoms are shortness of breath on exertion, jaw pain, back pain, or arm pain (especially on the left side, either during exertion or at rest), palpitations, dizziness, light-headedness or fainting, weakness on exertion or at rest, and irregular heartbeat. The most devastating sign of CHD is abrupt, unexpected cardiac arrest, while the opposite extreme is represented by the condition known as silent ischemia, in which no symptoms occur, even though an electrocardiogram (ECG, or heart tracing) and/or other tests show evidence of ischemia [4, 6].

Stroke is responsible for over 30 % of the global burden due to CVD; it is caused by the interruption of the blood supply to the brain because a blood vessel bursts (hemorrhagic stroke) or is blocked by a clot (ischemic stroke) [1]. In the first case, the cause is usually a rupture of a blood vessel as a result of an aneurysm or damage due to uncontrolled high blood pressure or atherosclerosis. In the second case, thrombus formation in an atherosclerotic cerebral blood vessel or traveling blood clots trapped in a cerebral blood vessel can block the blood flow to an area of the brain. These events cut off the supply of oxygen and nutrients, causing damage to the brain tissue. The symptoms depend on what part of the brain and how much of the brain tissue is affected. The most common are weakness in the arm or leg (or both) on the same side of the body, ranging from total paralysis to a very mild weakness; complete numbness or a pins-and-needles feeling that may be present on one side of the body or part of one side of the body; weakness in the muscles of the face, potentially associated with speech difficulties; coordination problems, leading to difficulty in walking or picking up objects; dizziness; vision problems; sudden severe headache; and loss of consciousness [4, 6].

Current Burden of Cardiovascular Disease

The evaluation and analysis of CVD burden and trends worldwide cannot be tackled without addressing the most important "key drivers" of rapid transition in global health [7]. The first pattern responsible for the growth in CVD burden is the demographic increase in both size and average age of the population. Clearly, an ageing population must contribute to the increment in these diseases, given that the first CVD event occurs at an average age of greater than 50 years. The second pattern of transition is the change in causes of death. From 1990 to 2010, the combined mortality and disability rates of all communicable, maternal, neonatal, and nutritional diseases decreased, due principally to better maternal education, prenatal care, and early-childhood interventions; improvements in preventive and medical care, where the use of new technologies has had a significant impact; improvements in socioeconomic status (SES); and increasing health expenditure, including greater provision for public health and medical care. At the same time, the burden of NCDs increased significantly, with only modest decreases in rates of NCDs and risk factor exposure in developed countries, and increasing rates of NCDs in the developing countries. The third element is the change in causes of disability, shifting from premature death to years lived with disability in the context of a significant increase in NCDs [2, 7].

Prevalence and Incidence

Information on the magnitude of CVD in high-income countries is available from three large longitudinal studies that collect multidisciplinary data from a representative sample of European and American individuals aged 50 and older [8, 9, 10]. Thus, according to the Health Retirement Survey (HRS) in the USA, almost one in three adults have one or more types of CVD [11, 12]. By contrast, the data of Survey of Health, Ageing and Retirement in Europe (SHARE), obtained from 11 European countries, and English Longitudinal Study of Aging (ELSA) show that disease rates (specifically heart disease, diabetes, and stroke) across these populations are lower (almost one in five) [11, 13, 14].

Among adults with one or more forms of CVD, the most prevalent conditions are, in decreasing order, hypertension, CHD, stroke, heart failure, and congenital heart defects. Although advancing age is the most powerful risk factor for CVD, in high-income countries, particularly in the USA and Europe, many adults with well-established CVD are younger than 65. Of particular concern are men and women aged 55–64: In this age-specific group, 52 % of men and 56.5 % of women live with one or more forms of CVD [9, 11].

Children and young adults also represent an important age group. Although the overall incidence is low, sudden cardiac death, due to congenital heart defects, accounts for one in five unexpected sudden deaths among children aged 1–13 and for one in three among those aged 14–21 [11]. Both congenital heart disease and acquired heart disease affect children and are particularly burdensome for children in low- and middle-income countries. Many of these children die prematurely because of late diagnosis and/or lack of access to appropriate treatment. Those who survive may face a lifetime of disability caused by a disease that is not well managed. In low- and middle-income countries, the problem of nutritional insufficiencies among infants and children, combined with greater access to nutrition-poor food, has been found to increase the risk of CVD later in life [1, 15].

Mortality

In 2008, the World Health Organization (WHO) reported that, with the exception of the African Region, NCDs mortality had surpassed the sum of the death rates of all communicable, maternal, neonatal, and nutritional diseases. In Europe, deaths of men from NCDs are 13 times higher than those of all other causes combined, while in the Western Pacific Region, they are estimated to be eight times higher [2, 4].

CVD causes 30 % of all deaths worldwide and almost half of deaths due to NCDs. The global distribution of age-adjusted CVD mortality is uneven and more than 80 % of these deaths occurred in low- and middle-income countries [1, 4]. The lowest mortality rates are now recorded in high-income countries and in parts of Latin America, whereas the highest rates are in Eastern Europe and in a number of low- and middle-income countries. Overall, age-adjusted CVD death rates are higher in most low- and middle-income countries than in developed countries [1, 4, 16]. CHD and stroke together are the first and third leading causes of death in developed and developing countries, respectively. In fact, excluding deaths from cancer, these two conditions were responsible for more deaths in 2008 than all remaining causes among the ten leading causes of death combined (including chronic diseases of the lungs, accidents, diabetes, influenza, and pneumonia) [1, 4, 16].

In Europe, CVD causes over four million deaths per year (52 % of deaths in women and 42 % of deaths in men), and they are the main cause of death in women in all European countries. Over a third of deaths are caused by CHD (1.8 million deaths each year) and just over a quarter are from stroke (almost 1.1 million deaths each year). Death rates from CHD and stroke are generally higher in Central and Eastern Europe than in Northern, Southern and Western Europe. CVD mortality is now falling in most European countries, including Central and Eastern European countries, which saw large increases until the beginning of the twenty-first century [16, 17].

Disability

In 1990, the major fraction of morbidity worldwide was due to communicable, maternal, neonatal, and nutritional disorders (47 %), while 43 % of disability adjusted life years (DALYs) lost were attributable to NCDs. Within two decades, these estimates had undergone a drastic change, shifting to 35 % and 54 %, respectively [18]. The global burden of disease is continuing to shift away from communicable to NCDs, as well as from premature death to years lived with disability. The increased disability rates due to CVD represent a significant loss of healthy life and an increasing cost for health care systems [7].

According to the Global Burden of Disease Study 2010 estimates, CVD is responsible for 18 % of DALYs in high-income countries and 10 % of DALYs in low- and middle-income countries [1, 19]. In 2010, CHD and stroke were the first and third cause, respectively, of disability worldwide, while in 1990, they were not among the first three major causes of morbidity. Compared to 1990, in 2010, the burden of CVD, in terms of DALYs, increased by 29 %, while the burden of stroke increased by 19 % [7, 18].

Disease Trends

The annual number of CVD deaths has increased from 14.4 million in 1990 to 18.5 million in 2010, of which 7.6 million are attributed to CHD and 5.7 million to stroke [19]. According to the WHO, this estimate will rise to 25 million in 2030, accounting for 30 % of all deaths worldwide. Over the next few decades, it is expected that NCDs will account for more than three quarters of deaths worldwide. CVD alone will be responsible for more deaths in low-income countries than infectious diseases (including HIV/AIDS, tuberculosis, and malaria), maternal and perinatal conditions, and nutritional disorders combined [16]. CVD will continue to be the largest single contributor to global mortality, dominating mortality trends in the future [4].

The US national academies (National Academy of Sciences, National Academy of Engineering, Institute of Medicine, and National Research Council) observed three different CHD mortality trends across a range of nations. The first is a rise-and-fall pattern, where mortality rates increase, peak, and then fall significantly. The second is a rising pattern, where rates are steadily increasing, indicating an ongoing epidemic. The third pattern is flat, i.e., CHD mortality rates are relatively low and stable. The rise-and-fall pattern is most notable in high-income countries (e.g., European countries, USA, and Australia), because in these countries, CHD mortality rates peaked in the 1960s or early 1970s and have since fallen precipitously, by an average of about 50 %. The rising pattern is notable in low- and middle-income countries, where mortality rates are increasing, sometimes to an alarming level. By contrast, CHD mortality rates in other countries (e.g., Japan and several European Mediterranean countries) are relatively low, following the flat pattern [16].

Economic Burden of CVD

The economic cost of CVD to families and society is high and escalating, caused not only by health care costs but also by production losses due to the death and illness of people of working age, as well as the financial impact on friends and relatives who act as informal carers of those with the disease [17, 20].

Estimates of the direct health care and nonhealth care costs attributable to CVD in many countries, especially in low- and middle-income countries, are unclear and fragmentary. In high-income countries (e.g., USA and Europe), CVD is the most costly disease both in terms of economic costs and human costs. Over half (54 %) of the total cost is due to direct health care costs, while one fourth (24 %) is attributable to productivity losses and 22 % to the informal care of people with CVD. Overall, CVD is estimated to cost the EU economy, in terms of health care, almost €196 billion per year, i.e., 9 % of the total health care expenditure across the EU and a cost per capita of €212 per annum. CHD is estimated to cost the EU economy €60 billion per year, while stroke costs over €38 billion per year, i.e., around one third and one fifth of the overall health care cost of CVD, respectively. Costs of inpatient hospital care for people who have CVD accounted for about 49 % of health care costs, and drugs for their treatment about 29 %. The health care costs for people with CVD varies widely across the EU, e.g., by tenfold in 2009, from €37 in Romania to €374 in Germany [17].

Major Risk Factors

In the past two decades, the contribution of different risk factors to the global disease burden has changed substantially, with a shift from risks for communicable towards those for NCDs. Factors associated with an increased risk of CVD are generally classified into two categories, i.e., either modifiable or nonmodifiable risk factors. Those of the first group can be controlled, treated, or modified through health interventions, while those of the second group relate to individual characteristics that cannot be changed [4, 21].

The Global Burden of Disease Study 2010, through an assessment of the leading risk factors across 187 countries, identified the risk factors that account for the leading cause of DALYs worldwide (Table 4.1). All modifiable risk factors associated with the development of CVD rank among the top 15 risk factors overall. The two leading risk factors for global disease burden are high blood pressure and tobacco smoking, including secondhand exposure to smoke. Other modifiable risk factors for CVD included alcohol abuse, high body mass index (BMI), high fasting plasma glucose level, high total cholesterol level, dietary risk factors (diets low in fruit and vegetables, and diets high in sodium), and physical inactivity [7, 18, 19].

Short History of CVD Risk Factors

The term *risk factor* appeared for the first time in a paper published in *Annals of Internal Medicine* and written by William B. Kannel, first director of the Framingham Heart Study [22]. The Framingham Heart Study, founded in 1948 under the direction of the National Heart Institute of Boston, analyzing the epidemiology of CVD in Framingham, a small town outside of Boston, has become the worldwide standard for cardiovascular epidemiology. At the beginning of the study, not much was known about the causes of CHD and stroke, at a time when the increasing death rates for CVD were becoming alarming. Therefore, the initial objective of the study was to identify the common environmental factors or personal characteristics that contribute to the development of CVD events by following a large multigenerational asymptomatic group over a long period of time [23]. This pioneering work, followed by the Seven Countries Study in the 1960s [24] and many others studies since then, including the WHO-MONICA Project [25] and the INTERHEART study [26], have resulted in the identification of the major factors and determinants

Table 4.1 Global DALYs attributable to the 25 leading risk factors in 1990 and 2010 (in bold the CVD risk factors). Results from Global Burden of Disease Study 2010 (GBD 2010) [7]

Risk factor	2010		1990	
	Rank	DALYs (95 % UI) *in thousands*	Rank	DALYs (95 % UI) *in thousands*
High blood pressure	1	173,556 (155,939–189,025)	4	137,017 (124,360–149,366)
Tobacco smoking (including exposure to secondhand smoke)	2	156,838 (136,543–173,057)	3	151,766 (136,367–169,522)
Household air pollution from solid fuels	3	108,084 (84,891–132,983)	2	170,693 (139,087–199,504)
Diet low in fruit	4	104,095 (81,833–124,169)	7	80,453 (63,298–95,763)
Alcohol use	5	97,237 (87,087–107,658)	8	73,715 (66,090–82,089)
High body mass index	6	93,609 (77,107–110,600)	10	51,565 (40,786–62,557)
High fasting plasma glucose level or diabetes	7	89,012 (77,743–101,390)	9	56,358 (48,720–65,030)
Childhood underweight	8	77,316 (64,497–91,943)	1	197,741 (169,224–238,276)
Exposure to ambient particulate matter pollution	9	76,163 (68,086–85,171)	6	81,699 (71,012–92,859)
Physical inactivity or low level of activity	10	69,318 (58,646–80,182)	–	–
Diet high in sodium	11	61,231 (40,124–80,342)	12	46,183 (30,363–60,604)
Diet low in nuts and seeds	12	51,289 (33,482–65,959)	13	40,525 (26,308–51,741)
Iron deficiency	13	48,225 (33,769–67,592)	11	51,841 (37,477–71,202)
Suboptimal breast-feeding	14	47,537 (29,868–67,518)	5	110,261 (69,615–153,539)
High total cholesterol level	15	40,900 (31,662–50,484)	14	39,526 (32,704–47,202)
Diet low in whole grains	16	40,762 (32,112–48,486)	18	29,404 (23,097–35,134)
Diet low in vegetables	17	38,559 (26,006–51,658)	16	31,558 (21,349–41,921)
Diet low in seafood n-3 fatty acids	18	28,199 (20,624–35,974)	20	21,740 (15,869–27,537)
Drug use	19	23,810 (18,780–29,246)	25	15,171 (11,714–19,369)
Occupational risk factors for injuries	20	23,444 (17,736–30,904)	21	21,265 (16,644–26,702)

Table 4.1 (continued)

Risk factor	2010		1990	
	Rank	DALYs (95 % UI) *in thousands*	Rank	DALYs (95 % UI) *in thousands*
Occupation-related low back pain	21	21,750 (14,492–30,533)	23	17,841 (11,846–24,945)
Diet high in processed meat	22	20,939 (6982–33,468)	24	17,359 (5137–27,949)
Intimate partner violence	23	16,794 (11,373–23,087)	–	–
Diet low in fiber	24	16,452 (7401–25,783)	26	13,347 (5970–20,751)
Lead exposure	25	13,936 (11,750–16,327)	31	5,365 (4534–6279)

DALYs disability-adjusted life years, *UI* uncertainty interval

correlated with CVD. The notion of CVD risk factor is today an integral part of the modern medical vocabulary and has led to the development of effective treatments in clinical practice and preventive strategies in public health.

Modifiable Risk Factors

High Blood Pressure

In 2008, the worldwide prevalence of high blood pressure, in adults over 25 years, was around 40 % and higher in the African Region (46 % for both sexes combined) [2, 4]. According to the Global Burden of Disease Study 2010, raised blood pressure is the first ranking risk factor contributing to the global burden of disease and the number of people with elevated blood pressure (systolic blood pressure ≥140 mmHg or diastolic blood pressure ≥90 mmHg) has increased from 600 million in 1980 to a billion in 2010 [7]. In 2010, high blood pressure was estimate to cause almost 9.4 million (95 % uncertainty interval (UI), 8.6 million to 10.1 million) of global deaths and 7 % of the total DALYs (Table 4.1) [7, 19].

The relationship between hypertension and CVD, especially CVD due to atherosclerosis, has been widely demonstrated and blood pressure levels are positively and continuously correlated with the risk of stroke and CHD. In some age groups, the CVD risk doubles for each increment of 20/10 mmHg of blood pressure, starting from 115/75 mmHg [2, 4]. In addition to CHD and stroke, complications of raised blood pressure include heart failure, PVD, renal impairment, retinal hemorrhage, and visual impairment [2, 4].

The major underlying risks for hypertension are sodium in the diet, body weight, and limited access to treatment. Therefore, nonpharmacological (sodium reduction, increase of fruit and vegetable intake, weight control) and pharmacological strategies can improve health outcomes of people with high blood pressure. Treating systolic blood pressure and diastolic blood pressure until they are less than 140/90 mmHg is associated with a reduction in complications, including CVD [2, 4, 19].

Tobacco Smoking

Worldwide, almost six million deaths each year are attributable to smoking, both from direct tobacco use and secondhand smoke [27]. By 2030, this number will increase to eight million [27]. Smoking is estimated to cause nearly 10 % of CVD and other important disorders such as lung cancer (71 %) and chronic respiratory disease (42 %) [27]. According to the Global Burden of Disease Study 2010, smoking, including secondhand smoke, is the second leading risk factor contributing to the burden of disease worldwide (6.3 million deaths and 6.3 % of DALYs; Table 4.1) [7]. Smoking prevalence is higher in high- and middle-income countries, but, within countries, there is an inverse relationship between income levels and prevalence of tobacco use [4].

The impact of smoking on increasing CVD incidence has been widely demonstrated and the estimated risk increases with the number of cigarettes smoked per day. The risk of a cardiovascular event in heavy smokers (greater than 40 cigarettes per day) is twice that of light smokers (fewer than 10 cigarettes per day) [28].

Smoking cessation has been shown to have a significant impact on the reduction of CHD mortality. Further, it leads to significantly lower rates of recurrent CVD events in people who have had a heart attack and reduces the risk of sudden cardiac death among people with well-established CHD. Although the specific time line of risk reduction depends on the number of years of smoking and the quantity of tobacco consumed daily, it is considered possible that, over time, the CVD risk among former smokers can drop to levels similar to that of the general population [29].

Unhealthy Diet

A healthy diet has a good balance of macronutrients (fats, proteins, and carbohydrates) to support energy needs without excessive weight gain from overconsumption, micronutrients to meet the needs for human nutrition without inducing toxicity, and an adequate amount of water. The leading problems of an unhealthy diet are an insufficient intake of fruit, vegetables, fish, legumes, whole grains, and nuts; an excessive intake of salt and total fats (exceeding 30 % of the total energy per day); and the consumption of saturated fat and trans-fatty acids. Low-income and socioeconomic levels are significant determinants of an unhealthy diet [4].

It has been widely demonstrated that a healthy diet is important for reducing many chronic health risks, such as obesity, high blood cholesterol, high blood pressure, and diabetes, which are closely related to excessive consumption of fatty, sugary, and salty foods [4].

According to the Global Burden of Disease Study 2010, a diet low in fruit is the fourth leading cause of DALYs worldwide, causing 4.9 million deaths and 4.2% of global DALYs (Table 4.1) [7]. Adequate consumption of fruit and vegetables reduces the risk not only of CVD but also of stomach and colorectal cancer.

Most populations consume much higher levels of salt than recommended by the WHO (5 g/day) and high salt consumption is an important determinant of high blood pressure and cardiovascular risk. A diet with high sodium intake is the 11th ranking risk factor contributing to the global burden disease worldwide and it is responsible for four million of deaths and 2.5% of global DALYs (Table 4.1) [7, 19]. It is estimated that even a modest reduction in salt intake, from levels of 9 to 12 g/day to the recommended level of 5 g/day, may significantly lower blood pressure [30].

High consumption of saturated fats and trans-fatty acids is strongly linked with CHD. The elimination of trans-fatty acids and the replacement of saturated fats with polyunsaturated vegetable oils have a positive impact on CVD risk. Available data suggest that fat intake has been rising rapidly in lower- and middle-income countries since the 1980s [4].

Other dietary risk factors, which have strong impact on the global burden of disease and are correlated with CVD events, are diets low in nuts and seeds (2.5 million of deaths in 2010, 2.1% of DALYs), low in whole grains (1.7 million of deaths, 1.6% of DALYs), and low in seafood omega-3 fatty acids (0.6 million of deaths, 0.5% of DALYs; Table 4.1) [7, 19].

Alcohol Use

Alcohol use is one of the most important avoidable risk factors, ranking fifth in the Global Burden of Disease Study 2010, which accounted for 4.9 million deaths and 5.5% of global DALYs (Table 4.1) [7]. While the adult per capita consumption is higher in high-income countries, alcohol use is also significant in some middle-income countries, and as a result is the leading risk factor in Eastern Europe, Andean Latin America, and southern sub-Saharan Africa [19]. Alcohol abuse is responsible for 3.8% of all deaths (half of which are due to CVD, cancer, and liver cirrhosis) and 4.5% of the global burden of disease [27].

The relationship between alcohol consumption and the development of CVD is complex. Excessive and hazardous alcohol intake is associated with increased risk of hypertension, stroke, CHD, and other forms of CVD. However, several epidemiological studies suggest a cardioprotective association for low or moderate average alcohol consumption, and the correlation may follow a "U" or "J" curve, with the lowest rates of CVD associated with light and moderate intakes of alcohol [31]. However, a cardioprotective relationship between alcohol use and CHD and stroke cannot be assumed for all drinkers, even at low levels of intake [31]. Moreover, alcohol may also contribute to overweight and obesity, since it is a significant source of daily calories in many countries. Finally, it is important to emphasize the association of alcohol misuse with many other diseases (neuropsychiatric disorders, cirrhosis, and cancer), which outweighs the potential and small cardioprotective effects [32].

Overweight and Obesity

Obesity is a CVD risk factor closely linked to diet and physical activity and it results when there is an imbalance between energy intake in the diet and energy expenditure. To achieve optimal health, the median BMI for adult populations should be in the range of 21–23 kg/m^2, while the goal for individuals should be to maintain a BMI in the range 18.5–24.9 kg/m^2 [4].

The incidence of high BMI has increased globally and at present 3.4 million people die prematurely each year as a result [19]. High BMI is responsible for 3.8 % DALYs worldwide, resulting as the sixth leading risk of global DALYs in 2010 [7, 19] (Table 4.1). It is the major risk factor in Australia, Asia, and southern Latin America, and it also ranks highly in other high-income regions, and in North Africa, the Middle East, and Oceania [7]. The prevalence of overweight is highest in upper-to-middle-income countries, but very high levels are also reported in some lower-to-middle-income countries. In the WHO European Region, the Eastern Mediterranean Region, and the Region of the Americas, over 50 % of women are overweight. The highest prevalence of overweight among infants and young children is in upper-to-middle-income populations, while the fastest rise in overweight is in the lower-to-middle-income group [19]. Globally, in 2008, 9.8 % of men and 13.8 % of women were obese compared to 4.8 % of men and 7.9 % of women in 1980 [27].

Obesity is strongly related to some of the major cardiovascular risk factors such as raised blood pressure, glucose intolerance, type 2 diabetes, and dyslipidemia [4]. Risks of heart disease, stroke, and diabetes increase steadily with increasing BMI [4].

Diabetes

Diabetes is defined as a group of metabolic diseases in which an individual have a fasting plasma glucose value of 7.0 mmol/l (126 mg/dl) or higher. Impaired glucose tolerance and fasting glycemia are categories of risk for the future development of diabetes [2]. In 2010, diabetes was responsible for 3.4 million deaths globally and 3.6 % of DALYs [7, 19] (Table 4.1). The prevalence is lower in low- and middle-income countries (8 %) compared to developed countries (10 %) [27].

There is a clear relationship between diabetes and CVD. Several studies showed a two- to threefold increased incidence of CVD in patients with diabetes compared to people without diabetes [33]. Furthermore, people with diabetes also have a poorer prognosis after cardiovascular events compared to people without diabetes [33]. In fact, CVD is by far the most frequent cause of death in both men and women with diabetes, accounting for about 60 % of all mortality [27]. Other severe complications resulting from lack of early detection and care of diabetes are renal failure, blindness, foot ulcers, and amputation.

It has been widely demonstrated that the risk of diabetes is increased with some conditions or types of behavior, such as obesity and overweight, which are the primary risk factors for type 2 diabetes, fat distribution, and physical inactivity [6].

Primary care with measurement of blood glucose levels and cardiovascular risk assessment, as well as the provision of essential medicines, including insulin, can significantly improve the health outcomes of people with diabetes [4].

Physical Inactivity

A low level of physical activity is defined as less than five episodes of 30 min of moderate activity per week, or less than three times of 20 min of vigorous activity per week [4]. In 2010, 3.2 million deaths and 2.8 % of global DALYs were due to insufficient physical activity (Table 4.1) [7, 19]. The prevalence of insufficient physical activity is higher in high-income countries (41 % of men and 48 % of women) compared to low-income countries (18 % of men and 21 % of women) as a likely consequence of the automation of work and overuse of vehicles [19]. Similarly to tobacco use and unhealthy diet, there is a relationship, in high-income countries, between physical inactivity and low-income level and SES [19].

According to the Global Burden of Disease Study 2010, physical inactivity or low physical activity is the tenth leading risk factor worldwide contributing to the global burden of disease (Table 4.1) [7]. In fact, physical activity plays a key role in regulating energy balance and weight control, and people who are insufficiently physically active have a 20–30 % increased risk of all-cause mortality [7]. Regular physical activity also reduces the risk of CVD through better control of high blood pressure and diabetes. This protective action is due to an improvement in endothelial function and, consequently, an enhancement in vasodilatation and vasomotor functions in the blood vessels. In addition, physical activity contributes positively to weight loss, glycemic control, lipid profile, and insulin sensitivity [4].

Dyslipidemia

The main functions of cholesterol are to assist in building and maintaining membranes in the body and to ensure membrane flexibility over a wide temperature range. Within membranes, cholesterol is needed for nerve and cell signaling and conduction. Moreover, cholesterol is stored in the adrenal glands, ovaries, and the testes and is converted to steroid hormones. It is also required for the manufacture of fat-soluble vitamins and bile acids. The lipid profile of body fat is composed of LDL cholesterol, which is also known as the "bad" cholesterol, high-density lipoprotein (HDL), known as the "good" cholesterol, and triglycerides [6, 34].

LDL levels are closely correlated with CVD. Raised cholesterol is considered the 15th leading risk factor for the global burden of disease and it is estimated to cause two million deaths and 1.6 % of total DALYs annually [7] (Table 4.1). The prevalence of raised total cholesterol varies according to the income level of the country. In low-income countries, around 25 % of adults have raised total cholesterol, while in high-income countries, over 50 % of adults have raised total cholesterol [4, 34]. Overall, one third of CHD disease is attributable to high cholesterol levels, and lowering blood cholesterol reduces the risk of heart disease [27].

Social Determinants

Social determinants of health represent the social conditions in which individuals live and work. They are shaped by the distribution of power, income, and access to resources, as much on a global and national level as on a local level. SES has been widely acknowledged as the most powerful social determinant of health [35].

While the relationship between CVD and the traditional risk factors described above has been widely studied, fewer studies have analyzed social determinants such as the level of education, working conditions, housing, or social relationships. Social determinants influence indirectly global health, as well as the cardiovascular health state, by impacting behavioral and metabolic cardiovascular risk factors, psychosocial status, and living conditions, and it is difficult to examine these underlying triggers [35].

Social determinants have been shown to be related to CVD in various ways. Work-related stress and depression have been linked to the development of cardiovascular risk factors, such as hypertension and atherosclerosis [35]. Negative social interactions were found to be related to higher blood pressure levels [35]. The poor have limited opportunities for healthy choices and have a high prevalence of smoking [2, 35]. Finally, also the access to health care may explain the link between SES and CHD [35].

Social determinants influence both the incidence and management of traditional risk factors and the management of CVD events [2, 35]. Thus, ignoring patients' social status, when scoring total cardiovascular risk using traditional models, may lead to the underestimation of the true cardiovascular risk for patients of low SES [35].

Nonmodifiable Risk Factors

Age

Age is a powerful cardiovascular risk factor, and the rapidly growing burden of CVD in low- and middle-income countries is accelerated by population ageing. The first CVD event occurs in the vast majority of people after the age of 55 years in males and 65 years in females [27]. As a person gets older, the heart undergoes subtle physiological changes, even in the absence of disease. The heart muscle of the aged heart may relax less completely between beats and, as a result, the pumping chambers become stiffer and may work less efficiently [6].

Gender

Males are at greater risk of CHD than females (premenopausal woman). After the menopause, the risk in women is similar to that in men [36]. Risk of stroke, however, is similar for men and women throughout life [36].

Family History

Family history is an independent predictor of CVD [37]. A positive family history for CVD captures the underlying complexities of gene–gene and gene–environment interactions by identifying families with combinations of risk factors, both measured and unmeasured, which lead to disease expression. Family history is a useful tool for identifying the relatively small subset of families in the population at highest risk of CVD who may benefit most from targeted screening and intensive interventions [37].

Reducing the Burden of Cardiovascular Disease: Strategies for Prevention

Prevention of CVD requires a stratified approach involving population-wide, high-risk, and secondary prevention strategies. These three strategies are not mutually exclusive, and indeed must be integrated for maximum CVD prevention [38].

The concepts of population-wide (or community-based) and high-risk prevention strategies were introduced into the public health arena by Geoffrey Rose in 1981 [39]. According to several reports published by the WHO on primary prevention of CVD, it is fundamental that the high-risk approach is complemented by a population-based strategy [40]. Without population-wide prevention efforts, CVD will continue to occur in people with low and moderate levels of risk, who represent the majority in any population. A community-based prevention strategy may also induce lifestyle changes in the high-risk population. The passage between primary and secondary prevention is correlated with the development of an established CVD and with a gradual increase in an individual's global risk. For this subgroup population, intensive behavioral interventions and drug treatments are recommended, and health care actions may switch from mainly nondrug interventions to drug interventions [38, 40].

Success in the prevention of CVD events is maximized when all three prevention strategies are applied simultaneously. The choice of the interventions to be implemented should depend on the proven effectiveness and cost-effectiveness of particular interventions and on the resources available.

Population-Wide Prevention Strategy

A community-based prevention strategy attempts to shift the distribution of exposure to risk factors in a population through lifestyle and environmental changes that affect the whole population, without requiring interventions at the individual level. The central concept behind this strategy is the recognition that exposure to risk factors reflects the functioning of society as a whole. A population-based prevention strategy is essential for the reduction of both the incidence and burden of CVD when there is a clear relationship between risk and exposure and the risk is widely distributed across the whole target population. This type of prevention strategy is mostly achieved by establishing health policies and community interventions. Rose in 1981 considered this approach more capable of preventing burden of disease than targeting the high-risk population because "a large number of people exposed to a low risk is likely to produce more cases than a small number of people exposed to a high risk" [39]. At present, it seems clear that, without a well-resourced national community strategy plan and without monitoring the major determinants, CVD will remain a leading cause of premature death and disability [18].

The European Society of Cardiology, the American Heart Association, and the WHO have identified several goals to be achieved through the implementation of national and international policies and community interventions: avoidance of tobacco, adequate physical activity, healthy food choices, avoidance of overweight, regulation of blood pressure (below 140/90 mmHg), and reduction of total cholesterol (below 200 mg/dl) [4]. Many of the interventions adopted in a population-wide prevention strategy are relatively inexpensive and easy to implement. They have a relevant public health impact and are highly cost-effective and, therefore, they are considered to be "best buys" for investors [5]. Examples of these types of actions are tobacco control measures (raising taxes on tobacco, protecting people from tobacco smoke, warning messages on cigarettes packs, enforcing bans on tobacco advertising, etc.), control measures against the harmful use of alcohol (raising taxes on alcohol, restricting access to alcohol demand, enforcing bans on alcohol advertising, etc.), and measures that promote a healthy diet and physical activity (reducing salt intake in foods, replacing trans-fat with polyunsaturated fat, promotion of physical activity, etc.). In addition to health policy interventions such as taxes, subsidies and regulation of price, availability, and marketing, the WHO identified also the main elements of the urban environment for preventing chronic diseases, such as providing bicycles and cycleways as well as parks and green spaces to increase physical activity [41] The main limitation of the population strategy is the small benefit perceived at individual level, but if healthy behaviors become social norms, it is easier for individuals not to initiate, or to change, risky behaviors [38].

High-Risk Primary Prevention Strategy

A high-risk primary prevention strategy is a clinically oriented approach that focuses efforts at an individual level, dealing with healthy population subgroups with high absolute risk of future CVD. The aim is to reduce the total cardiovascular risk of healthy individuals belonging to the upper part of the risk distribution, and it represents the natural approach for medical practitioners who are concerned with the occurrence of CVD in individuals [39, 42].

The probability that an individual could develop CVD in a given period of time (absolute risk) depends more on the combination of multiple cardiovascular risk factors than on the presence of any single risk factor, because the cumulative effect of causal factors is additive or synergistic. It is reasonable to expect that a primary prevention strategy based on estimating the total cardiovascular absolute risk would be more effective and cost-effective than a clinical approach based on identifying and correcting single risk factors [42].

Electronic and paper-based tools, tailored to each specific population (American, European, Australian, African, etc.), are available to calculate the individual risk of CVD in people who do not have established CHD, stroke, or other atherosclerotic disease. These risk charts, and the relative guidelines for intervention, are based on risk equations derived from large prospective cohort studies (Framingham, PROCAM—Munster, Seven Countries Study, SCORE, CUORE Project, etc.) and include the following variables: age, sex, blood pressure, cigarette smoking, total cholesterol and HDL cholesterol, and diabetes. To estimate the absolute risk, expressed as a percentage, it is necessary, as a first step, to select the appropriate chart depending on the gender (male/female tables) and on the presence or absence of diabetes. Then, after indicating an individual's smoking habits, systolic blood pressure (mmHg), and total blood cholesterol level (mmol/l), an output is obtained showing level of risk. When adjusted for the different thresholds used in each country, the risk is graded as low, moderate, or severe [4, 42].

The main strengths of this strategy are that it provides high-risk individuals with a strong motivation to change their behavior and it allows health professionals to promote change on an individual basis through direct communication. Moreover, the selectivity of the interventions may increase the likelihood that resources are used cost-effectively. By contrast, this strategy's main weaknesses are that (a) it underestimates the fact that a large number of people exposed to a small risk may generate more cases of CVD than a small number of individuals exposed to a large risk; (b) it results in a higher propensity for pharmacological intervention; (c) individual-level strategies tend to be either palliative or temporary, and are not focused on influencing behavior.

Secondary Prevention Strategy

A secondary prevention strategy focuses on the rapid initiation of treatments to stop the progression of disease in individuals with well-established CVD. Since the cardiovascular risk is a continuum, the transition between primary (first step) and secondary (second step) prevention represents the passage from interventions on high-risk groups (with asymptomatic evidence of CVD) to those on highest-risk groups (with symptomatic CVD). Secondary prevention involves identifying, treating, and rehabilitating these patients to reduce their risk of recurrence, to decrease their need for interventional procedures, to improve their quality of life, and to extend their overall survival [38, 39].

Programs for secondary prevention have proven to be effective in improving recovery and functional status, and in reducing readmissions to hospital. Several studies have demonstrated the effectiveness of secondary prevention strategies in the control of CVD, such as the WHO-MONICA study that from the early 1980s monitored trends in CHD over 10 years, across 38 populations, and in 21 countries. Data from this study indicate that secondary prevention interventions and changes in coronary care are strongly linked with declining CVD end points [25].

Making Choices to Reduce the Burden of Cardiovascular Disease

This section provides an overview of reviews and systematic reviews on the effectiveness and cost-effectiveness of CVD-preventive interventions. Clinical guidelines and reports of authoritative institutions were also reviewed to detect the "best buy" interventions and to provide examples of best practices. The section follows the conceptual framework set out earlier, following the three levels of prevention, components of a comprehensive approach that systematically integrates policy, and action (identifying population-level health promotion and disease prevention program, targeting groups and individuals at high risk, maximizing population coverage with effective treatment and care).

Box 1. Characteristics of included studies

The initial search yielded 635 results from all databases investigated (Cochrane Database, PubMed–Medline, NHS Economic Evaluation Database, SCOPUS), of which 62 were retrieved as full text after review of title and abstract. Fifty-three studies were included and analyzed (Fig. 4.1).

Publication date of the retrieved reviews range from 1998 to 2013, with the majority (29/53) published within the past 5 years. The large majority of the reviews (43/53) reported both effectiveness and cost-effectiveness information.

Twenty-two reviews were focused on community-based interventions. Seventeen evaluated only community-based interventions, while five reviews also evaluated interventions at the individual level. Different CVD risk factors were evaluated: unhealthy diet [43–52], physical inactivity [44, 45, 49, 50, 52–55], smoking [20, 45, 50, 56, 57], obesity, especially in childhood [49, 58–62], and alcohol [63]. In general, reviews on population-based prevention reported evidence on cost-effectiveness for the interventions considered in the setting/s of interest.

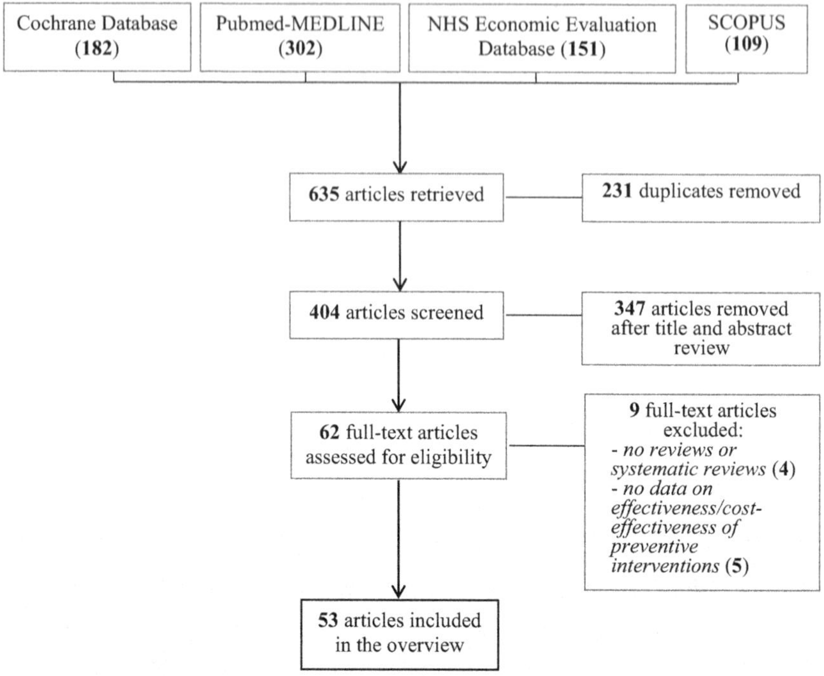

Fig. 4.1 Study selection process for the identification of reviews and systematic reviews on effectiveness and cost-effectiveness of CVD-preventive interventions

Twenty-nine reviews on primary prevention were identified. Eighteen considered only primary prevention, while another five and six also evaluated community-based interventions and secondary prevention, respectively. Different types of interventions were evaluated, specific to different risk factors: high blood pressure [64–74], dyslipidemia [64–69, 71, 73–75], smoking [20, 45, 50, 57, 68, 69, 76–78], physical inactivity [45, 50, 54, 77, 79], diabetes [57, 70, 80–83], unhealthy diet [45, 50, 77], obesity [45, 84, 85], and alcohol [77]. Three reviews, using the absolute risk-based approach, evaluated the effectiveness or cost-effectiveness of providing preventive lifestyle interventions and/or medication on the basis of absolute risk determined from risk charts [85–87]. Many of the primary prevention interventions examined in the reviews have been reported to be effective or cost-effective in the setting/s analyzed.

Thirteen papers evaluated pharmacological interventions within a secondary prevention strategy, and six of these also in a primary prevention context. In the vast majority of cases, preventive therapy was against high blood pressure [64, 71, 73, 88–94], high blood cholesterol [45, 64, 71, 73, 88, 94], and diabetes [80, 82]. Drugs to lower high blood pressure were found to be in the "very cost-effective" or "cost-effective" range in all studies.

Effectiveness and Cost-Effectiveness of Population-Wide Interventions

Reducing the rate of tobacco use worldwide is one of the most important health care goals for the prevention of chronic diseases, including CVD. Tobacco control and prevention policies described in the literature as population-wide prevention strategies have proved very cost-effective. Although the estimates in the literature are subject to local variations and each country is guided by local policies, increasing taxes on cigarettes and tobacco has been found to be the most cost-effective antismoking intervention [20, 45, 50, 56, 57]. Furthermore, interventions based on tobacco taxation have a proportionally greater effect on smokers of lower SES and younger smokers, who might otherwise be difficult to influence. Several studies suggest that the application of a 10 % rise in price could lead to as much as a 2.5–10 % decline in smoking [20, 45, 50, 56]. Other public health actions reported as cost-saving are the creation of completely smoke-free environments in indoor workplaces, public places, and transportation; warning the population of the dangers of tobacco through educational campaigns; and the banning tobacco advertising, promotion, and sponsorship [20, 45, 50, 56, 57]. All preventive actions evaluated in the reviews retrieved are included in the important treaty "WHO Framework Convention for Tobacco Control", embraced by 173 countries and covering almost 90 % of the world's population. This treaty identifies several actions and policies that each country must implement, including increased taxation, legislated restrictions on smoking in public places, comprehensive bans on advertising of tobacco products, information dissemination through health warning labels, counter advertising, various consumer information packages, the creation of national tobacco control program, and the protection of public health policies from commercial and other interests of the tobacco industries [95]. According to WHO data, the total expenditure for implementation of tobacco control policies would range from US$ 0.10 to US$ 0.23/person/year in low- and middle-income countries, and from US$ 0.11 to US$ 0.72/person/year in upper-middle-income countries [4, 96]. An important fraction of this expenditure is attributed to educational media campaigns, while other measures come at a lower cost (e.g., increasing taxes, completely smoke-free indoor environments, health warnings, banning tobacco advertising).

Preventive interventions aimed at the avoidance of an unhealthy diet, at controlling overweight and obesity, and at the promotion of physical activity could achieve a downward shift in the distribution of blood pressure, cholesterol level, and diabetes risk across a population, thus potentially reducing morbidity, mortality, and the lifetime risk of developing CVD. Nutrition policies evaluated by the literature are mainly focused on programs aiming to reduce salt, saturated fats and trans-fatty acids, and free sugars in the diet [43–52]. The current literature on reducing salt intake suggests that all correlated interventions are very cost-effective [43, 45–48, 51, 52]. The most valued intervention reported, especially in studies from high-income countries, is the lowering of salt levels in processed food and condiments by manufacturers. Other studies have estimated the cost-effectiveness of a sustained mass media campaign aimed at encouraging dietary change within households and communities [47, 52]. These interventions appear to be the best choices for encouraging people to use less salt in rural areas in low- and middle-income countries, where most of the sodium intake comes from salt added during cooking or from sauces and additives. The evidence on the cost-effectiveness of reducing the marketing of foods with high levels of saturated fats, trans-fatty acids, or sugar-free is less convincing, but these interventions are also likely to be very cost-effective [48, 49, 59]. The maximum benefit of interventions for the implementation of a healthy diet would be achieved by targeting early stages of life (childhood and adolescence) [49, 58–61]. Relevant programs include the use of economic regulation (e.g., taxes or subsidies) to reduce the marketing to children and adolescents of foods and nonalcoholic beverages with high levels of salt, fats, and sugar. Nationwide and international food markets that comply with healthy dietary guidelines based on compelling evidence are potentially the basis for large health gains, and cost-effectiveness studies tend to support their adoption [4, 58–61]. Physical activity could play a substantial role in reducing overweight and obesity [44, 45, 49, 50, 53–55]. Intersectoral and multidisciplinary action is required to improve physical activity levels. Appropriate actions include the combination of social support in a variety of setting (e.g., school-based programs, activities at worksites, community walking events), transport policies (e.g., creating walking and cycling trains, providing easy access to weight and aerobic fitness places, facilities and equipment in community centers), primary care support (e.g., counseling and seminars provided by physicians), and community-wide campaigns (e.g., increasing public awareness through mass media and social networks). All these physical activity programs appear to be very cost-effective compared to other well-accepted preventive strategies. The WHO, according to the existing evidence [53–55], reported that creating an enabling environment, providing appropriate information, and ensuring the wide accessibility of venues for physical activity are critical actions that influence behavior changes, regardless of the setting [4].

Another category of effective and cost-effective population-based measures is the reduction of alcohol-related harms. There is substantial evidence in the literature of systematic reviews and meta-analyses informing alcohol policies, not only for the prevention of CVD but also to control other chronic diseases such as cancer, liver cirrhosis, and injuries [32]. Particular alcohol-related policies include restrictions on the availability of alcoholic beverages (e.g., state monopolies and licensing systems, restrictions in off-premise retail sale, age requirements for purchase and consumption of alcoholic beverages), drink driving legislation, price and taxation of alcoholic beverages, advertising and sponsorship (e.g., restrictions on sponsorship, enforcement of advertising), and alcohol-free environments [63]. All these population-based interventions represent a cost-effective use of resources and compare favorably with treatment strategies for disease and injury. An unclear result was obtained for school-based education interventions, because this approach seems unable to reduce alcohol consumption [63].

Effectiveness and Cost-Effectiveness of Individual High-Risk Primary Prevention Interventions

Primary prevention is characterized by measures that decrease the likelihood of a first occurrence of CVD through health promotion, screening for risk factors, and risk factor modification with an individual approach. The most cost-effective route of action is often attained by choosing interventions targeted at the risk profile of a specific population group. Therefore, knowledge of the risk profile is essential for a targeted delivery of intensive lifestyle interventions and appropriate drug therapy. Specific risk prediction charts, providing approximate estimates of CVD risk in people without established CVD, are available. The use of these tools to identify subjects at higher cardiovascular risk, to motivate them to introduce behavioral changes, and, where appropriate, to prescribe antihypertensive therapy, lipid-lowering drugs, and aspirin, is an effective and, depending on the setting, cost-effective measure [85–87].

Primary prevention interventions include both lifestyles changes and pharmacological treatments. The evidence suggests that counseling by physicians to reduce intake of total fat, saturated fat intake, and daily salt, and to increase fruit and vegetable intake, is very cost-effective, leading to dietary changes, improved weight control, and increased physical activity [64–69]. The threshold for the introduction of drugs in preventive programs is not defined, but, generally, when people belong to the high-risk profile subgroup, the use of drugs may be cost-effective [71–73]. Reduction of serum cholesterol levels of high-risk subjects has been shown to lower the risk of adverse cardiovascular events [74, 75]. Statins and dietary modifications are effective tools in lowering levels of serum LDL cholesterol, although different settings and comparators were considered in literature. The role of statins as a cost-effective means of preventing CVD depends on the risk profile and the drug price is the main determinant of cost-effectiveness within a given risk group. As more statin drugs become generic, patients at low risk for coronary disease may be treated cost-effectively [69]. However, there is no universal consensus on the use of statins for primary prevention of CHD for persons at high risk but with no symptoms [74, 75].

A medical solution aimed at reducing the CVD risk by attacking several biological processes simultaneously, and that could be viewed potentially as the therapy of the future, is the "polypill," containing a fixed dose of aspirin, a statin to lower cholesterol, and one or two blood pressure-lowering drugs [97]. Our systematic review did not include the studies on the polypill use, because this kind of treatment has not been marked anywhere in the world to date, and the full benefits of such pill remain unclear. However, it is important to mention this kind of multidrug strategy for the extensive discussion about its use in the primary prevention and the future next marketing in USA [98, 99]. Polypill has been proposed as a public health intervention for use by all adults more than 55 years of age regardless of risk factor levels. Multiple different polypill formulations have been developed over the past 5 years, with randomized controlled trials of their benefit currently underway [100]. Preliminary results reported the efficacy of this pill in high-risk populations and the enormous potential for developing countries, where principal barriers are both the cost and complexity of multiple drug use [101].

Drug therapy was also found to be cost-effective for moderate and high-risk profile subgroups with persistent raised blood pressure (≥130/80 mmHg) that are unable to lower blood pressure through lifestyle changes. Drugs evaluated for first-line therapy and primary prevention are thiazide-like diuretics, angiotensin-converting enzyme (ACE) inhibitors, and calcium channel blockers. The beta-blockers are considered more suitable for secondary prevention [86, 88–90].

According to the available scientific evidence, smoking cessation with health care professional counseling and nicotine replacement treatment is highly cost-effective in high-risk populations. Health care providers play a central role in creating dedicated places for antismoking counseling and in educating physicians to discourage people, especially the young, from becoming smokers, to strongly encourage all high-risk subgroups to stop smoking and to support those who decide to quit with pharmaceutical and psychological interventions. Nicotine replacement therapy and/or nortriptyline or amfebutamone (bupropion) should be offered to moderate and high-risk subgroups who fail to quit with counseling [20, 45, 57, 76]. By contrast, the mass media promotion of smoking cessation was found to be less cost-effective than physician counseling and nicotine replacement treatment, especially in subjects with more than one risk factor [76–78].

In conclusion, a wide range of evidence-based individual interventions have been demonstrated to be effective, with a significant impact on the health outcomes of people at high risk of CVD. Improved access to highly cost-effective interventions at the primary health care level will have the greatest potential in reversing the progression of the disease, preventing complications and reducing hospitalizations, health care costs, and out-of-pocket expenditures. However, individual interventions need to be targeted to subjects at high total cardiovascular risk based on the presence of combinations of risk factors. If interventions are aimed at single risk factor levels above traditional thresholds, such as hypertension and hypercholesterolemia, they become less cost-effective.

Effectiveness and Cost-Effectiveness of Secondary Prevention

Interventions for secondary prevention of CVD include both modification of risk behaviors (smoking cessation, promotion of healthy diet, and physical activity) and the use of medication. The vast majority of secondary prevention interventions deal with several pharmacological treatments, including aspirin and other oral antiplatelet drugs (dipyridamole, clopidogrel), ACE inhibitors, lipid-lowering drugs, and beta-blockers; these treatments reduce raised blood pressure and cholesterol levels [64, 70, 73, 80, 82, 88–94]. The target population is generally represented by individuals with well-established CVD or people with very high-risk profile but with no established CVD, and different protocols of treatment are compared. However, pharmacological interventions were always delivered in association with nonpharmacological interventions. In all reviews, this combination is considered a key contribution to the reduction of recurrences and cardiovascular mortality in people with established CVD.

The benefits of aspirin for the secondary prevention of CVD are well established among patients at high risk of cardiovascular events [88, 89]. Several recent studies have documented the effectiveness of dipyridamole for the secondary prevention of stroke, and clopidogrel for the treatment of symptomatic CVD [91–93]. The cost-effectiveness of these antiplatelet drugs is correlated with the price of the treatment and can be optimized by individualizing the treatment decision on the basis of the patient risk profile and the expected risk reduction [88–94].

Strong evidence for the efficacy of these drugs has been obtained from studies that were mostly carried out in affluent societies, while few studies were performed in low- and middle-income countries. Therefore, many recommended medical interventions evaluated in developed countries may cause economic hardship when applied in developing nations [71]. In low- and middle-income countries, there are major gaps in the implementation of secondary prevention interventions for CVD, which could be best delivered at the primary care level.

Best Buys for Prevention and Control of Cardiovascular Disease

The decision to allocate resources for implementing a particular health intervention depends not only on the strength of the evidence (effectiveness of intervention) but also on the cost of achieving the expected health gain. Cost-effectiveness analysis is the primary tool for evaluating health interventions on the basis of the magnitude of their incremental net benefits in comparison with others, which allows the economic attractiveness of one program over another to be determined [102]. If an intervention is both more effective and less costly than the existing one, there are compelling reasons to implement it. However, the majority of health interventions do not meet these criteria, being either more effective but more costly, or less costly but less effective, than the existing interventions. Therefore, in most cases, there is no "best" or absolute level of cost-effectiveness, and this level varies mainly on the basis of health care system expenditure and needs [102]. Furthermore, cost-effectiveness information indicates solutions, but not their feasibility, affordability, and acceptability.

The "best buy" is defined as a highly cost-effective intervention for which there is compelling evidence that it is also feasible, low cost, and appropriate to implement within the constraints of a national health system [2, 5]. Policymakers can consider "best buys" the best investment for governments and a core set of essential health programs. Interventions that do not meet the above criteria, but which still offer good value for money and other features that recommend their use, can be defined as highly cost-effective programs although not as "best buys," and they can be considered part of an expanded set of measures to be made available if resources allow it. The "best buy" is a very pragmatic concept, and evidence has demonstrated that, even in the poorest countries with absence of income growth, deaths and illnesses can be reduced using existing knowledge and strategies [5]. The derived health improvements will help countries to achieve their development goals: Low-income countries need not wait until they are wealthy before becoming healthier [5].

This overview highlights the literature evidence in favor of the implementation of "best buys." The vast majority of "best buys" are community-based interventions and the target is the whole population. Concerning tobacco control, four interventions, included in the WHO Framework Convention on Tobacco Control (increasing taxes, legislation for smoke-free indoor workplaces and public places, health information and warnings about the effects of tobacco, and bans on advertising, promotion, and sponsorship), constitute "best buys" [20, 41, 46, 52, 53]. The available evidence, based on the analysis of the implementation of all four programs in 23 low- and middle-income countries, quantifies five million deaths avoided at an average cost of US$ 0.20/person/year [96]. Enhanced taxation of alcoholic beverages and bans on their marketing also show favorable cost-effectiveness and feasibility and are recommended as "best buys" [59]. Reducing salt intake through mass media campaigns and regulation of processed food, and substitution of hydrogenated trans-fat with polyunsaturated fats in packaged food, are the "best buys" for improving the diet [43, 45–49, 51, 52, 58–61]. In combination with these interventions, promoting physical activity through the media to combat obesity, high blood pressure, dyslipidemia, and diabetes is reported to be both cost-effective and feasible [53–55]. Individual high-risk interventions that could be considered best buys include providing aspirin to people with high-risk profile or who have already suffered a heart attack; reducing the cardiovascular risk (controlling blood pressure, blood cholesterol, and blood sugar; reducing tobacco use) in people, including those with diabetes, who are at high risk of heart attacks and strokes; and controlling glucose levels in people with diabetes, preventing complications such as blindness and kidney failure [4, 5]. These preventive actions can be combined with more targeted approaches to improve health, depending on the resources available.

In conclusion, the association between behavioral risk factors and CVD has been widely demonstrated in the past 50 years and a great amount of evidence on effectiveness and cost-effectiveness interventions for preventing CVD has been provided. As WHO advocates, we have now the required bases of science and technology to effectively reduce the public health impact of CVD [2].

Lifestyle and behavioral interventions, mainly referred to a population-wide approach, appear generally to be very cost-effective, while pharmacological interventions have an impact of greater certainty and magnitude in both primary and secondary prevention. The two strategies of interventions can thus be seen as complementary. They have to be implemented together, taking into account that the nature of policy-making is increasingly interdependent and multidimensional. The fact that health is affected by policies of other sectors has been recognized for a long time, and the need to cooperate with sectors such as those of education, social affairs, transport, environment, housing, agriculture, and nutrition is widely recognized [41].

Box 2. Examples of best practices

In 1972, Finland had the world's highest CVD mortality rate. Planners examined existing policies and major factors contributing to CVD and introduced appropriate changes (low-fat dairy products, antismoking legislation, and healthy school meals), providing one of the best-documented examples of community intervention [103]. They used mass media, courses in schools and worksites, and spokespersons from sports, education, and agriculture to educate residents. After 5 years, significant improvements were documented in smoking, cholesterol, and blood pressure. In 1995, CHD mortality rates for men aged 35–64 years were reduced by 65 %. The program was so successful that it was expanded, including other lifestyle-related diseases. Twenty years later, major reductions in CVD risk factor levels, morbidity, and premature mortality were attributed to the project [103].

In 2003, Denmark introduced mandatory compositional restrictions on trans-fatty acids in fats and oils to less than 2 % of total fatty acids. A 2006 survey indicated that industrially produced trans-fatty acids in Denmark had been virtually eliminated from the food supply and that both the population average and the high-risk groups consume less than 1 g of industrially produced trans-fatty acids per day [104].

In 2006, the Massachusetts health care system reformed the law on tobacco cessation for the Massachusetts Medicaid population. For Medicaid subscribers, two 90-day courses per year, medications like nicotine replacement therapy, and individual or group counseling sessions were available. A total of 37 % of all Medicaid smokers used the newly available benefit between 2006 and 2008. After implementation, in just over 2 years, 26 % of Medicaid smokers quit smoking, and there was a decline in the use of other costly health care services (38 % decrease in hospitalizations for CHD, 17 % drop in emergency room and clinic visits for asthma, and a 17 % drop in claims for adverse maternal birth complications). Additional research showed that comprehensive coverage led to reduced hospitalizations for CHD and net savings of US$ 10.5 million or a US$ 3.07 return on investment for every dollar spent [50].

Despite some preventive approaches are so cost-effective that country income levels could not be perceived as major barriers to actual implementation, the cost-effectiveness analyses of CVD-preventive interventions and strategies should be performed taking into account the local contexts, such as the prevailing burden of disease, the existing health interventions, and the financial capacity of the health system. Since each community is unique, every country should develop its own health policy to win the battle against CVD [2, 41].

References

1. World Health Organization (2013) World Health Statistics 2013. In: Global Health Observatory (GHO). http://www.who.int/gho/publications/world_health_statistics/en/. Accessed 28 June 2013
2. Alwan A (ed) (2011) Global status report on noncommunicable diseases 2010. World Health Organization Press, Geneva
3. Omran AR (1971) The epidemiologic transition: a theory of the epidemiology of population change. Milbank Meml Fund Q 49:509–538
4. Mendis S, Puska P, Norrving B (eds) (2011) Global atlas on cardiovascular disease prevention and control. World Health Organization Press, Geneva
5. World Health Organization, World Economic Forum (eds) (2011) From burden to "Best Buys": reducing the economic impact of non-communicable diseases in low and middle income countries. World Health Organization Press, Geneva
6. Longo DL, Fauci AS, Kasper DL et al (eds) (2011) Harrison's principles of internal medicine. McGraw-Hill Medical Publishing Division, New York
7. Murray CJL, Phil D, Lopez AD (2013) Measuring the global burden of disease. N Engl J Med 369:448–457
8. Banks J, Marmot M, Oldfield Z et al (2006) Disease and disadvantage in the United States and in England. J Am Med Assoc 295:2037–2045
9. Banks J, Muriel A, Smith JP (2010) Disease prevalence, disease incidence, and mortality in the United States and in England. Demography 47:S211–S231
10. Laslett LJ, Alagona P, Clark BA et al (2012) The worldwide environment of cardiovascular disease: prevalence, diagnosis, therapy, and policy issues: a report from the American College of Cardiology. J Am Coll Cardiol 60:S1–S49
11. Mensah GA, Brown DW (2007) An overview of cardiovascular disease burden in the United States. Health Aff 26:38–48
12. HRS—Health and Retirement Study (2013) A longitudinal study of heath, retirement, and aging sponsored by the National Institute on Aging. http://hrsonline.isr.umich.edu/index.php. Accessed 9 Aug 2013
13. ELSA—English Longitudinal Study of Aging (2013) Department of Epidemiology and Public Health University College, London. http://www.ifs.org.uk/ELSA. Accessed 9 Aug 2013
14. SHARE—Survey of Health, Ageing and Retirement in Europe (2013) Munich Center for the Economics of Aging, Munich. http://www.share-project.org/home0.html. Accessed 9 Aug 2013
15. Smith S, Ralston J, Taubert K (2012) Urbanization and cardiovascular disease: raising heart-healthy children in today's cities. The World Heart Federation. http://www.worldheart.org/urbanization. Accessed 9 Aug 2013
16. Fuster V, Kelly BB (eds) (2010) Promoting cardiovascular health in the developing world: a critical challenge to achieve global health. Institute of Medicine (US) Committee on preventing the global epidemic of cardiovascular disease: meeting the challenges in developing countries. National Academies Press, Washington DC
17. Nichols M, Townsend N, Luengo-Fernandez R et al (2012) European cardiovascular disease statistics 2012. European Heart Network, Brussels and European Society of Cardiology, Sophia Antipolis
18. Murray CJL, Vos T, Lozano R et al (2012) Disability-adjusted life years (DALYs) for 291 diseases and injuries in 21 regions, 1990–2010: a systematic analysis for the global burden of disease study 2010. Lancet 380:2197–2223
19. Lim SS, Vos T, Flaxman AD et al (2012) A comparative risk assessment of burden of disease and injury attributable to 67 risk factors and risk factor clusters in 21 regions, 1990–2010: a systematic analysis for the Global burden of disease study 2010. Lancet 380:2224–2260
20. Gaziano TA (2007) Reducing the growing burden of cardiovascular disease in the developing world. Health Aff 26:13–24

21. Soler EP, Ruiz VC (2010) Epidemiology and risk factors of cerebral ischemia and ischemic heart diseases: similarities and differences. Curr Cardiol Rev 6:138–149
22. Kannel WB, Dawber TR, Kagan A et al (1961) Factors of risk in the development of coronary heart disease—six year follow-up experience. The Framingham Study. Ann Intern Med 55:33–50
23. Framingham Heart Study (2013) A project of the National Heart, Lung and Blood Institute and Boston University. http://www.framinghamheartstudy.org/index.html. Accessed 6 June 2013
24. Keys A (ed) (1980) Seven countries: a multivariate analysis of death and coronary heart disease. Harvard University Press, Cambridge
25. The WHO MONICA Project (2013) Multinational MONItoring of trends and determinants in Cardiovascular disease. http://www.thl.fi/monica. Accessed 6 June 2013
26. INTER-HEART (2002) A global case-control study of risk factors for acute myocardial. http://www.phri.ca/interheart. Accessed 6 June 2013
27. World Health Organization (2009) Global health risks: mortality and burden of disease attributable to selected major risks. World Health Organization Press, Geneva
28. Wolf PA, D'Agostino RB, Kannel WB et al (1988) Cigarette smoking as a risk factor for stroke. The Framingham Study. J Am Med Assoc 259:1025–1029
29. Doll R, Boreham J, Sutherland I (2004) Mortality in relation to smoking: 50 years' observations on male British doctors. Br Med J 328:1519–1522
30. Strazzullo P et al (2009) Salt intake, stroke, and cardiovascular disease: meta-analysis of prospective studies. Br Med J 339:b4567
31. Roerecke M, Rehm J (2012) The cardioprotective association of average alcohol consumption and ischaemic heart disease: a systematic review and meta-analysis. Addiction 107:1246–1260
32. Møller L, Galea G, Brummer J (2013) Status report on alcohol and health in 35 European countries 2013. World Health Organization Press, Geneva
33. Levitan B et al (2004) Is non-diabetic hyperglycaemia a risk factor for cardiovascular disease? A meta-analysis of prospective studies. Arch Intern Med 164:2147–2155
34. Farzadfar F et al (2011) National, regional, and global trends in serum total cholesterol since 1980: systematic analysis of health examination surveys and epidemiological studies with 321 country-years and 3.0 million participants. Lancet 337:578–586
35. Lang T, Lepage B, Schieber AC, Lamy S, Kelly-Irving M (2012) Social determinants of cardiovascular diseases. Public Health Rev 33:601–622
36. Jousilahti P, Vartiainen E, Tuomilehto J, Puska P (1999) Sex, age, cardiovascular risk factors, and coronary heart disease: a prospective follow-up study of 14,786 middle-aged men and women in Finland. Circulation 99:1165–1172
37. Hunt SC, Gwinn M, Adams TD (2003) Family history assessment: strategies for prevention of cardiovascular disease. Am J Prev Med 24:136–142
38. Doyle YG, Furey A, Flowers J (2006) Sick individuals and sick populations: 20 years later. J Epidemiol Commun Health 60:396–398
39. Rose G (1981) Strategy of prevention: lessons from cardiovascular disease. Br Med J (Clin Res Ed) 282:1847–1851
40. Beaglehole R, Le Galès-Camus C (eds) (2005) Cardiovascular disease prevention. Translating evidence into action. World Health Organization Press, Geneva
41. Stuckler D, Siegel K (eds) (2011) Sick societies: responding to the global challenge of chronic disease. Oxford University Press, Oxford
42. National Health and Medical Research Council (eds) (2009) Guidelines for the assessment of absolute cardiovascular disease risk. http://www.heartfoundation.org.au/SiteCollection-Documents. Accessed 27 June 2013
43. Brunner E, Cohen D, Toon L (2001) Cost effectiveness of cardiovascular disease prevention strategies: a perspective on EU food based dietary guidelines. Public Health Nutr 4:711–715
44. Matson-Koffman DM, Brownstein JN, Neiner JA et al (2005) A site-specific literature review of policy and environmental interventions that promote physical activity and nutrition for cardiovascular health: what works? Am J Health Promot 19:167–193

45. Gaziano TA, Galea G, Reddy KS (2007) Scaling up interventions for chronic disease prevention: the evidence. Lancet 370:1939–1946
46. Mohan S, Campbell NR (2009) Salt and high blood pressure. Clin Sci 117:1–11
47. He FJ, MacGregor GA (2009) A comprehensive review on salt and health and current experience of worldwide salt reduction programmes. J Hum Hypertens 23:363–384
48. Dall TM, Fulgoni VL, Zhang Y et al (2009) Potential health benefits and medical cost savings from calorie, sodium, and saturated fat reductions in the American diet. Am J Health Promot 23:412–422
49. Cecchini M, Sassi F, Lauer JA, et al (2010) Tackling of unhealthy diets, physical inactivity, and obesity: health effects and cost-effectiveness. Lancet 376:1775–1784
50. Weintraub WS, Daniels SR, Burke LE et al (2011) Value of primordial and primary prevention for cardiovascular disease: a policy statement from the American Heart Association. Circulation 124:967–990
51. Barton P, Andronis L, Briggs WR et al (2011) Effectiveness and cost effectiveness of cardiovascular disease prevention in whole populations: modeling study. Br Med J 343:d4044
52. He FJ, Macgregor GA (2012) Salt intake, plasma sodium, and worldwide salt reduction. Ann Med 44:S127–S137
53. Roux L, Pratt M, Tengs TO et al (2008) Cost effectiveness of community-based physical activity interventions. Am J Prev Med. 35:578–588
54. Garrett S, Elley CR, Rose SB et al (2011) Are physical activity interventions in primary care and the community cost-effective? A systematic review of the evidence. Br J Gen Pract 61:e125–e133
55. Bock C, Jarczok MN, Litaker D (2013) Community-based efforts to promote physical activity: a systematic review of interventions considering mode of delivery, study quality and population subgroups. J Sci Med Sport pii:S1440–S2440
56. Ranson MK, Jha P, Chaloupka FJ et al (2002) Global and regional estimates of the effectiveness and cost-effectiveness of price increases and other tobacco control policies. Nicotine Tob Res 4:311–319
57. Ortegón M, Lim S, Chisholm D et al (2012) Cost effectiveness of strategies to combat cardiovascular disease, diabetes, and tobacco use in sub-Saharan Africa and South East Asia: mathematical modelling study. Br Med J 344:e607
58. Wolfenden L, Wiggers J (2012) Strengthening the rigour of population-wide, community-based obesity prevention evaluations. Public Health Nutr 19:1–15
59. Hollingworth W, Hawkins J, Lawlor DA, Brown M, Marsh T, Kipping RR (2012) Economic evaluation of lifestyle interventions to treat overweight or obesity in children. Int J Obes 36:559–566
60. Moodie M, Sheppard L, Sacks G, Keating C, Flego A (2013) Cost-effectiveness of fiscal policies to prevent obesity. Curr Obes Rep 2:211–24
61. Bleich SN, Segal J, Wu Y, Wilson R, Wang Y (2013) Systematic review of community-based childhood obesity prevention studies. Pediatrics 132:e201–e210
62. Anderson P (2008) Reducing overweight and obesity: closing the gap between primary care and public health. Fam Pract 25:i10–i16
63. Janssen MM, Mathijssen JJ, van Bon-Martens MJ et al (2013) Effectiveness of alcohol prevention interventions based on the principles of social marketing: a systematic review. Subst Abuse Treat Prev Policy 8:18
64. Brown AD, Garber AM (1998) Cost effectiveness of coronary heart disease prevention strategies in adults. Pharmacoeconomics 14:27–48
65. Grieve R, Hutton J, Green C (2003) Selecting methods for the prediction of future events in cost-effectiveness models: a decision-framework and example from the cardiovascular field. Health Policy 64:311–324
66. Ward S, Lloyd Jones M, Pandor A et al (2007) A systematic review and economic evaluation of statins for the prevention of coronary events. Health Technol Assess 11:1–160

67. Lim SS, Gaziano TA, Gakidou E et al (2007) Prevention of cardiovascular disease in high-risk individuals in low-income and middle-income countries: health effects and costs. Lancet 370:2054–2062
68. Schwappach DLB, Boluarte TA, Suhrcke M (2007) The economics of primary prevention of cardiovascular disease—a systematic review of economic evaluations. Cost Eff Resour Alloc 5:5
69. Franco OH, der Kinderen AJ, De Laet C et al (2007) Primary prevention of cardiovascular disease: cost-effectiveness comparison. Int J Technol Assess Health Care 23:71–79
70. Saha S, Gerdtham UG, Johansson P (2010) Economic evaluation of lifestyle interventions for preventing diabetes and cardiovascular diseases. Int J Environ Res Public Health 7:3150–3195
71. Suhrcke M, Boluarte TA, Niessen L (2012) A systematic review of economic evaluations of interventions to tackle cardiovascular disease in low- and middle-income countries. BMC Public Health 12:2
72. Cadilhac DA, Carter R, Thrift AG et al (2012) Organized blood pressure control programs to prevent stroke in Australia: would they be cost-effective? Stroke 43:1370–1375
73. Shroufi A, Chowdhury R, Anchala R et al (2013) Cost effective interventions for the prevention of cardiovascular disease in low and middle income countries: a systematic review. BMC Public Health 13:285
74. Scotti L, Baio G, Merlino L et al (2013) Cost-effectiveness of enhancing adherence to therapy with blood pressure-lowering drugs in the setting of primary cardiovascular prevention. Value Health 16:318–324
75. Mitchell AP, Simpson RJ (2012) Statin cost effectiveness in primary prevention: a systematic review of the recent cost-effectiveness literature in the United States. BMC Res Notes 5:373
76. Ronckers ET, Groot W, Ament AJ (2005) Systematic review of economic evaluations of smoking cessation: standardizing the cost-effectiveness. Med Decis Making 25:437–448
77. Gordon L, Graves N, Hawkes A et al (2007) A review of the cost-effectiveness of face-to-face behavioural interventions for smoking, physical activity, diet and alcohol. Chronic Illn 3:101–129
78. Müller-Riemenschneider F, Bockelbrink A, Reinhold T et al (2008) Long-term effectiveness of behavioural interventions to prevent smoking among children and youth. Tob Control 17:301–302
79. Lowensteyn I, Coupal L, Zowall H et al (2000) The cost-effectiveness of exercise training for the primary and secondary prevention of cardiovascular disease. J Cardiopulm Rehabil 20:147–155
80. Vijgen SM, Hoogendoorn M, Baan CA et al (2006) Cost effectiveness of preventive interventions in type 2 diabetes mellitus: a systematic literature review. Pharmacoeconomics 24:425–441
81. Buse JB, Ginsberg HN, Bakris GL et al (2007) Primary prevention of cardiovascular diseases in people with diabetes mellitus: a scientific statement from the American Heart Association and the American Diabetes Association. Diabetes Care 30:162–172
82. Li E, Zhang P, Barker LE et al (2010) Cost-effectiveness of interventions to prevent and control diabetes mellitus: a systematic review. Diabetes Care 33:1872–1894
83. Anderson P, Chisholm D, Fuhr DC (2009) Effectiveness and cost-effectiveness of policies and programmes to reduce the harm caused by alcohol. Lancet 373:2234–2246
84. Gandjour A (2012) Cost-effectiveness of preventing weight gain and obesity: what we know and what we need to know. Expert Rev Pharmacoecon Outcomes Res 12:297–305
85. Willis A, Davies M, Yates T et al (2012) Primary prevention of cardiovascular disease using validated risk scores: a systematic review. J R Soc Med 105:348–356
86. Labrunée M, Pathak A, Loscos M et al (2012) Therapeutic education in cardiovascular diseases: state of the art and perspectives. Ann Phys Rehabil Med 55:322–341
87. Stevanovic J, Postma MJ, Pechlivanoglou P (2012) A systematic review on the application of cardiovascular risk prediction models in pharmacoeconomics, with a focus on primary prevention. Eur J Prev Cardiol 19:42–53

88. McAlister FA, Lawson FM, Teo KK et al (2001) Randomised trials of secondary prevention programmes in coronary heart disease: systematic review. Br Med J 323:957–962
89. Ho WK, Hankey GJ, Eikelboom JW (2004) Prevention of coronary heart disease with aspirin and clopidogrel: efficacy, safety, costs and cost-effectiveness. Expert Opin Pharmacother 5:493–503
90. Gaziano TA, Opie LH, Weinstein MC (2006) Cardiovascular disease prevention with a multidrug regimen in the developing world: a cost-effectiveness analysis. Lancet 368:679–686
91. Heeg B, Damen J, Van Hout B (2007) Oral antiplatelet therapy in secondary prevention of cardiovascular events: an assessment from the payer's perspective. Pharmacoeconomics 25:1063–1082
92. Plosker GL, Lyseng-Williamson KA (2007) Atorvastatin: a pharmacoeconomic review of its use in the primary and secondary prevention of cardiovascular events. Pharmacoeconomics 25:1031–1053
93. Cheng JW (2007) Pharmacoeconomic analysis of clopidogrel in secondary prevention of coronary artery disease. J Manage Care Pharm 13:326–336
94. Soini EJ, Davies G, Martikainen JA et al (2010) Population-based health-economic evaluation of the secondary prevention of coronary heart disease in Finland. Curr Med Res Opin 26:25–36
95. World Health Organization (2003) WHO framework convention on tobacco control. World Health Organization Press, Geneva
96. Asaria P, Chisholm D, Mathers C, Ezzati M, Beaglehole R (2007) Chronic disease prevention: health effects and financial costs of strategies to reduce salt intake and control tobacco use. Lancet 370:2044–2053
97. Sanz G, Fuster V (2009) Fixed-dose combination therapy and secondary cardiovascular prevention: rationale, selection of drugs and target population. Nat Clin Pract Cardiovasc Med 6:101–110
98. Nguyen C, Cheng-Lai A (2013) The polypill: a potential global solution to cardiovascular disease. Cardiol Rev 21:49–54
99. Wald DS, Wald NJ (2010) The polypill in the primary prevention of cardiovascular disease. Fundam Clin Pharmacol 24(1):29–35
100. Carey KM, Comee MR, Donovan JL, Kanaan AO (2012) A polypill for all? Critical review of the polypill literature for primary prevention of cardiovascular disease and stroke. Ann Pharmacother 46:688–695
101. Lafeber M, Spiering W, Singh K, Guggilla RK, Patil V, Webster R (2012) The cardiovascular polypill in high-risk patients. Eur J Prev Cardiol 19:1234–1242
102. Laupacis A, Feeny D, Detsky AS et al (1992) How attractive does a new technology have to be to warrant adoption and utilization? Tentative guidelines for using clinical and economic evaluations. Can Med Assoc J 146:473–481
103. Puska P, Vartiainen E, Tuomilehto J et al (1998) Changes in premature deaths in Finland: successful long-term prevention of cardiovascular diseases. Bull World Health Organ 76:419–425
104. Willett WC, Koplan JP, Nugentet R et al (2006) Prevention of chronic disease by means of diet and lifestyle changes. In: Jamison DT, Breman JG, Measham AR et al (eds) Disease control priorities in developing countries, 2nd edn. The World Bank, Washington DC. http://www.ncbi.nlm.nih.gov/books/NBK11795. Accessed 17 July 2013.

Chapter 5
Epidemiology of Cancer and Principles of Prevention

Stefania Boccia, Carlo La Vecchia and Paolo Boffetta

Introduction

Neoplasms include several hundreds of diseases, which can be distinguished by localization, morphology, clinical behaviour and response to therapy [1]. They are classified according to the International Classification of Diseases—Oncology [2] into topographical categories (according to the organ where the neoplasm arises) and morphological categories (according to the characteristics of the cells).

Benign neoplasms represent localized growths of tissue with predominantly normal characteristics: In most cases, they cause relatively minor symptoms and are amenable to surgical therapy. Benign tumours, however, can become clinically important when they occur in organs in which compression is possible and surgery cannot be easily performed (e.g. the brain), and when they produce hormones or other substances with a systemic effect (e.g. epinephrine produced by benign pheochromocytoma) [2].

Malignant neoplasms are characterized by progressive growth of tissue with structural and functional alterations with respect to the normal tissue. A peculiarity of most malignant tumours is the ability to migrate and colonize other organs (metastatization) via blood and lymph vessel penetration [2].

S. Boccia (✉)
Section of Hygiene, Institute of Public Health,
Università Cattolica del Sacro Cuore, L.go F. Vito 1, 00168 Rome, Italy
e-mail: sboccia@rm.unicatt.it

C. La Vecchia
Department of Clinical Sciences and Community Health,
Universitá degli Studi di Milano, Via Augusto Vanzetti 5, 20122 Milan, Italy
e-mail: carlo.lavecchia@unimi.it, lavecchia@marionegri.it

P. Boffetta
Mount Sinai School of Medicine Tisch Cancer Institute,
1190 5th Avenue, 10029 New York, NY, USA
e-mail: paolo.boffetta@gmail.com

S. Boccia et al. (eds.), *A Systematic Review of Key Issues in Public Health*,
DOI 10.1007/978-3-319-13620-2_5

Knowledge about the causes and consequently the possible preventive strategies for malignant neoplasms has greatly advanced during the past decades. This has been largely based on the development of cancer epidemiology. Indeed, the identification of the determinants of cancer relies on two complementary approaches, the epidemiological and the experimental, and the epidemiological one has produced both general and specific evidence for the role of different types of agents in cancer causation.

Genetic determinants of cancer have also been demonstrated. Several inherited conditions carry a very high risk of one or several cancers. High-penetrance genes are identified through family-based and other linkage studies. These conditions are rare and explain only a small proportion of human cancers. Genetic factors are also likely to play an important role in interacting with non-genetic factors to determine individual susceptibility to cancer, although the observation of changes of incidence in migrant groups after they have moved to a new living environment suggests a major role of non-genetic factors.

In parallel to the identification of the causes of cancer, primary preventive strategies have been developed. Secondary preventive approaches have also been proposed and in some cases their effectiveness has been evaluated. A careful consideration of the achievements of cancer research, however, suggests that the advancements in knowledge about the causes of cancer have not been followed by an equally important reduction in the burden of cancer. Part of this paradox is explained by the long latency occurring between exposure to carcinogens and development of the clinical disease. Thus, changes in exposure to risk factors are not followed immediately by changes in disease occurrence. The main reason for the gap between knowledge and public health action, however, rests with the cultural, societal and economic aspects of exposure to most carcinogens.

Epidemiology

Global Burden of Disease

The number of new cases of cancer worldwide in 2008 has been estimated at about 12,700,000 [3]. Of these, 6,600,000 occurred in men and 6,000,000 in women. About 5,600,000 cases occurred in high-resource countries (North America, Japan, Europe including Russia, Australia and New Zealand) and 7,100,000 in low- and middle-income countries. Among men, lung, stomach, colorectal, prostate and liver cancers are the most common malignant neoplasms (Fig. 5.1), while breast, colorectal, cervical, lung and stomach are the most common neoplasms among women (Fig. 5.2). The number of deaths from cancer was estimated at about 7,600,000 in 2008 [3]. No global estimates of survival from cancer are available: Data from selected cancer registries suggest wide disparities between high- and low-income

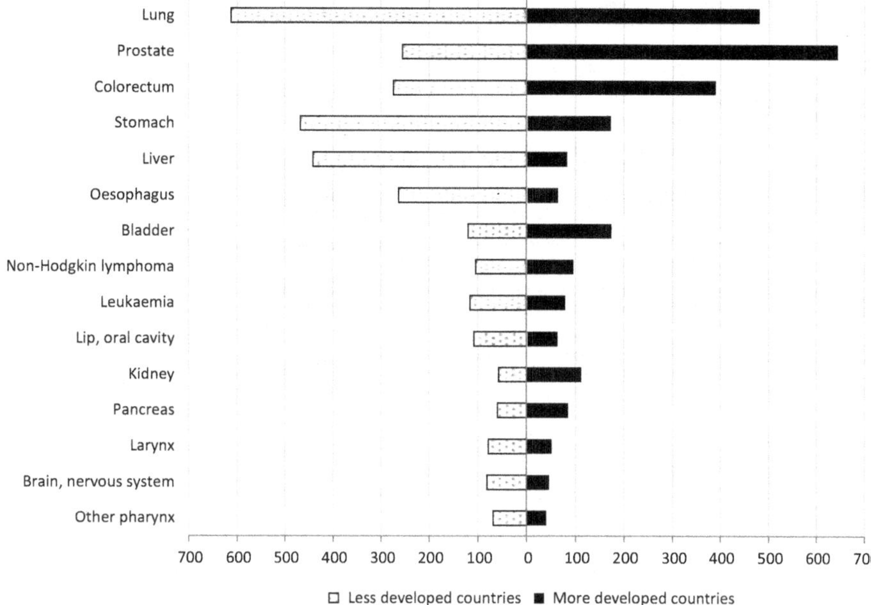

Fig. 5.1 Estimated number of new cancer cases (× 1000), 2008—men [3]

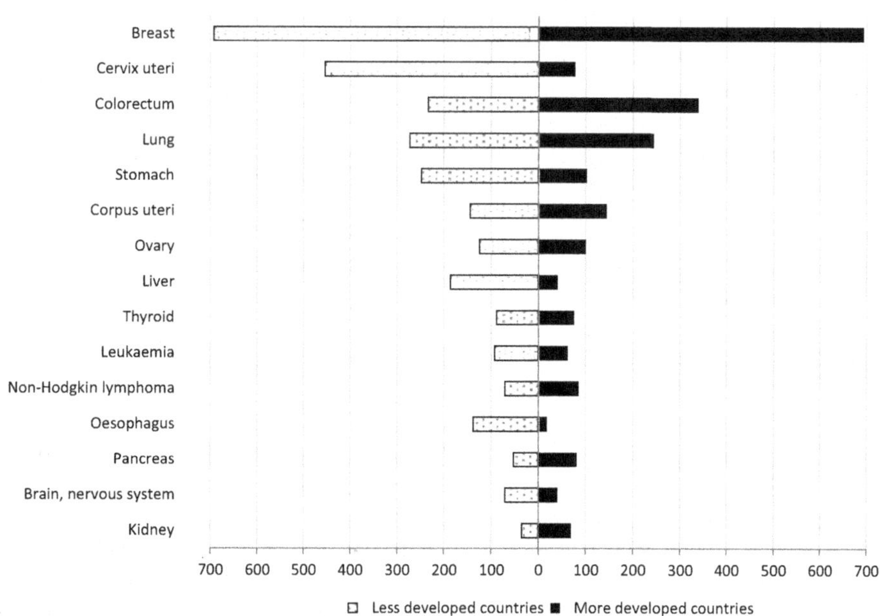

Fig. 5.2 Estimated number of new cancer cases (× 1000), 2008—women [3]

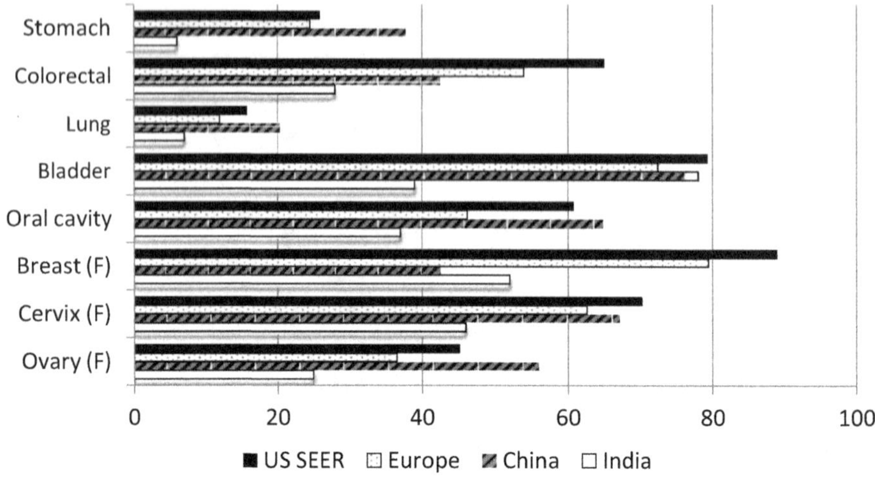

Fig. 5.3 Five-year relative survival from cancer in selected populations [4–6]

countries for neoplasms with effective but expensive treatment, such as leukaemia, while the gap is narrow for neoplasms without an effective therapy, such as lung cancer (Fig. 5.3) [4–6]. The overall 5-year survival of cases diagnosed during 1995–1999 in 23 European countries was 49.6 % [5]. A complementary approach in assessing the global burden of neoplasms is to estimate the loss in disability-adjusted life-years (DALYs). This indicator weighs the years of life with disability and adds them to the years lost because of premature death. An estimate for 2008 resulted in about 169,000,000 DALYs lost worldwide because of malignant neoplasms. In absolute terms, Asia and Europe contributed to 73 % of DALYs lost because of cancer, and China for 25 %. Lung, liver, breast, stomach, colorectal, cervical and oesophageal cancers and leukaemia had the highest proportion of DALYs, with a combined contribution of 65 % to the total cancer burden [7].

Risk Factors

Tobacco Smoking

Tobacco smoking is the main single cause of human cancer worldwide [8] and the largest cause of death and disease. It is the key cause of lung cancer, and a major cause of cancers of the oral cavity, pharynx, nasal cavity, larynx, oesophagus, stomach, pancreas, uterine cervix, kidney and bladder, as well as of myeloid leukaemia. In high-income countries, tobacco smoking causes approximately 30 % of all human cancers [9]. In many middle- and low-income countries, the burden of tobacco-related cancer is still lower, given the relatively recent start of the epidemics of smoking, which will however result in a greater number of cancers in the future, in the absence of adequate intervention to control tobacco.

A benefit of quitting tobacco smoking in adulthood has been shown for all major cancers causally associated with the habit. Smokers who stop around age 50 avoid over 50 % of overall excess mortality from all causes [10–12], from lung cancers [13] as well as from other tobacco-related cancers [14], and those who stop around age 40 or earlier avoid most of their tobacco-related cancer risk.

This emphasizes the need to devise anti-smoking strategies that address avoidance of the habit among the young, as well as reduction of smoking and quitting among adults. In fact, the decline in tobacco consumption that has taken place during the past half century among men in North America and several European countries, and which has resulted in decreased incidence of and mortality from lung cancer [15–17], was caused primarily by quitting at middle age. The great challenge for the control of tobacco-related cancers, however, lies today in middle- and low-income countries, in particular in China and other Asian countries: The largest increase in tobacco-related cancers has been forecasted in this region of the world [18]. The control of tobacco-related cancers in the first half of this century is essentially due to stopping in middle age, since diseases and deaths in adolescents who stand now with occur in the second half of the century. Despite growing efforts from medical and public health institutions and the growing involvement of non-governmental organizations, the fight against the spread of tobacco smoking among women and in middle-low-income countries remains the biggest and most difficult challenge of cancer prevention in the next decades. In 2008, the World Health Organization (WHO) established the MPOWER policy package highlighting priority interventions towards tobacco control [19]. The evidence base for the effect of the MPOWER recommendations is still limited, though the prevalence of tobacco smoking has declined across the WHO regions. Modelling suggests, however, that it will be difficult to achieve rates below 10 % within a 20-year time horizon [20].

Use of smokeless tobacco products has been associated with increased risk of cancer of the head and neck and the pancreas [8], though the data remain open to discussion [21]. Chewing of tobacco-containing products is particularly prevalent in Southern Asia, where it represents a major cause of oral and pharyngeal cancer.

Dietary Factors

The role of dietary factors in causing human cancer remains largely obscure. For no dietary factor other than alcohol and aflatoxin (a carcinogen produced by some fungi in certain tropical areas), there is sufficient evidence of an increased or decreased risk of cancer. In particular, a role of intake of fat in determining breast and colorectal cancer risk has not been confirmed by recent meta-analyses [22, 23]. A high intake of red and processed meat, instead, has been associated with an increased risk of colorectal cancer in a meta-analysis of prospective studies [24], and a protective effect has been reported for fish intake [25], milk and total dairy products [26] and magnesium intake [27].

Thus, the World Cancer Research Foundation 2007 [28] recommends the population average consumption of red meat to be no more than 300 g (11 oz) a week, very little if any of which is processed.

Concerning vegetable intake, the World Cancer Research Foundation 2007 report [28] gave probable evidence of risk reduction with cancers of the mouth and pharynx, larynx, oesophagus and stomach, and limited evidence for nasopharynx, lung, colorectum, ovary and endometrium. With reference to fruit, it gave probable evidence of risk reduction for mouth and pharynx, larynx, oesophagus, lung and stomach, and limited for nasopharynx, pancreas, liver and colorectum.

A number of vitamins and other micronutrients or food components (including carotenoids, lycopene and flavonoids) showed an inverse relation with cancer risk. With reference to flavonoids, there are suggestions for a protective role of flavanones on upper aerodigestive tract, proanthocyanidins on gastric cancer, flavonols and proanthocyanidins on colorectal, flavonols and flavones on breast and isoflavones on ovarian cancers [29].

There is evidence of lack of cancer-preventive activity for preformed vitamin A [30] and for ß-carotene when used at high doses [31], and a lack of evidence of increased cancer risk associated with vitamin D status [32]. Systematic reviews have concluded that nutritional factors may be responsible for about one fourth of human cancers in high-income countries, although, because of the limitations of the current understanding of the precise role of diet in human cancer, the proportion of cancers known to be avoidable in practicable ways is much smaller [9]. The only justified dietary recommendation for cancer prevention is to reduce the total caloric intake, which would contribute to a decrease in overweight and obesity, an established risk factor for human cancer.

Obesity and Physical Exercise

There is sufficient evidence for a cancer-preventive effect of avoidance of weight gain, with reference to risk of cancers of the colon, gallbladder, postmenopausal breast, endometrium, kidney and oesophagus (adenocarcinoma) [33]. The recommendation number one of the World Cancer Research Foundation 2007 report [28] suggests to "be as lean as possible within the normal range of body weight".

It is likely that obesity exerts a carcinogenic effect in conjunction with other factors such as insulin resistance, low physical activity and menopausal status. The magnitude of the excess risk is not very high (for most cancers, the relative risk (RR) ranges between 1.5 and 2 for body weight higher than 35 % above the ideal weight). Estimates of the proportion of cancers attributable to overweight and obesity in Europe range from 2 % [9] to 5 % [34]. However, this figure is likely to be larger in North America, where the prevalence of overweight and obesity is higher.

Increasing physical activity should be a part of any comprehensive cancer prevention strategy. Increased workplace or recreational physical activity decreased the risk of colon and breast cancers and that of endometrial and prostate cancers [33]. The RR of colon and breast cancers for regular versus no activity is in the order of 1.5–2. Worldwide, physical inactivity (defined as do not engage in any brisk walking for at least 30 min every day) causes 10 % (5.6–14.1) of breast cancer and 10 % (5.7–13.8) of colon cancer cases [35].

Alcohol Drinking

Alcohol drinking increases the risk of cancers of the oral cavity, pharynx, larynx, oesophagus and liver, colorectum and female breast [36]. For all cancer sites, risk is a function of the amount of alcohol consumed. Alcohol drinking and tobacco smoking show an interactive (i.e. multiplicative) effect on the risk of cancers of the head and neck.

Heavy alcohol consumption (i.e. ≥4 drinks/day) is significantly associated with an about fivefold increased risk of oral and pharyngeal cancer and oesophageal squamous cell carcinoma (SqCC), 2.5-fold for laryngeal cancer, 50 % for colorectal and breast cancers and 30 % for pancreatic cancer [37]. These estimates are based on a large number of epidemiological studies, and are generally consistent across strata of several covariates. The evidence suggests that at low doses of alcohol consumption (i.e. ≤1 drink/day) the risk is also increased by about 20 % for oral and pharyngeal cancer and 30 % for oesophageal SqCC. While consumption of less than three alcoholic drinks/week is not associated with an increased risk of breast cancer, an intake of 3–6 drinks/week might already yield a (small) increase in risk. On the other hand, intakes up to one drink/day are not associated with the risk of laryngeal, colorectal and pancreatic cancer [38].

The positive association between alcohol consumption and the risk of head and neck cancers is independent from tobacco exposure [37]. The global burden of cancer attributable to alcohol drinking has been estimated at 3.6 and 3.5 % of cancer deaths [39], although this figure is higher in high-income countries (e.g. the figure of 6 % has been proposed for UK [9] and 9 % in Central and Eastern Europe).

These included over 5 % of cancers and cancer deaths in men and about 1.5 % of cancers and cancer deaths in women. Restriction of alcohol drinking to the limits indicated by the European Code Against Cancer [40] (20 g/day for men and 10 g/day for women) would avoid about 90 % of alcohol-related cancers and cancer deaths in men and over 50 % of cancers in women, i.e. about 330/360,000 cancer cases and about 200/220,000 cancer deaths. Avoidance or moderation of alcohol consumption to 2 drinks/day in men and 1 drink/day in women is therefore a global public health priority.

Infectious Agents

There is growing evidence that chronic infection with some viruses, bacteria and parasites represents a major risk factor for human cancer, in particular in low-income countries. A number of infectious agents have been evaluated within the International Agency for Research on Cancer (IARC) Monograph programme, and the evidence of a causal association has been classified as sufficient for several of them. A global burden of cancers attributable to infections in 2008 has been published in 2012 [41]. The population attributable fraction for infectious agents was 16.1 % in 2008, meaning that around two million new cancer cases were attributable to infections. Hepatitis B virus (HBV)- and hepatitis C virus (HCV)-related liver cancer, human papillomavirus (HPV)-related cervical cancer and *Helicobacter pylori*-related stomach cancer overall are responsible for 95 % of the total number of infection-related cancers. The estimate of the attributable fraction is higher in low- and middle-income countries than in high-income countries (22.9 % of total cancer vs. 7.4 %).

Use of safe, effective (and ideally cheap) vaccines represents the best preventive strategy for cancers caused by viruses, and HBV and HPV infection can be effectively prevented today. Chronic infection with *H. pylori* can be prevented by eradication treatment and sanitation measures, and changes in dietary practices (e.g. avoidance of raw fish) can prevent infection by carcinogenic parasites.

Occupation and Pollution

Approximately 40 occupational agents, groups of agents and mixtures have been classified as carcinogenic by IARC. While some (e.g. bis-chloromethythes) represent today a historic curiosity, exposure is still present for carcinogens such as asbestos, silica, arsenic and polycyclic aromatic hydrocarbons (PAHs). Estimates of the global burden of cancer attributable to occupation in high-income countries result in the order of 1–5 % [9, 42]. In the past, almost 50 % of these were due to asbestos alone, while in recent years the impact of asbestos on lung cancer (but not yet mesothelioma in several populations) is levelling off [43]. However, these cancers concentrate in some sectors of the population (mainly male blue-collar workers), among whom they may represent a sizable proportion of total cancers. Furthermore, unlike lifestyle factors, exposure is involuntary. An appreciable reduction of exposure to occupational and environmental carcinogens has taken place in high-income, but also in several middle-income, countries during recent decades. Still, further efforts should be made to further control exposure, particularly in low- and middle-income countries.

The available evidence suggests, in most populations, a small role of air, water and soil pollutants. Global estimates are in the order of 1 % or less of total cancers [9, 42]. This is in striking contrast with public perception, which often identifies pollution as a major cause of human cancer. However, in selected areas (e.g.

residence near asbestos processing plants or in areas with drinking water contaminated by arsenic), environmental exposure to carcinogens may represent an important cancer hazard.

Reproductive Factors and Exogenous Hormones

There is a strong association between reproductive history and risk of cancer of the breast, ovary and endometrium. However, the role played by specific hormones and the mechanisms by which they act are still unclear. The reproductive factors with the strongest effect on breast cancer risk are parity and age at first full-term pregnancy. Nulliparity or low parity is also related to increased risk of endometrial and ovarian cancer. In contrast, high parity is associated with an increased risk of cervical cancer. Oestrogenic stimulation is probably a major cause of breast cancer, as shown by the strong reduction in breast cancer risk among women enrolled in randomized trials of tamoxifen and other antioestrogenic drugs. Exogenous oestrogens and progestins given in combination as hormone replacement therapy (HRT) in menopause and in steroid contraceptives increase the risk of breast cancer [44]. The risk is present, but considerably smaller, for use of oestrogen-only HRT. In contrast, unopposed oestrogens are strongly related to endometrial cancer. Oral contraceptives (OCs) exert a consistent and long-term protection against ovarian and endometrial cancer, but current use of OCs is associated with an increased risk of breast and cervical cancer [44]. Current OC use has also been associated with an excess risk of benign liver cancer and a modest increase of liver cancer [45]. No detailed estimates are available of the contribution of reproductive factors to the global burden of cancer, and given the uncertainties in the definition of the relevant circumstances of exposure, proposed figures for high-income countries range from 3 % [46] to 15 % [9].

An effect of sex hormones on testicular and prostate cancer is plausible, but the epidemiological evidence is currently inadequate to draw any conclusion.

Perinatal and Growth Factors

Excess energy intake early in life is probably associated with an increased risk of breast and colon cancer [47]. The role of attained height, growth factors and other factors such as insulin resistance is unclear. In addition, high birth weight is possibly associated with an increased risk of breast, prostate cancer and head and neck cancer. The implications of these findings for preventive strategies should be clarified by a more complete understanding of the underlying carcinogenic mechanisms.

Ionizing and Nonionizing Radiation

Ionizing radiation causes several neoplasms, including in particular acute lymphocytic leukaemia, acute and chronic myeloid leukaemia and cancers of the breast, lung, bone, brain and thyroid [48]. Theoretical considerations and extrapolations from high doses lead to the conclusion that a threshold below which no excess cancer risk is present is unlikely, although the quantification of the excess risk at low doses, at which most people are commonly exposed, is difficult. For most individuals, the main exposure is natural radiation, including indoor radon, although artificial sources (e.g. radiotherapy) might be important in particular cases. The estimates of the contribution of ionizing radiation to human cancer in high-income countries are in the order of 3 % [46] to 5 % [9].

Solar (ultraviolet, UV) radiation is carcinogenic to the skin. Over 90 % of skin neoplasms are attributable to sunlight; because of the low fatality of non-melanocytic skin cancer, solar radiation is responsible for about 1 % of total cancer deaths [9]. Avoidance of sun exposure, in particular during childhood, is an important cancer-preventive behaviour. The evidence of a carcinogenic effect of other types of nonionizing radiations, in particular electric and magnetic fields, is inconclusive and likely negligible, if any [49].

Medical Procedures and Drugs

The drugs that may cause or prevent cancer fall into several groups. Many cancer chemotherapy drugs are active on the DNA, which might also result in damage to normal cells. The main neoplasm associated with chemotherapy treatment is leukaemia, although the risk of solid tumours might also be increased. A second group of carcinogenic drugs includes immunosuppressive agents, notably used in transplanted patients. Non-Hodgkin's lymphoma (NHL) is the main neoplasm caused by these drugs. The effects of HRT and OCs are discussed above. Phenacetin-containing analgesics increase the risk of cancer of the renal pelvis.

No precise estimates are available for the global contribution of drug use to human cancer. It is unlikely, however, that they represent more than 1 % in high-resource countries [9]. Furthermore, the benefits of therapies are usually much greater than the potential cancer risk.

Use of ionizing radiation for diagnostic purposes is likely to carry a small risk of cancer, which has been demonstrated only for childhood leukaemia following intrauterine exposure. Radiotherapy increases the risk of cancer in the irradiated organs. There is no evidence of an increased cancer risk following other medical procedures, including surgical implants.

Chemoprevention can also be considered for primary and secondary prevention of cancer, but data are negative or inconsistent for most micronutrients or other substances considered.

Data are however more promising for aspirin. In fact, aspirin has been associated with a reduced risk of colorectal and possibly of a few other common cancers, but quantification remains open to discussion [50]. A meta-analysis of observational studies on aspirin and 12 cancer sites published up to September 2011 included a total of 139 studies [51]. Regular aspirin is associated with a reduced risk of colorectal cancer (summary RR based on more than 30,000 cases = 0.73, 95 % confidence interval (CI) 0.67–0.79) and of other digestive tract cancers (RR = 0.61, 95 % CI = 0.50–0.76 for squamous cell oesophageal cancer; RR = 0.64, 95 % CI = 0.52–0.78 for oesophageal and gastric cardia adenocarcinoma; and RR = 0.67, 95 % CI = 0.54–0.83 for gastric cancer). Modest inverse associations were also observed for breast (RR = 0.90, 95 % CI = 0.85–0.95) and prostate cancer (RR = 0.90, 95 % CI = 0.85–0.96), while lung cancer was significantly reduced in case–control studies (0.73, 95 % CI = 0.55–0.98) but not in cohort ones (RR = 0.98, 95 % CI = 0.92–1.05). No meaningful associations were observed for cancers of the pancreas, endometrium, ovary, bladder and kidney. Thus, a large number of observational studies, but also evidence from prospective clinical trials [52], indicate a beneficial role of aspirin on colorectal and other digestive tract cancers; modest risk reductions were also observed for breast and prostate cancer.

Genetic Factors

A number of inherited mutations of a high-penetrance cancer gene increase substantially the risk of some neoplasms (see sections on specific neoplasms). However, these are rare conditions in most populations and the number of cases attributable to them is rather small.

Familial aggregation has been shown for most types of cancers, also in noncarriers of known high-penetrance genes. This is notably the case for cancers of the breast, colon, prostate and lung. The RR is in the order of 2–4, and is higher for cases diagnosed at young age. Although some of the aggregations can be explained by shared risk factors among family members, it is plausible that a true genetic component exists for most human cancers. This takes the form of an increased susceptibility to endogenous and exogenous carcinogens. The effect on cancer risk of common genetic variants with a small to moderate risk of cancer (approximately twofold) responsible for such susceptibility has been extensively studied in the past two decades within genetic association studies. Some synopses have been published mostly regarding genes involved in the DNA repair, encoding for metabolic enzymes and cell cycle control [53]. Despite many years of candidate gene studies testing for gene–environment interaction, however, there are only few notable replicated and widely agreed-upon examples of success (e.g. *N*-acetyltransferase 2 (NAT2), smoking and bladder cancer; aldehyde dehydrogenase 2 (ALDH2), alcohol, head and neck and oesophageal cancer), as publication bias and false-positive findings largely affected the literature in this field.

In recent years, genome-wide association studies (GWAS) that use an agnostic approach identified new genes that might confer cancer susceptibility, though their clinical utility is currently very limited [54].

Best Practices for Cancer Prevention

In the following paragraphs, we describe some principles of primary and secondary prevention, with the strategies of prevention for the most common malignant neoplasms.

Principles of Primary Prevention

The main goal of primary prevention of cancer is to reduce the incidence through the reduction of exposure to risk factors for cancer at the population level. Where feasible, primary prevention programmes are demonstrated to be largely cost-effective, i.e. the reduction of the burden of disease is achieved with a reasonable money investment, while this is not always the case for secondary prevention programmes. Many determinants of malignant neoplasms, including tobacco smoking, alcohol drinking, a number of viruses and parasites, UV radiation, ionizing radiation and a number of chemicals, industrial processes and occupational exposures, are sufficiently well established to constitute logical priorities for preventive action. Two more reasons add weight to this priority: Some of the agents are responsible for sizeable proportions of the cancers occurring today, and for many agents it is in principle feasible to reduce or even to completely eliminate exposure. If this is taken as the objective of preventive action, some practical points are helpful in guiding such action.

First, although epidemiological data in most cases do not allow a direct estimate of the risk of cancer at low doses, it is reasonable (at least from a preventive point of view) to assume that the dose (exposure)–risk relationship for agents acting through damage to DNA is linear with no threshold [55]. Second, the carcinogenic effect is not equally dependent on the dose rate (dose per unit of time) and on duration of exposure. For example, in regular smokers, the incidence rate of lung cancer depends more strongly on duration of exposure, increasing with the fourth power of it, than on dose rate, increasing only with the first or second power of it [56].

The attribution of population attributable risks to specific agents (as done when, for instance, smoking is said to be the cause of some 30 % of all cancer deaths) is complicated by their interactive effects. This is particularly relevant when considering the relative effectiveness of removing (or reducing) exposure to one of two (or more) jointly acting agents. Whenever a positive interaction (synergism) occurs between two (or more) hazardous exposures, there is an enlarged possibility of preventive action; the effect of the joint exposure can be attacked in two (or more) ways, each requiring the removal or reduction of one of the exposures; moreover, the larger the size of the interaction relative to the total effect, the more these ways of attack tend to become equal in effectiveness. Finally, reducing exposure to carcinogens can be implemented in two major ways: by elimination of the carcinogen or its substitution with a noncarcinogen or by impeding by various means the contact with the carcinogen. Reduction of exposure depends in each case on technical and economical considerations. Cancer prevention strategies have evolved from a predominant environmental and lifestyle approach to a model that matches individual-oriented actions with public health interventions. Advances in identifying, developing and testing agents with the potential either to prevent cancer initiation or to inhibit or reverse the progression of initiated lesions support this approach. Encouraging laboratory and epidemiologic studies, along with studies of secondary end points in prevention trials, have provided a scientific rationale for the hypothesis and promising results have been reported for various types of cancer, in particular among high-risk individuals [57–59].

Principles of Secondary Prevention

Given the limitations still constraining the primary prevention of many cancers, early detection needs to be considered as a secondary and alternative option, based on the reasonable expectation that the earlier the diagnosis and the stage at which a malignancy is discovered, the better the prognosis. This implies that an effective treatment for the disease exists and that the less advanced the cancer at the preclinical stage, the better the scope for treatment, and the better the prognosis. This latter aspect cannot be taken for granted.

Before a screening programme can be adopted on a large scale, a number of other requirements need to be fulfilled. First of all, a screening test (that is, a relatively simple and rapid test aimed at the presumptive identification of preclinical disease) must be available that is capable of correctly identifying cases and non-cases. In other words, both sensitivity and specificity should be high, approaching 100 %. While high sensitivity is obviously important, given that the very purpose of screening is to pick up, if possible, all cases of a cancer in its detectable preclinical phase, it is specificity that plays a dominant role in the practical utilization of the test within a defined population. As the prevalence of a preclinical cancer to be screened in well-defined populations is often in the range of 1–10 per 1000, if a test is used with a specificity of 95 %, then at least 5 % of results will be false positives. In other words, for every case which will turn out at the diagnostic workup to be a true cancer (assuming 100 % sensitivity), there will be 5–50 cases falsely identified as such and ultimately found not to be cancers. This situation is likely to prove unacceptable due to too high psychological and economical costs. One solution is an increase in specificity, for example, by developing better tests or combinations of tests, or by changing the criterion of positivity of a given test to make it more stringent (this necessarily decreases sensitivity). In addition, one might select populations with relatively high prevalence of the cancer ('high-risk' groups), so as to increase the number of the true positives. Whatever the group on which the programme operates, additional requirements are that the test is safe, easily and rapidly applicable, and acceptable in a broad sense to the population to be examined. It has also to be cheap, but what is or is not cheap is better evaluated within a cost-effectiveness analysis of different ways of preventing a cancer case or death, an issue not further discussed here. If these requirements are met, still little is known about the possible net benefit in outcome deriving from the screening programme (in fact, screening test plus diagnostic workup plus treatment, as applied in a given population). To evaluate benefit, several measures of outcome can be assessed. An early one, useful but not sufficient, is the distribution by stage of the detected cancer cases which, if the programme is ultimately to be beneficial, should be shifted to earlier, less invasive stages of the disease in comparison with the distribution of the cases discovered through ordinary medical care. A second measure of outcome is the survival of cases detected at screening compared with the survival of cases detected through ordinary medical care. This is a superficially attractive but usually equivocal criterion, to the extent that a screening may only advance the time of diagnosis (and therefore the apparent survival time), without postponing the time of death ('lead-time bias'). A final outcome (and the main test of the programme) is the site-specific cancer mortality in the screened population compared with the mortality in the unscreened population.

Correct, unbiased comparison of this outcome, and thus unbiased measure of the effect of the screening programme, should in principle be made within the framework of a randomized controlled trial (RCT), in which two groups of subjects are randomly allocated to the screening programme and to no screening (that is, receiving the existing medical care) or to two alternative screening programmes, for instance, entailing different tests or different intervals between periodical examinations. However, largely due to pressures to adopt on a large scale screening programmes hoped to be effective, a situation has often arisen where withholding screening to a group has been regarded as unethical or socially unacceptable, thus preventing the conduct of a proper experiment. Only a few randomized trials evaluating the effectiveness of screening programmes are available and comparisons made through non-randomized experiments or through observational studies. In addition to lead-time bias, three types of biases are peculiar to the assessment of screening programmes. Because of self-selection, persons who elect to receive early detection may be different from those who do not: For instance, they may belong to better educated classes, be generally healthier and health conscious, and this could produce a longer survival independent of any effect of early detection. In addition, cancers with longer preclinical phases, which may mean less biological aggressiveness and better prognosis, are, in any case, more likely to be intercepted by a programme of periodical screening than cancers with a short preclinical phase, and a rapid, aggressive clinical course (length bias). Finally, because of criteria of positivity adopted to maximize yield of early time cases, a number of lesions which in fact would never become malignant growths are included as 'cases', thus falsely improving the survival statistics (overdiagnosis bias). Chemoprevention can also be considered for primary and secondary prevention of cancer, but data are negative or inconsistent for most micronutrients or other substances considered. Data are however more promising for aspirin.

Prevention of Lung Cancer

Control of tobacco smoking remains the key strategy for the prevention of lung cancer. Reduction in exposure to occupational and environmental carcinogens (in particular indoor pollution and radon) as well as increase in consumption of fruits and vegetables are additional preventive opportunities. Spiral computed tomography (CT) scan has been shown to reduce lung cancer mortality [60], although this effect needs to be assessed with respect to potential overdiagnosis of lung nodules with low malignant potential.

Prevention of Breast Cancer

Primary prevention of breast cancer has been attempted via nutritional intervention, involving reduction of energy intake, reduction of proportion of calories from fat and increase in fruit and vegetable consumption. No evidence of efficacy has been produced so far. However, control of weight gain and of overweight and obesity or postmenopausal women would have favourable implications in breast cancer risk. Tamoxifen, an antioestrogen drug used in chemotherapy, has shown a chemopreventive action against breast cancer, although its use is recommended in women with a previous breast cancer only. Aspirin and other nonsteroidal anti-inflammatory drugs might also have a chemopreventive effect on breast cancer risk, although results from epidemiological studies are heterogeneous [51]. The most suitable approach for breast cancer control is secondary prevention through mammography. Breast cancer screening began to be implemented in the late 1980s. The effectiveness of screening by mammography in women older than 50 years has been demonstrated, and programmes have been established in various countries, although some controversies remain in the interpretation of the available evidence [61]. The reduction in mortality, typically of the order of 25 % seen in RCTs, are not replicated in routine screening where the reductions are more often in the range of 10–15 % in the general population 15–20 years after full rollout of the programme [62, 63]. The effectiveness in women younger than 50 has not been demonstrated. Other screening techniques, including breast self-examination, have not been proven to reduce breast cancer mortality.

Prevention of Prostate Cancer

The wide geographical variability of prostate cancer (i.e. a twofold higher mortality in Sweden than in Italy) suggests that environmental factors, likely related to diet and other lifestyle factors, such as physical activity, are important determinants of the disease. Primary prevention, however, is hampered by the fragmentary knowledge of its precise causes. Secondary prevention has been proposed, based on measurement of prostate-specific antigen (PSA) and digital rectal examination. There is little evidence from controlled trials that either procedure decreases the mortality from prostate cancer [64, 65]. Despite this lack of evidence, these procedures, in particular the PSA testing, have gained popularity in many countries, and are the reasons for the steep increase in number of diagnosed cased since the mid-1980s in North America and other high-income countries. It is unclear how much of the decrease in mortality reported since the mid-1990s in the USA and in Western Europe can be attributed to a beneficial effect of (unorganized) use of PSA testing, but it is likely due mainly to improved management and treatment of the disease, including better surgery, radiotherapy and medical therapy.

Prevention of Cancer of the Uterine Cervix

Cytological examination of exfoliated cervical cells (the Papanicolaou smear (PAP) test) is effective in identifying precursor lesions, resulting in a substantial decrease in incidence of and mortality from invasive cancer. Cytological smears are not largely applicable, however, in countries with limited availability of cytologists and pathologists, including many countries with high prevalence of HPV infection and high incidence of invasive cancer. Alternative approaches for secondary prevention have therefore been proposed, including visual inspection of the cervix with possible enhancement of precursor lesions by acetic acid, but their efficacy on cervical cancer prevention remains unquantified. Use of HPV testing appears now however to be more specific and sensible than the PAP test, and is therefore likely to replace PAP smear as the first screening method in the near future. The primary method for prevention of cervical cancer for future generations, however, is HPV vaccination. One vaccine against HPV 16, 18 (as well 6 and 11, linked to genital warts) and another against HPV 16 and 18 only have been available for a few years now [66]. Vaccines including larger numbers of HPV strains (i.e. eight strains) are in the late stage of testing. The final impact of the effect of such vaccination is complicated by the geographical variations in the distribution of HPV types [67].

Prevention of Colorectal Cancer

Increased physical activity and avoidance of overweight and obesity are the main tools for the primary prevention of colorectal cancer. Chemopreventive strategies other than aspirin cannot be recommended at present. Control of HPV infection, possibly via vaccination in new generations, represents the main preventive measure for anal cancer. Surveillance via flexible colonoscopy, involving removal of adenomas, is a secondary preventive measure. An additional approach consists in the detection of faecal occult blood. The method suffers from low specificity and, to a lesser extent, low sensitivity, in particular in the ability to detect adenomas. However, trials have shown a reduced mortality from colorectal cancer after the annual test, although this is achieved at a high cost due to an elevated number of false-positive cases. Current recommendations for individuals aged 50 and over include either annual faecal occult blood testing or once colonoscopy [68]. The WHO endorsed in 2011 the recommendations of the Council of The European Union of 2003, that advice for population-based screening of colorectal cancer, though the cost-effectiveness remains somewhat underlined [69].

Prevention of Stomach Cancer

Primary prevention of stomach cancer by dietary means is feasible by encouraging high-risk populations to decrease consumption of cured meats and salt-preserved foods. Prevention may also be feasible through eradication of *H. pylori* infection, particularly in childhood and adolescence, by avoiding mother-to-child transmission. Screening and early detection of stomach cancer have been developed in Japan with use of X-ray photofluorography to identify possible lesions, followed by gastroscopy. Screen-detected cases are more likely to be early-stage localized disease and have a greater survival than other cases. Screening and early detection are not considered cost-effective in populations outside high-incidence areas.

Prevention of Liver Cancer and Biliary Tract Cancers

The strong role in liver carcinogenesis of infection with HBV, a virus for which effective and cheap vaccines are available, indicates that a large proportion of liver cancers are preventable. In high-prevalence areas, HBV vaccination should be introduced in the perinatal period. In the past decades, many countries from Asia, Southern Europe and, to a lesser extent, Africa have expanded the national childhood vaccination programme to include HBV. A similar primary preventive approach is not available for HCV. Control of transmissions is however feasible and medical treatment of carriers with newer and more effective interferon-free treatment schemes might represent an alternative approach (which is also available for HBV carriers).

Control of aflatoxin contamination of foodstuffs represents another important preventive measure. While this has been achieved in high-income countries and some middle-income ones, its implementation is limited by economic and logistic factors in many high-prevalence regions. Control of tobacco smoking and excessive alcohol drinking represents additional primary preventive measures.

Ultrasound has been proposed as a screening method for liver cancer, but its effectiveness has not been proven. In general, population-based studies are currently available showing a decreased mortality from liver cancer in screened populations.

Cholecystectomy is an obvious means of preventing gallbladder cancer. The removal of the gallbladder in asymptomatic patients, however, is not justified, with the possible exception of high-risk circumstances such as large stones and calcified gallbladder.

Prevention of Oesophageal Cancer

Avoidance of tobacco smoking and elevated alcohol drinking remains the main preventive approach in reducing the burden of oesophageal SqCC in Western populations. Improved diet, in particular increase in consumption of fresh fruits and vegetables, might also contribute to oesophageal cancer prevention. The incomplete understanding of the role of other factors complicates the elaboration of preventive strategies in many high-risk regions, although a decrease in intake and temperature of hot drink might be important.

Prevention of Lymphoid Neoplasms

The limited knowledge of the causes of lymphatic and haematopoietic neoplasms limits the opportunity for prevention. Avoidance of known risk factors (e.g. unnecessary radiation exposure, benzene) is likely to result in the prevention of a small proportion of these neoplasms in several populations.

Prevention of Oral and Pharyngeal Cancers

Avoidance of tobacco smoking, chewing and snuffing and avoidance of excessive alcohol drinking represent the main preventive measures for cancer of the oral cavity and pharynx. The fact that HPV vaccination will contribute to the prevention of oropharyngeal cancer is an important argument to extend the existing programme to boys. It is possible that additional benefits are obtained from increase in fruit and vegetable intake and improvement of oral hygiene. Avoidance of excessive exposure to solar radiation would represent the main preventive approach for lip cancer. In populations at high risk of nasopharyngeal cancer from China and possibly other countries, avoidance of salted fish, pickled vegetables and other preserved food, in particular as weaning food, should be recommended.

Oral inspection aimed to identify pre-neoplastic lesions is an effective approach for secondary prevention of oral cancer [70]. The inspection can be performed by medically certified professionals, but also, in particular in high-risk areas from middle- and low-income countries such as India (where oral cancer incidence is very high), by specifically trained health workers.

Prevention of Non-melanocytic Skin Cancer

Avoidance of sun exposure, in particular during the middle of the day, is the primary preventive measure to reduce the incidence of skin cancer. There is no adequate evidence of a protective effect of sunscreens, possibly because use of sunscreens is associated with increased exposure to the sun. The possible benefit in reducing skin cancer risk by reduction of sun exposure, however, should be balanced against possible favourable effects of UV radiation in promoting vitamin D metabolism. Control of occupational skin carcinogens has taken place in many industries, although high-exposure circumstances still take place in a few low-income countries. Control of exposure to sunshine is still largely inadequate. Avoidance of drinking water with a high arsenic level should be a priority in contaminated areas for skin, but also for several other neoplasms, including lung and bladder [71]. Secondary prevention can be achieved by regular skin examination, in particular for high-risk individuals: However, there is a lack of controlled trials on skin cancer screening.

Prevention of Malignant Melanoma

Reducing of solar and other sources of UVB exposure, especially in childhood, is the major primary preventive measure. Early diagnosis, in particular of thin lesions, is associated with better survival: Screening via medical examination is justified in high-risk individuals, defined according to familial history, type of skin and reaction to solar radiation.

Conclusions

Neoplasms are a group of diverse diseases with complex distributions in human populations and with different aetiological factors. A comprehensive strategy for cancer control might lead to the avoidance of a sizeable proportion of human cancers, and the greatest benefit can be achieved via tobacco control. However, such a strategy would imply major cultural, societal and economic changes. More modest objectives for cancer prevention should focus on the neoplasms and the exposures that are prevalent in any given population. For example, vaccination of children against HBV and adolescent women against HPV are likely to be the most cost-effective cancer prevention action in many countries of Africa and Asia.

Neoplasms will continue to be a major source of human disease and death. Considerable efforts are made in the public and private domains and here have been able to develop effective therapeutic approaches for a wide number of important neoplasms. Even if further advances in the clinical management of cancer patients will be accomplished in the near future, the changes will mainly affect the affluent part of the world population. Prevention of the known causes of cancer remains the most promising approach in reducing the consequences of cancer, in particular in countries with limited resources. Control of tobacco smoking and of smokeless tobacco products, reduced overweight and obesity, moderation in alcohol intake, increased physical activity, avoidance of exposure to solar radiation in central hours of the days in summer and control of known occupational and environmental [49] carcinogens remain the main approaches; we currently have to reduce the burden of human neoplasms.

References

1. Boffetta P, Boccia S, La Vecchia C (2014) A quick guide to cancer epidemiology. Springer Switzerland
2. WHO (1990) International classification of diseases for oncology (ICD-O), 2nd edn. Springer brief in cancer research, World Health Organization, Geneva
3. Ferlay J, Shin HR, Bray F, Forman D, Mathers C, Parkin DM (2010) Estimates of worldwide burden of cancer in 2008: GLOBOCAN 2008. Int J Cancer 127:2893–2917
4. Baili P, Micheli A, De Angelis R et al (2008) Life tables for world-wide comparison of relative survival for cancer (CONCORD study). Tumori 94:658–668
5. Sant M, Allemani C, Santaquilani M, Knijn A, Marchesi F, Capocaccia R (2009) EUROCARE-4. Survival of cancer patients diagnosed in 1995–1999. Results and commentary. Eur J Cancer 45:931–991
6. Sankaranarayanan R, Swaminathan R, Jayant K, Brenner H (2011) An overview of cancer survival in Africa, Asia, the Caribbean and Central America: the case for investment in cancer health services. IARC Sci Publ (162):257–291
7. Soerjomataram I, Lortet-Tieulent J, Parkin DM et al (2012) Global burden of cancer in 2008: a systematic analysis of disability-adjusted life-years in 12 world regions. Lancet 380:1840–1850
8. IARC (2004) Tobacco smoke and involuntary smoking. In: IARC monographs on the evaluation of the carcinogenic risks to humans, vol 83. IARC, Lyon, pp 51–1187
9. Doll R, Peto R (2005) Epidemiology of cancer. In: Warell DA, Cox TM, Firth JD (eds) Oxford textbook of medicine, vol 3, 4th edn. Oxford University Press, New York, pp 193–218
10. Doll R, Peto R, Boreham J, Sutherland I (2004) Mortality in relation to smoking: 50 years' observations on male British doctors. Br Med J 328:1519
11. Jha P, Ramasundarahettige C, Landsman V et al (2013) 21st-century hazards of smoking and benefits of cessation in the United States. N Engl J Med 368:341–350
12. Pirie K, Peto R, Reeves GK, Green J, Beral V (2013) The 21st century hazards of smoking and benefits of stopping: a prospective study of one million women in the UK. Lancet 381:133–141
13. Peto R, Darby S, Deo H, Silcocks P, Whitley E, Doll R (2000) Smoking, smoking cessation, and lung cancer in the UK since 1950: combination of national statistics with two case-control studies. Br Med J 321:323–329
14. Bosetti C, Gallus S, Peto R et al (2008) Tobacco smoking, smoking cessation, and cumulative risk of upper aerodigestive tract cancers. Am J Epidemiol 167:468–473

15. La Vecchia C, Bosetti C, Lucchini F et al (2010) Cancer mortality in Europe, 2000–2004, and an overview of trends since 1975. Ann Oncol 21:1323–1360
16. Bosetti C, Malvezzi M, Rosso T et al (2012) Lung cancer mortality in European women: trends and predictions. Lung Cancer 78:171–178
17. Malvezzi M, Bosetti C, Rosso T et al (2013) Lung cancer mortality in European men: trends and predictions. Lung Cancer 80:138–145
18. Peto J, Decarli A, La Vecchia C, Levi F, Negri E (1999) The European mesothelioma epidemic. Br J Cancer 79:666–672
19. Song Y, Zhao L, Palipudi KM et al (2013) Tracking MPOWER in 14 countries: results from the Global Adult Tobacco Survey, 2008–2010. Glob Health Promot
20. Mendez D, Alshanqeety O, Warner KE (2013) The potential impact of smoking control policies on future global smoking trends. Tob Control 22:46–51
21. Bertuccio P, La Vecchia C, Silverman DT et al (2011) Cigar and pipe smoking, smokeless tobacco use and pancreatic cancer: an analysis from the International Pancreatic Cancer Case-Control Consortium (PanC4). Ann Oncol 22:1420–1426
22. Alexander DD, Morimoto LM, Mink PJ, Lowe KA (2010) Summary and meta-analysis of pro-spective studies of animal fat intake and breast cancer. Nutr Res Rev 23:169–179
23. Liu L, Zhuang W, Wang RQ et al (2011) Is dietary fat associated with the risk of colorectal cancer? A meta-analysis of 13 prospective cohort studies. Eur J Nutr 50:173–184
24. Chan DS, Lau R, Aune D et al (2011) Red and processed meat and colorectal cancer incidence: meta-analysis of prospective studies. PLoS One 6:e20456
25. Wu S, Feng B, Li K et al (2012) Fish consumption and colorectal cancer risk in humans: a systematic review and meta-analysis. Am J Med 125:551–559.e5
26. Aune D, Lau R, Chan DS et al (2012) Dairy products and colorectal cancer risk: a systematic review and meta-analysis of cohort studies. Ann Oncol 23:37–45
27. Chen GC, Pang Z, Liu QF (2012) Magnesium intake and risk of colorectal cancer: a meta-analysis of prospective studies. Eur J Clin Nutr 66:1182–1186
28. WCRF (2007) World Cancer Research Fund/American Institute for Cancer Research. Food, nutrition, physical activity, and the prevention of cancer: a global perspective. AICR, Washington, DC
29. Pelucchi C, Bosetti C, Rossi M, Negri E, La Vecchia C (2009) Selected aspects of Mediterranean diet and cancer risk. Nutr Cancer 61:756–766
30. IARC (1998) Vitamin A. In: IARC handbooks of cancer prevention, vol 3. pp 1–261. IARC Publications, IARC, Lyon
31. IARC (1998) Carotenoids. In: IARC handbooks of cancer prevention, vol 2. pp 1–326. IARC Publications, IARC, Lyon
32. IARC (2008) Vitamin D and cancer/a report of the IARC working group on vitamin D, vol 5. IARC, Lyon
33. IARC (2002) Weight control and physical activity. In: IARC handbooks of cancer prevention, vol 6. pp 1–315. IARC Publications, IARC, Lyon
34. Bergstrom A, Pisani P, Tenet V, Wolk A, Adami HO (2001) Overweight as an avoidable cause of cancer in Europe. Int J Cancer 91:421–430
35. Lee IM, Shiroma EJ, Lobelo F, Puska P, Blair SN, Katzmarzyk PT (2012) Effect of physical inactivity on major non-communicable diseases worldwide: an analysis of burden of disease and life expectancy. Lancet 380:219–229
36. Baan R, Straif K, Grosse Y et al (2007) Carcinogenicity of alcoholic beverages. Lancet Oncol 8:292–293
37. Pelucchi C, Tramacere I, Boffetta P, Negri E, La Vecchia C (2011) Alcohol consumption and cancer risk. Nutr Cancer 63:983–990
38. Bagnardi V, Rota M, Botteri E et al (2013) Light alcohol drinking and cancer: a meta-analysis. Ann Oncol 24:301–308
39. Boffetta P, Hashibe M (2006) Alcohol and cancer. Lancet Oncol 7:149–156
40. Boyle P, Autier P, Bartelink H et al (2003) European Code Against Cancer and scientific justification: third version (2003). Ann Oncol 14:973–100

41. de Martel C, Ferlay J, Franceschi S et al (2012) Global burden of cancers attributable to infections in 2008: a review and synthetic analysis. Lancet Oncol 13:607–615
42. Schottenfeld D, Beebe-Dimmer JL, Buffler PA, Omenn GS (2013) Current perspective on the global and United States cancer burden attributable to lifestyle and environmental risk factors. Annu Rev Public Health 34:97–117
43. La Vecchia C, Boffetta P (2012) Role of stopping exposure and recent exposure to asbestos in the risk of mesothelioma. Eur J Cancer Prev 21:227–230
44. IARC (2007) Combined estrogen-progestogen contraceptives and combined estrogen progestogen menopausal therapy. In: IARC monographs on the evaluation of carcinogenic risks to humans, vol 91. IARC monographs, IARC, Lyon
45. Cibula D, Gompel A, Mueck AO et al (2010) Hormonal contraception and risk of cancer. Hum Reprod Update 16:631–650
46. Harvard Center for Cancer Prevention (1996) Harvard report on cancer prevention. Volume 1: causes of human cancer. Cancer Causes Control 7(Suppl 1):S3–59
47. Trichopoulos D (1990) Hypothesis: does breast cancer originate in utero? Lancet 335:939–940
48. IARC (2000) X-radiation and y-radiation. In: IARC monographs on the evaluation of carcinogenic risks to humans. Ionizing radiation, part 1: X- and Gamma (y)-radiation, and neutrons, vol 75. pp 121–362, IARC monographs, IARC, Lyon
49. Chang E, Adami HO, Bailey WH et al (2014) Validity of geographically modeled environmental exposure estimates. Critical Rev Toxicol
50. Cuzick J, Otto F, Baron JA et al (2009) Aspirin and non-steroidal anti-inflammatory drugs for cancer prevention: an international consensus statement. Lancet Oncol 10:501–507
51. Bosetti C, Rosato V, Gallus S, Cuzick J, La Vecchia C (2012) Aspirin and cancer risk: a quantitative review to 2011. Ann Oncol 23:1403–1415
52. Rothwell PM, Fowkes FG, Belch JF, Ogawa H, Warlow CP, Meade TW (2011) Effect of daily aspirin on long-term risk of death due to cancer: analysis of individual patient data from randomized trials. Lancet 377:31–41
53. Vineis P, Manuguerra M, Kavvoura FK et al (2009) A field synopsison low-penetrance variants in DNA repair genes and cancer susceptibility. J Natl Cancer Inst 101:24–36
54. Stadler ZK, Thom P, Robson ME et al (2010) Genome-wide association studies of cancer. J Clin Oncol 28:4255–4267
55. Peto R, Gray R, Brantom P, Grasso P (1991) Effects on 4080 rats of chronic ingestion of N-nitrosodiethylamine or N-nitrosodimethylamine: a detailed dose-response study. Cancer Res 51:6415–6451
56. Peto R (1977) Epidemiology, multistage models and short-term mutagenicity tests. In: Hiatt HH, Watson JD, Winsten JA (eds) Origins of human cancer. Cold Spring Harbor Laboratory, Cold Spring Harbor, pp 1403–1428
57. Greenwald P (2005) Lifestyle and medical approaches to cancer prevention. Recent Results Cancer Res 166:1–15
58. Boffetta P, La Vecchia C (2009) Neoplasms. In: Detels R, Beaglehole R, Lansang MA, Gulliford M (eds) The practice of public health. Oxford textbook of public health, vol 3, 5th edn. Oxford University Press, New York, pp 997–1020
59. Zhang Z-F, Boffetta P, Neugut AI, La Vecchia C (2014) Cancer epidemiology and public health. In: Oxford textbook of public health. Oxford University Press, Oxford
60. Aberle DR, Adams AM, Berg CD et al (2011) Reduced lung-cancer mortality with low-dose computed tomographic screening. N Engl J Med 365:395–409
61. IUKPBCS (2012) The benefits and harms of breast cancer screening: an independent review. Lancet 380:1778–1786
62. Anttila A, Sarkeala T, Hakulinen T, Heinavaara S (2008) Impacts of the Finnish service screening programme on breast cancer rates. BMC Public Health 8:38
63. Kalager M, Zelen M, Langmark F, Adami HO (2010) Effect of screening mammography on breast-cancer mortality in Norway. N Engl J Med 363:1203–1210

64. Boyle P, Brawley OW (2009) Prostate cancer: current evidence weighs against population screening. CA Cancer J Clin 59:220–224
65. Welch HG, Albertsen PC (2009) Prostate cancer diagnosis and treatment after the introduction of prostate-specific antigen screening: 1986–2005. J Natl Cancer Inst 101:1325–1329
66. FUTURE II Study Group (2007) Quadrivalent vaccine against human papillomavirus to prevent high-grade cervical lesions. N Engl J Med 356:1915–1927
67. Cuzick J (2010) Long-term cervical cancer prevention strategies across the globe. Gynecol Oncol 117:S11–S14
68. Smith RA, Brooks D, Cokkinides V, Saslow D, Brawley OW (2013) Cancer screening in the United States, 2013: a review of current American Cancer Society guidelines, current issues in cancer screening, and new guidance on cervical cancer screening and lung cancer screening. CA Cancer J Clin 63:88–105
69. Sigurdsson JA, Getz L, Sjonell G, Vainiomaki P, Brodersen J (2013) Marginal public health gain of screening for colorectal cancer: modelling study, based on WHO and national databases in the Nordic countries. J Eval Clin Pract 19:400–407
70. Sankaranarayanan R, Ramadas K, Thara S, et al (2013) Long term effect of visual screening on oral cancer incidence and mortality in a randomized trial in Kerala, India. Oral Oncol 49:314–321
71. Steinmaus CM, Ferreccio C, Romo JA, et al (2013) Drinking water arsenic in northern Chile: high cancer risks 40 years after exposure cessation. Cancer Epidemiol Biomarkers Prev 22:623–630

Chapter 6
Obesity and Diabetes

Anna Maria Ferriero and Maria Lucia Specchia

Overweight and Obesity

Definition

Overweight and obesity, defined as abnormal or excessive fat accumulation that presents a risk to health, are both labels for ranges of weight that are greater than what is generally considered healthy for a given height. The terms also identify ranges of weight that have been shown to increase the likelihood of certain diseases and other health problems [1, 2]. As shown in the literature and suggested also by the Centers for Disease Control and Prevention (CDC), overweight and obesity could be caused by genetic factors, environmental factors and some diseases or drugs. Regarding environmental ones, the major factors are quantity and quality of the food consumed and lack of physical activity. Nowadays, furthermore, among factors considered at high risk for obesity, great importance is given also to socio-economic status [3]. There is a large literature that has demonstrated inequalities in obesity in both high- and low-income contexts worldwide; however, the direction of this association differs by economic context. In high-income contexts, there is a strong inverse association between socioeconomic status and obesity, whereas in low-income countries socioeconomic status and obesity are directly associated [4]. Recent studies, such as that of Akil and colleagues, have confirmed that an increased rate of obesity may be linked to several socioeconomic factors, such as poverty and low income [3]. Another important risk factor for obesity seems to be the level of education; indeed, overall, there is a significant inverse relationship between obesity prevalence and education of household head [5].

A. M. Ferriero (✉) · M. L. Specchia
Section of Hygiene, Institute of Public Health, Università Cattolica del Sacro Cuore,
L.go F. Vito 1, 00168 Rome, Italy
e-mail: annamariaferriero@hotmail.it

M. L. Specchia
e-mail: marialucia.specchia@rm.unicatt.it

S. Boccia et al. (eds.), *A Systematic Review of Key Issues in Public Health*,
DOI 10.1007/978-3-319-13620-2_6

Classification of Overweight and Obesity

For adults, the most commonly used measure for overweight and obesity is the body mass index (BMI): it is defined as the weight in kilograms divided by the square of the height in meters (kg/m^2). The BMI is the same for both genders and for all ages of adults. However, it should be considered as a rough guide because it may not correspond to the same body fat percentage in different individuals [6]. BMI is used because, for most people, it correlates with their amount of body fat [1]. To achieve optimum health, the median BMI for an adult population should be in the range from 21 to 23 kg/m^2, while the goal for individuals should be to maintain BMI in the range from 18.5 to 24.9 kg/m^2. There is an increased risk of comorbidities for BMI values from 25.0 to 29.9, and a moderate to severe risk of comorbidities for BMI > 30 [7]. An adult who has a BMI between 25 and 29.9 is considered overweight and an adult who has a BMI ≥ 30 is considered obese (Table 6.1) [1].

Although correlating with the amount of body fat, BMI does not directly measure body fat. As a result, some people, such as athletes, may have a BMI that identifies them as overweight even though they do not have excess body fat [1].

Other methods of estimating body fat and body fat distribution include measurements of skinfold thickness and waist circumference, calculation of waist-to-hip circumference ratios, and techniques such as ultrasound, computed tomography, and magnetic resonance imaging (MRI) [1].

BMI is just one indicator of potential health risks associated with being overweight or obese. For assessing someone's likelihood of developing overweight- or obesity-related diseases, the National Heart, Lung, and Blood Institute guidelines recommend looking at two other predictors:

- Waist circumference (because abdominal fat is a predictor of risk for obesity-related diseases)
- Other risk factors for diseases and conditions associated with obesity (e.g., high blood pressure or physical inactivity) [1]

Regarding childhood, the BMI chart is not yet usable for children and it is difficult to develop one simple index for the measurement of overweight and obesity in children and adolescents because their bodies undergo a number of physiological

Table 6.1 Body mass index (BMI) classification. (Adapted from: WHO 2013. Global strategy on diet, physical activity and health) [6]

Underweight	< 18.5
Normal range	18.5–24.9
Overweight	≥ 25.0
Preobese	25.0–29.9
Obese	≥ 30.0
Obese class I	30.0–34.9
Obese class II	35.0–39.9
Obese class III	≥ 40.0

changes as they grow. Depending on age, different methods to measure a body's healthy weight are available [6]:

- For children and adolescents, aged 2–19 years:
  - *Overweight* is defined as a BMI≥85th percentile and <95th percentile for children of the same age and gender
  - *Obesity* is defined as a BMI≥95th percentile for children of the same age and gender [8]
- For children aged 0–5 years: the World Health Organization (WHO) Child Growth Standards, launched in April 2006, include measures for overweight and obesity for infants and young children up to age 5.
- For individuals aged 5–19 years: WHO developed the growth reference data for 5–19 years. It is a reconstruction of the 1977 National Center for Health Statistics (NCHS)/WHO reference and uses the original NCHS data set supplemented with data from the WHO child growth standards sample for young children up to age 5 [6].

Current Burden of the Disease

Epidemiology

Nowadays, obesity is the most frequently encountered metabolic disease [9]. The worldwide prevalence of obesity has nearly doubled during the past 30 years [7]; indeed, in 2008 10 % of men and 14 % of women in the world were obese compared with 5 % for men and 8 % for women in 1980, this means that a total of more than half a billion adults worldwide are obese (205 million men and 297 million women) [7]. On account of this, the WHO has termed the increased prevalence of obesity and diabetes as a "twenty-first-century epidemic" [9].

The prevalence of overweight and obesity is different in the different world regions: it is highest in the WHO Regions of the Americas (62 % for overweight in both sexes, and 26 % for obesity) and lowest in the WHO Region for Southeast Asia (14 % overweight in both sexes and 3 % for obesity). Moreover, differences in prevalence rates, as talked about above, are shown also with regard to the income level. The prevalence of overweight in high-income and upper middle-income countries is more than double than the prevalence in low-income and lower middle-income countries and, as for obesity, the difference is more than tripled, with prevalence ranging from 7 % in both genders in lower middle-income countries to 24 % in upper middle-income countries. Regarding gender, women's obesity is significantly higher, approximately double, than men's in low and lower middle-income countries, but in high-income countries it is similar [7] (Fig. 6.1).

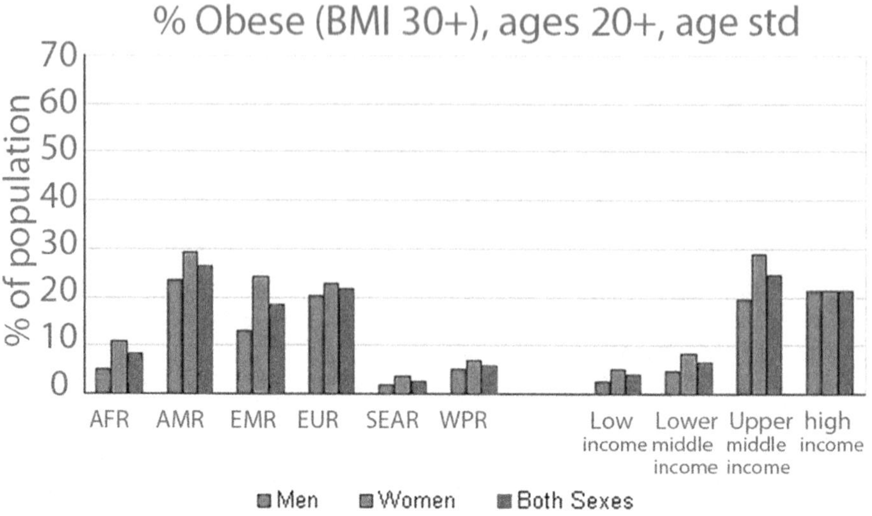

Fig. 6.1 Prevalence of overweight and obesity. (Adapted from WHO 2013. Global Health Observatory. Obesity—situation and trends) [7]

Epidemiology of Childhood Obesity

In 2011, more than 40 million children under 5 years were overweight [10]. The number of overweight adolescents has tripled since 1980 and the prevalence of obesity in younger children has more than doubled [11].

Health Consequences of Overweight and Obesity

Overweight and obesity are the fifth leading risk for global deaths [10]. Being overweight or obese, indeed, constitutes a health risk as it is associated with several comorbidities including type 2 diabetes (T2D) mellitus, cardiovascular diseases, hypertension, dyslipidemia, hyperuricemia, respiratory diseases, osteoarthritis, and depression [1, 2, 9]. Raised BMI also increases the risk of cancer of the breast, colon, prostate, endometrium, kidney, and gall bladder and mortality rates increase with increasing degrees of overweight, as measured by BMI [7]. Worldwide, 44 % of the diabetes burden, 23 % of the ischemic heart disease burden, and between 7 and 41 % of certain cancer burdens are attributable to overweight and obesity and at least 2.8 million adults die each year as a result of being overweight or obese and an estimated 35.8 million (2.3 %) of global disability-adjusted life years (DALYs) are caused by overweight or obesity [7, 10]. Overweight and obesity are linked to more deaths worldwide than underweight. For example, 65 % of the world's population lives in countries where overweight and obesity kill more people than underweight (this includes all high-income and most middle-income countries) [10].

Consequences of Childhood Obesity

Even more serious are the consequences of childhood obesity, which can have a harmful effect on the body in a variety of ways. Obese children are more likely to have:

- High blood pressure and high cholesterol, which are risk factors for cardiovascular disease
- Increased risk of impaired glucose tolerance, insulin resistance, and T2D
- Hypertension
- Breathing problems, such as sleep apnea and asthma
- Joint problems and musculoskeletal discomfort
- Increased risk of fractures
- Fatty liver disease, gallstones, and gastroesophageal reflux (i.e., heartburn)
- Higher chance of obesity, premature death, and disability in adulthood
- Greater risk of social and psychological problems, such as discrimination and poor self-esteem, which can continue into adolescence and adulthood [8, 10]

Health Policy Programs Available

In view of what has been said, the increasing rate of obesity has raised serious concerns for governments and public health organizations and, worldwide, several strategies have been carried out to face this problem. Many countries have implemented intervention programs with the aim of reducing the burden of disease due to obesity and its consequences. Some examples of these programs against obesity are shown below.

The USA

Nutrition and Physical Activity Program to Prevent Obesity and Other Chronic Diseases

In the USA, the Division of Nutrition, Physical Activity, and Obesity (DNPAO) of the CDC currently funds 25 states to address the problems of obesity and other chronic diseases through statewide efforts coordinated with multiple partners. The main goal of the program is to improve the health of Americans by changing environments where people live, work, learn, and play. The plan also aims to address obesity and other chronic diseases through a variety of evidence-based nutrition and physical activity strategies [12]. Therefore, the program has different objectives: some are outcome objectives, such as decrease prevalence of obesity, increase physical activity, and improve dietary behaviors. Others are impact objectives:

- Increase the number and the quality of evidence-based strategies to support healthful eating and physical activity in various settings

- Increase access and use of environments to support healthful eating and physical activity in various settings
- Increase the number and the quality of social and behavioral approaches to promote healthful eating and physical activity

The program has different target areas, of which the principal are increase physical activity, increase the consumption of fruits and vegetables, decrease the consumption of sugar-sweetened beverages; increase breast-feeding initiation, duration, and exclusivity; reduce the consumption of high-energy-dense foods; and decrease television viewing [13].

DNPAO developed six guidance documents to provide assistance and direction regarding each of the principal target areas. The guidance document, developed to increase physical activity, includes the following strategies:

- Community-wide campaigns
- Point-of-decision prompts to encourage use of stairs
- Individually adapted health behavior change programs
- Enhanced school-based physical education
- Social support interventions in community settings
- Enhanced access to places for physical activity combined with informational outreach activities
- Active transport to school (e.g., walking, bicycling, and skating)
- Urban design and transportation policies and practices:
  - Street-scale urban design and land-use policies
  - Community-scale urban design and land-use policies
  - Transportation and travel policies and practices

These types of policies and practices can encourage active transportation by facilitating walking, bicycling, and public transportation use [14].

Communities Putting Prevention to Work

The US Department of Health and Human Services (HHS) awarded more than US$ 119 million to states and US territories to support public health efforts to reduce obesity, increase physical activity, improve nutrition, and decrease smoking. This initiative is funded under the American Recovery and Reinvestment Act of 2009 [15].

To help address these health issues, the US Department of HHS created Communities Putting Prevention to Work (CPPW), which is led by CDC. CPPW is a locally driven initiative supporting 50 communities to tackle obesity and tobacco use. Through CPPW, communities—including urban, small, rural, and tribal areas—are implementing environmental changes to make healthy living easier, such as improving means for safe active transportation for pedestrians, bicyclists, and mass transit users; ensuring provision of healthy food and beverage options in schools; limiting exposure to secondhand smoke; and increasing available tobacco cessation resources. These efforts will produce broad, high-impact, sustainable health outcomes for the communities [16].

Europe

EU Platform on Diet, Physical Activity and Health

In response to the dramatic increase of obesity across Europe, in March 2005, the European Union (EU) Commission launched the "EU Platform on Diet, Physical Activity and Health" [17], which is one of the tools for implementing the European strategy on nutrition, overweight and obesity-related health issues. This platform is an action-oriented cooperative process aimed at helping to reverse the obesity trend and consists of a forum of European-level umbrella organizations, that includes food industry advertisers, retailers, fast-food restaurants, the cooperative movement, consumer groups, and health nongovernmental organizations (NGOs), willing to commit to tackling current trends in diet and physical activity with concrete actions that are termed "commitments." The platform has been in existence since 2005 and during that time its members have bought to action more than 300 commitments [18].

The focal areas for the actions cover promotion for a healthy lifestyle, education, nutritional information and labeling, dissemination, advertising/marketing, product redevelopment/reformulation/portion size, and policy development (Table 6.2) [17].

Since the platform was also launched to exchange experiences and to learn from their own and other actions, continuous monitoring and appropriate evaluation are a crucial need to identify best practices. In May 2006, the newsletter on food safety, health, and consumer policy from the European Commission's Health and Consumer Protection Directorate General announced that "the projects will be monitored and overall progress will be evaluated by the beginning of 2007" [17].

In the program, some key areas to be taken into account were defined:

1. Improving the nutritional value of school meals and home meals:
   - Education programs on healthy diet for children as well as for parents
   - Offering free or subsidized fruit, vegetables, and drinking water
   - Training of kitchen staff
   - General guidelines and/or standards for school meals including regular control and enforcement
2. Good practice for the provision of physical activity in schools on a regular basis:
   - Physical education classes at least three times or more than 3 h per week
   - Stimulation of sport projects between schools and local sport clubs or associations
   - Safe walking or biking to school
3. Good practice for fostering healthy dietary choices at schools:
   - Banning energy-dense snacks and sugar-sweetened drinks from the school
   - A "whole school food approach" with a focus on explaining the concept of labeling

Table 6.2 European Union (EU) platform on diet, physical activity and health: some examples for commitments. (Adapted from: Fussenegger et al. 2008) [17]

Advertising to children	The Union of European Beverages Associations has committed to a voluntary restriction on advertisements targeting children. Several major soft drink manufacturers, including Pepsi and Coca-Cola, agreed to the ban on advertisements in print media, on websites, and on television shows targeted at children below the age of 12 years. Moreover, Kraft has pledged not to market certain products directly to children unless they meet specific nutritional criteria
Nutritional information	Members of the European Modern Restaurant Association, including McDonalds, have committed to providing nutritional information on leaflets, wrappers, and tray mats on the amount of fat, sugar, salt, and calories contained in their meals as a percentage of the maximum daily allowance
Food composition	Members of the European Snacks Association have committed to developing healthier products, such as snacks reduced in calories, fat, salt, and sugar. For the purpose of improving portion control, different packing sizes will be offered. Unilever, for example, expressed their commitment to reformulate products
Promoting a healthy lifestyle	The multinational packaged food giant Nestlé has supported a study in two French towns and developed a following innovative prevention program with special attention on obese children
Education	The "Food Dude Healthy Eating Programme" by the Irish Food Board aims at improving children's long-term consumption of fruits and vegetables by providing free fruits and vegetables at school for 16 days along with videos and rewards based on the "Food Dude" characters. The program will be carried out from 2005 to 2008 in 150 primary schools across Ireland and will involve approximately 31,000 children
Physical activity	"Fit am Ball—Der Schul-Cup von funny-frisch" ("Fit on the ball—the funny-frisch School Cup") is a soccer-based project organized by the German Sports University Cologne and sponsored by the German snack manufacturer Intersnack. The program will be implemented in 1000 schools, reaching 35,000 children aged 8–12 years

   - Involvement of dietitians and nutritionists at school
   - Involvement of parents

4. Supporting health education efforts made by schools:

   - Financial support, e.g., by the food sector
   - Evaluation of school interventions and exchange of best practices, supported by public administrations
   - Involvement of all stakeholders
   - Assistance of the media in providing consistent and clear health messages, e.g., by using role models or cartoons. Restriction for advertising in the media [17]

Across Europe, a broad range of activities and initiatives are currently being implemented to control pediatric and adult obesity. But still for most of these measures, clear evidence is lacking so far that they affect indicators of health behavior and obesity prevalence. As appropriate monitoring and evaluation are widely considered as a basic principle to identify best practices and strategies, there is an urgent need to assess the impact of those actions and programs. Only then target-group-oriented and cost-effective interventions can be implemented. A wider knowledge of impact, respectively, successful interventions, might also support health ministries to convince their finance ministries to provide adequate funding for counteracting the public health crisis [17].

Identification of the Best Practices

More than half of the adult population is overweight or obese and a large proportion needs help with weight management. Prevention and management of overweight and obesity are complex problems to address, with no easy answers. To achieve substantial results, it is necessary to act on lifestyles and modify risk behaviors and to do this advice needs to be tailored for different groups, with well-planned interventions for target groups. This is particularly important for people from black and minority ethnic groups, vulnerable groups (such as those on low incomes), and people at life stages with increased risk for weight gain (such as during and after pregnancy, at the menopause, or when stopping smoking) [19].

It is unlikely that the problem of obesity can be addressed through primary care management alone, so public health and clinical audiences need evidence-based and cost-effective solutions to improve health. Although there is no simple solution, the most effective strategies for prevention and management share similar approaches. The clinical management of obesity cannot be viewed in isolation from the environment in which people live, so barriers to lifestyle change should be explored [19]. Possible barriers include: lack of knowledge about buying and cooking food, and how diet and exercise affect health; the cost and availability of healthy foods and opportunities for exercise; safety concerns, for example about cycling; lack of time; personal tastes; the views of family and community members; low levels of fitness, or disabilities; low self-esteem and lack of assertiveness [19].

In conclusion, prevention and management of obesity should be a priority for all, because of the considerable health benefits of maintaining a healthy weight and the health risks associated with overweight and obesity. Managers and health professionals in all primary care settings should ensure that preventing and managing obesity is a priority, at both strategic and delivery levels and dedicated resources should be allocated for action. It is also necessary that the public health recommendations must be divided according to their key audiences and the settings they apply to: the public, the National Health Service (NHS), local authorities and partners in the community, early years settings, schools, workplaces, self-help, and commercial and community programs [19].

Key Elements for Decision Makers

- Worldwide obesity has nearly doubled since 1980.
- In 2008, more than 1.4 billion adults, 20 and older, were overweight. Of these, more than 200 million men and nearly 300 million women were obese.
- Thirty-five percent of adults, aged 20 and over, were overweight in 2008 and 11 % were obese.
- Sixty-five percent of the world's population lives in countries where overweight and obesity kills more people than underweight.
- More than 40 million children under the age of 5 were overweight in 2011.
- Obesity is preventable.
- The prevention and management of obesity should be a priority for all, because of the considerable health benefits of maintaining a healthy weight and the health risks associated with overweight and obesity.
- Several programs have been launched worldwide, nevertheless preventing and managing overweight and obesity are complex problems, with no easy answers.
- Managers and health professionals in all primary care settings should ensure that preventing and managing obesity is a priority, at both strategic and delivery levels. Dedicated resources should be allocated for action.

Diabetes

Definition

The term "diabetes mellitus" describes a metabolic disorder of multiple etiology characterized by chronic hyperglycemia with disturbances of carbohydrate, fat, and protein metabolism resulting from defects in insulin secretion, insulin action, or both. The effects of diabetes mellitus include long-term damage, dysfunction, and failure of various organs [20].

There are two main types of diabetes:

- *Type 1 diabetes (T1D)*: Usually develops in childhood and adolescence and patients require lifelong insulin injections for survival.
- *Type 2 diabetes T2D:* Usually develops in adulthood and is related to obesity, lack of physical activity, and unhealthy diets [20].

Other categories of diabetes include gestational diabetes (a state of hyperglycemia which develops during pregnancy) and other rarer causes (genetic syndromes, acquired processes such as pancreatitis, diseases such as cystic fibrosis, exposure to certain drugs, viruses, and unknown causes) [20].

Type 1 Diabetes

T1D is formerly known as insulin-dependent diabetes mellitus (IDDM) [20]. It is caused by an autoimmune reaction, where the body's defense system attacks the insulin-producing beta cells in the pancreas. As a result, the body can no longer produce the insulin it needs. Why this occurs is not fully understood. The disease can affect people of any age, but usually occurs in children or young adults. People with this form of diabetes require lifelong insulin injections for survival [21, 22]. Patients with this type of diabetes are usually not obese, but obesity is not incompatible with the diagnosis and, such as patients with T2D, they are at increased risk of developing microvascular and macrovascular complications [21].

Type 2 Diabetes

T2D is the most common type of diabetes, representing 90 % of cases worldwide and it is named non-insulin-dependent diabetes mellitus (NIDDM). There are several important risk factors for T2D, such as obesity, poor diet, physical inactivity, advancing age, family history of diabetes ethnicity, and high blood glucose during pregnancy [20, 22]. Especially obesity is generally considered to be a strong risk for the later development of T2D. Obesity and T2D frequently occur together: statistics show that 60–90 % of all patients with T2D are or have been obese and the relative risk for a given obese patient to develop T2D is tenfold for women and 11.2-fold for men. T2D is characterized by hyperglycemia due to a defect in insulin secretion usually with a contribution from insulin resistance and patients usually do not require lifelong insulin but can control blood glucose with diet and exercise alone, or in combination with oral medications, or with the addition of insulin. This type of diabetes, unlike T1D, usually develops in adulthood [9, 21]. In contrast to people with T1D, the majority of those with T2D usually does not require daily doses of insulin to survive but many people are able to manage their condition through a healthy diet and increased physical activity or oral medication. However, if they are unable to regulate their blood glucose levels, they need insulin [22].

Current Burden of the Disease

Epidemiology

Diabetes mellitus is undoubtedly one of the most challenging health problems in the twenty-firstcentury. It is one of the most common noncommunicable diseases globally and the fourth or fifth leading cause of death in most high-income countries and there is substantial evidence that it is epidemic in many economically developing and newly industrialized countries [22]. The number of people who develop both the T1D and the T2D is increasing. The reasons for the rise of T1D are still unclear but may be due to changes in environmental risk factors, early events in the womb, diet early in life,

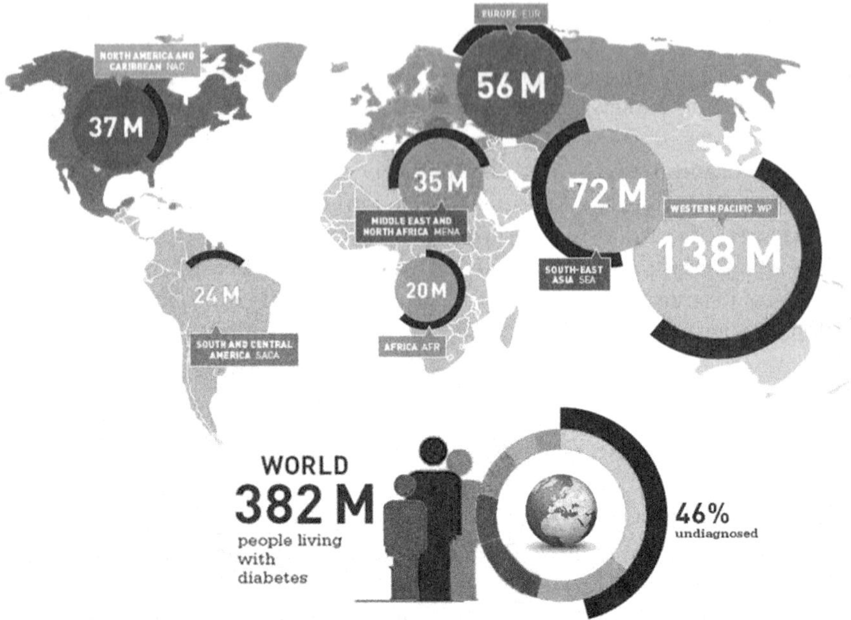

Fig. 6.2 Worldwide epidemiology of diabetes. (Adapted from IDF Diabetes Atlas. 6th edn. 2013) [22]

Table 6.3 Prevalence of diabetes mellitus (DM) in 2013 and projections for 2035. (Adapted from International Diabetes Federation (IDF) Diabetes Atlas. 6th edn. 2013) [22]

	2013	2035
Total world population (billions)	7.2	8.7
Adult population (20–79 years, billions)	4.6	5.9
Diabetes (20–79 years)		
Global prevalence (%)	8.3	10.1
Comparative prevalence (%)	8.3	8.8
Number of people with diabetes (millions)	382	592

or viral infections. This rise of T2D, on the other hand, is associated with economic development, aging populations, increasing urbanization, dietary changes, reduced physical activity, and changes in other lifestyle patterns [22], which are all risk factors also for obesity. This explains why the vertiginous rise in obesity triggers a parallel upward swing in T2D statistics [9]. Nowadays, 382 million people have diabetes, with the greatest number of patients aged between 40 and 59 and 80% living in low- and middle-income countries (Fig. 6.2). By 2035, this number will rise to 592 million and, in particular, the number of people with T2D will increase by 55%. Prevalence of the disease was 8.3% in 2013 and projections estimate that it will be 10.1% in 2035 (Table 6.3) [22]. Moreover, people with T2D can remain undiagnosed for many years, unaware of the long-term damage being caused by the disease: it is estimated that currently 175 million people with diabetes, 46% of cases, are undiagnosed [22].

Burden of Disease

Diabetes and its complications are major causes of early death in most countries [23]. Complications are divided into microvascular (due to damage to small blood vessels) and macrovascular (due to damage to larger blood vessels). Microvascular ones are diabetic retinopathy, diabetic nephropathy, and diabetic neuropathy; macrovascular ones are cardiovascular diseases (such as heart attacks, strokes and insufficiency in blood flow to legs) [24]. Cardiovascular disease is one of the leading causes of death for people with diabetes and can account for 50%-80% of deaths due to diabetes in some populations [23, 25].

Estimating the number of deaths due to diabetes is challenging because more than a third of countries do not have any data on diabetes-related mortality and also because existing routine health statistics underestimate the number of deaths due to this disease [23]. However, it is clear that the burden of disease, in human as well as financial terms, is enormous [22]. Approximately 5.1 million people aged between 20 and 79 years died from diabetes in 2013, accounting for 8.4% of global all-cause mortality among people in this age group. This number of deaths in 2013 showed an 11% increase over estimates for 2011. This increase was largely due to rises in the number of deaths due to the disease in the Africa, Western Pacific, and Middle East and North Africa Regions [22]. Diabetes imposes also a large economic burden on individuals and families, national health systems, and countries. Health spending on diabetes accounted for 10.8% of the total health expenditure worldwide in 2013. Global health spending to treat diabetes and manage complications totaled at least US$ 548 billion in 2013, an estimated average of US$ 1437 per person, and by 2035, this number is projected to exceed US$ 627 billion [22].

Health Policy Programs Available

In consideration of the unsustainable burden of the disease so far discussed, diabetes is getting its place on the global health agenda and political leaders are seeking solutions to tackle the problem. Some of the strategies implemented worldwide are shown below.

United Nations

Global Diabetes Plan 2011–2021. International Diabetes Federation

International Diabetes Federation (IDF) brought together world diabetes experts and consulted widely to provide solutions to face the disease. The result of those deliberations, the first ever Global Diabetes Plan, presents the evidence and proposes cost-effective solutions in a coherent framework for action [26].

The aims of the Global Diabetes Plan are to:

1. Reframe the debate on diabetes to further raise political awareness of its causes and consequences and the urgent need for action at the global and country level to prevent and treat diabetes
2. Set out a generic, globally consistent plan to support and guide the efforts of governments, international donors and IDF member associations to combat diabetes
3. Propose proven interventions, processes, and partnership for reducing the personal and societal burden of diabetes
4. Support and build on existing policies and initiatives such as the WHO 2008–2013 Action Plan for the global strategy for the prevention and control of non-communicable diseases
5. Strengthen the global movement to combat the diabetes epidemic and to improve the health and lives of people with diabetes [27]

The plan aims at improving the health outcomes of people with diabetes, preventing the development of T2D, and stopping discrimination against people with the disease [26].

To ensure objectives set out above are achieved, the plan also proposes that:

- The UN and its agencies work intensively with national governments to reorient health systems from the traditional focus on acute care to a more proactive and preventative continuing care model, including training and equipping health professionals to manage diabetes more effectively
- Countries develop a prioritized national research agenda that fills knowledge gaps which currently hamper the prevention and control of diabetes, improves diabetes medicines and technologies for easier delivery especially in remote, resource-poor communities, and supports the search for a cure
- Governments ensure that robust monitoring and data collection is performed and communicated and underpins continuing improvements to care delivery
- Procurement and supply systems are reviewed and streamlined to ensure the effective distribution of essential diabetes medicines and technologies
- Innovative, sustained, and predictable financing is secured to implement the plan and accelerate progress towards international development goals
- Governments, the private sector, and civil society work together to foster innovation such as improving building design for greater physical activity, spark new thinking, and build new financing streams [26]

Europe

Also the EU has been supporting diabetes research for several years through its research programs, such as IMAGE project, SWEET project, DIAMAP project, and Horizon 2020, which is the EU Framework Program for Research and Innovation for 2014–2020.

The IMAGE Project

The IMAGE project (2007–2010), which stands for the "Development and Implementation of a European Guideline and Training Standards for Diabetes Prevention," was an EU-funded project that was established to improve the ability of EU countries to prevent T2D [28].

The objectives of IMAGE were to develop:

- European practice-oriented guidelines for the primary prevention of T2D to improve information and knowledge about public health strategies to prevent T2D and its comorbidities
- An European curriculum for the training of prevention managers to enhance the ability of health-care professionals to respond swiftly to the drastic increase of T2D and its burden to society
- European standard for quality control in order to monitor and report these systematically in the member states and at EU level using comparative data
- An European e-health training portal for prevention managers to improve availability of evidence-based health information for health-care professionals Diabetes Prevention Forum [28]

Final results of the project were an European evidence-based guideline for the prevention of T2D, a toolkit for the prevention of T2D in Europe, and quality and outcome indicators for the prevention of T2D in Europe [28].

The SWEET Project

The SWEET project (2008–2011), which stands for "Better control in paediatric and adolescent diabetes in the EU: working to create centres of reference," was an EU-funded project with the main objective being to improve secondary prevention, diagnosis, and control of T1D and T2D in children and adolescents by supporting the development of centers of reference (CORs) for pediatric and adolescent diabetes services across the EU [29].

The project had five specific objectives:

1. Strengthen the knowledge base regarding the status of pediatric and adolescent diabetes and related care in the EU
2. Enhance and promote equal standards of treatment and care in pediatric and adolescent diabetes and related care in the EU
3. Improve control of diabetes and prevent complications by means of age-appropriate patient education programs
4. Support health-care professionals in providing high-quality specialized care to children and adolescents with diabetes
5. Stimulate the development of centers of reference for pediatric and adolescent diabetes services in Europe [29]

The SWEET project produced a Paediatric Diabetes Toolbox including recommendations for minimum treatment and care, for patient education programs, and for training programs for health professionals. It also supplied definition and criteria for centers of references for pediatric and adolescent diabetes [29].

DIAMAP Project

In April 2008, EURADIA (Alliance for European Diabetes Research) was awarded a Seventh Framework Programme (FP7) grant from the European Commission for an innovative 2-year project to guide a Road Map for Diabetes Research in Europe, called DIAMAP. This project was the first ever publicly funded research road mapping exercise in Europe focused on a single disease and it has served as the model for subsequent FP7 research road map projects [30, 31]. The mission of DIAMAP (2008–2010) was to undertake a wide survey of the current European diabetes research landscape from which expert opinion could identify gaps and highlight strengths, to guide a road map strategy for diabetes research in Europe [30].

The objectives of the project were to:

- Perform a survey of research activities and funding for diabetes research, both public and private, at the regional, national, and European level
- Create a diabetes research database from survey of European and limited worldwide data
- Identify gaps, strengths, weaknesses, and opportunities in diabetes research in Europe by expert analysis
- Develop final road map report by an overarching Expert Advisory Board to outline strategy for diabetes research in Europe, taking into account different scenarios, including the Innovative Medicines Initiative [32]

The most significant recommendation of DIAMAP was the creation of the European Platform for Clinical Research in Diabetes (EPCRD) that would coordinate European efforts in this clinical research space, offering common resources, training, and standardized protocols [33].

Horizon 2020

Horizon 2020 is a new EU Framework Program for Research and Innovation for 2014–2020, for €80 billion [34, 35]. The Program aims to ensure a steady stream of world-class research to secure Europe's long-term competitiveness and is structured around three pillars:

- Excellent science
- Industrial leadership
- Societal challenges [34]

Health is addressed under Horizon 2020's third pillar on societal challenges which allocates €9077 billion to tackle "Health, demographic change and wellbeing" [36]. In the first pillar "Excellent Science—Research Infrastructure," and the third pillar "Societal Challenges—Health, Demographic Change and Wellbeing," the program will tackle noncommunicable diseases such as diabetes [37].

In the current economic context and given the rising cost of health and social care, the Commission highlights the need for an appropriate European level response to research and innovation in the area of chronic diseases. Diabetes is mentioned as one of the chronic conditions, which are major causes of disability, ill health, and premature death, and presents considerable social and economic costs [36].

Identification of the Best Practices

There is now extensive evidence on the optimal management of diabetes, offering the opportunity of improving the immediate and long-term quality of life of people with the disease [38]. Unfortunately, such optimal management does not reach many, perhaps the majority, of the people who could benefit. This could be explained by different reasons such as size and complexity of the evidence-based interventions and the complexity of diabetes care itself. A lack of proven cost-effective resources for diabetes care and diversity of standards of clinical practice are the results of this situation [38]. A help could derive from guidelines, which are one part of a process which seeks to address those problems. Many guidelines have appeared internationally, nationally, and more locally in recent years; however, many countries around the world do not have the resources, either in expertise or financially, that are needed to develop diabetes guidelines, because published national guidelines come from relatively resource-rich countries, and may be of limited practical use in poorer countries [38].

As a key part of the effort to stop diabetes, the American Diabetes Association each year identifies legislative priorities and policy goals which could be considered as best practices for the management of the disease at the central level [39]. These priorities include:

- Federal funding for diabetes research and programs
- Health insurance
- Prevention (primary prevention of T2D focused on individuals with prediabetes as well as in the general public, including efforts to reduce obesity and improve nutrition and physical activity)
- Health disparities
- (support proposals specifically focused on reducing the disparate impact of diabetes on minority communities)
- Research and surveillance
- Discrimination issues (oppose proposals resulting in discrimination against people with diabetes)
- Bills related to complications and comorbidities of diabetes

- National Diabetes Clinical Care Commission Act (creation of a commission to better coordinate and evaluate clinical care for diabetes and developing of recommendations on diabetes care)
- Reducing sugar-sweetened beverage consumption [39]

Key Element for Decision Makers

- Prevalence of diabetes was 8.3 % in 2013 and projections estimate that it will be 10.1 % in 2035.
- In 2013, 382 million people had diabetes; in 2035, they could be 592 million.
- The number of people with diabetes is increasing in every country.
- Almost half of the people with diabetes are undiagnosed.
- 5.1 million people died due to diabetes in 2013.
- During 2013, about US$ 548 billion were spent on health care for diabetes.
- Management of the disease is not optimal and does not reach many, perhaps the majority, of the people who could benefit.
- There is now extensive evidence on the optimal management of diabetes, offering the opportunity of improving the immediate and long-term quality of life of patients and avoiding complications which are major causes of early death in most countries.
- Several programs have been launched worldwide and they could help managers and clinicians for the prevention and management of the disease.

References

1. CDC (2013) Overweight and obesity. http://www.cdc.gov/obesity/adult/defining.html. Accessed 23 Jul 2013
2. WHO (2013) Health Topics: Obesity. http://www.who.int/topics/obesity/en/. Accessed 17 July 2013
3. Akil L, Ahmad HA (2011) Effects of socioeconomic factors on obesity rates in four southern states and Colorado. Ethn Dis Winter 21(1):58–62
4. El-Sayed AM, Scarborough P, Galea S (2012) Socioeconomic inequalities in childhood obesity in the United Kingdom: a systematic review of the literature. Obes Facts 5(5):671–692. Epub 2012 Oct 6
5. Ogden CL, Lamb MM, Carroll MD, Flegal, KM (2010) Obesity and socioeconomic status in children: United States 1988–1994 and 2005–2008. NCHS data brief no 51. National Center for Health Statistics, Hyattsville
6. WHO (2013) Global strategy on diet, physical activity and health. http://www.who.int/dietphysicalactivity/childhood_what/en/index.html. Accessed 23 July 2013
7. WHO (2013) Global health observatory. obesity – situation and trends. http://www.who.int/gho/ncd/risk_factors/obesity_text/en/. Accessed 23 July 2013
8. CDC (2013) Basics about childhood obesity. http://www.cdc.gov/obesity/childhood/basics.html. Accessed 23 Jul 2013

9. Golay A, Ybarra J (2005) Link between obesity and type 2 diabetes. Best Pract Res Clin Endocrinol Metab 19(4):649–663.
10. WHO (2013) Obesity and overweight. Fact sheet N°311. Updated March 2013. http://www.who.int/mediacentre/factsheets/fs311/en/index.html. Accessed 24 July 2013
11. Pelone F, Specchia ML, Veneziano MA, et al (2012) Economic impact of childhood obesity on health systems: a systematic review. Obes Rev 13(5):431–440.
12. CDC (2013) Overweight and obesity. State programs funded by CDC. http://www.cdc.gov/obesity/stateprograms/fundedstates.html. Accessed 25 July 2013
13. CDC (2013) Overweight and obesity. Program goal and objectives. http://www.cdc.gov/obesity/stateprograms/programGoal.html. Accessed 25 July 2013
14. CDC (2013) DNPAO state program highlights. Active transport to school. http://www.cdc.gov/obesity/downloads/ActiveTransporttoSchool.pdf. Accessed 25 July 2013
15. CDC (2013) Overweight and obesity. communities putting prevention to work: states and territories initiative. http://www.cdc.gov/obesity/stateprograms/programGoal.html. Accessed 25 July 2013
16. CDC (2013) Communities putting prevention to work. http://www.cdc.gov/CommunitiesPuttingPreventiontoWork/index.htm. Accessed 25 July 2013
17. Fussenegger D, Pietrobelli A, Widhalm K (2008) Childhood obesity: political developments in Europe and related perspectives for future action on prevention. Obes Rev 9(1):76–82
18. John Griffiths J, Vladu C, George E (2012) DG SANCO—Monitoring the EU Platform for Action on Diet, Physical Activity and Health Activities—Special Report (reference period 2006–2012). http://ec.europa.eu/health/nutrition_physical_activity/docs/eu_platform_special_report_2006_2012_en.pdf. Accessed 5 May 2014
19. NICE (2006) Clinical guideline 43. Obesity guidance on the prevention, identification, assessment and management of overweight and obesity in adults and children. http://www.nice.org.uk/nicemedia/pdf/CG43NICEGuideline.pdf. Accessed 5 May 2014
20. WHO (2013) About diabetes. http://www.who.int/diabetes/action_online/basics/en/index.html. Accessed 29 July 2013
21. WHO (2013) About diabetes. Types of diabetes. http://www.who.int/diabetes/action_online/basics/en/index1.html. Accessed 29 July 2013
22. IDF (2014) Diabetes atlas. 6th edn. http://www.idf.org/sites/default/files/EN_6E_Atlas_Full_0.pdf. Accessed 7 May 2014
23. IDF (2013) Diabetes atlas. 5th edn. Mortality. http://www.idf.org/diabetesatlas/5e/mortality. Accessed 31 July 2013
24. WHO (2013) Diabetes programme. http://www.who.int/diabetes/action_online/basics/en/index3.html. Accessed 1 Aug 2013
25. WHO (2013) 10 Facts about diabetes. http://who.int/features/factfiles/diabetes/facts/en/index1.html. Accessed 31 July 2013
26. IDF (2013) Diabetes atlas, 5th edn. Global solutions to a global problem. http://www.idf.org/diabetesatlas/5e/global-solutions-to-a-global-problem. Accessed 31 July 2013
27. IDF (2013) Global Diabetes Plan 2011–2021. International Diabetes Federation. http://www.idf.org/sites/default/files/Global_Diabetes_Plan_Final.pdf. Accessed 31 July 2013
28. IDF Europe (2013) IMAGE project. http://diabetespreventionforum.org/index.php/projects/6-image-project. Accessed 31 July 2013
29. IDF Europe (2013) SWEET project. http://diabetespreventionforum.org/index.php/projects/7-sweet-project. Accessed 31 July 2013
30. IDF Europe (2013) DIAMAP project. http://diabetespreventionforum.org/index.php/projects/8-diamap-project. Accessed 31 July 2013
31. DIAMAP Road Map for Diabetes Research in Europe (2010) Road Map Report. http://www.diamap.eu/uploads/pdf/DIAMAP-Road-Map-Report-Sept2010.pdf. Accessed 31 July 2013
32. DIAMAP Objectives (2013) http://www.diamap.eu/about-us/diamap-objectives. Accessed 31 July 2013
33. EURADIA (2013) Newsletter May 2013. http://www.euradia.org/uploads/EURADIA_newsletter_May2013_final.pdf. Accessed 31July 2013

34. EU (2013) Research and Innovation. Horizon 2020. http://ec.europa.eu/research/horizon2020/index_en.cfm. Accessed 31 July 2013
35. EU (2013) Horizon 2020. http://ec.europa.eu/research/horizon2020/pdf/press/horizon2020-presentation.pdf. Accessed 31 July 2013
36. EURADIA (2013) Research advocacy. High-level advocacy for diabetes research in Horizon 2020. http://www.euradia.org/research-advocacy/advocacy. Accessed 1 Aug 2013
37. EURADIA Position on Horizon 2020 (2013) http://www.euradia.org/uploads/EURADIA%20Position%20Paper%20Horizon%202020.pdf. Accessed 31 July 2013
38. IDF (2013) Global Guideline For Type 2 Diabetes http://www.idf.org/global-guideline-type-2-diabetes-2012. Accessed 31 July 2013
39. American Diabetes Association (2013) Legislative Priorities. http://www.diabetes.org/assets/pdfs/advocacy/2013-legislative-priorities.pdf. Accessed 31 July 2013

Chapter 7
Respiratory Diseases and Health Disorders Related to Indoor and Outdoor Air Pollution

Francesco Di Nardo and Patrizia Laurenti

Introduction

Among all the diseases of the lungs and airways, chronic respiratory diseases are the major concern to public health. Chronic respiratory diseases are a group of chronic conditions that can affect all age groups, last many years, and greatly limit the physical abilities of people suffering from them. Together, asthma and chronic obstructive pulmonary disease (COPD), the two most important respiratory diseases, are likely to affect more than 500 million people all over the world. For the control of these diseases, which have extremely high direct and indirect costs, the most cost-effective interventions are often represented by the removal of the risk factors and by people health education. Tobacco smoke is the most important risk factor, accounting for about 42 % of all cases. Indoor and outdoor air pollutants also account for an important part of the burden of respiratory diseases and are discussed extensively, together with their effects on health, given their important role in the pathogenesis of these diseases (especially in Africa and Asia), and the growing concern worldwide for the environmental pollution. The most common air pollutants are typical of the crowded urban areas and the poorly ventilated indoor environments and are different from the airborne toxic substances that are historically linked to the work-related COPD (although occupational exposure still causes about 12 % of all the cases of the disease). Also, allergic conditions, which are a risk factor for asthma, and respiratory allergens, which are among the most dangerous asthma triggers, are discussed in this chapter. Here, we lastly discuss an emerging disease, the obstructive sleep apnea syndrome (OSAS), which is estimated to affect more than 100 million people worldwide. Lung cancer and tuberculosis are other

F. Di Nardo (✉) · P. Laurenti
Institute of Public Health, Section of Hygiene, Università Cattolica del Sacro Cuore,
L.go F. Vito 1, 00168 Rome, Italy
e-mail: francesco_pope84@hotmail.com

P. Laurenti
e-mail: plaurenti@rm.unicatt.it

S. Boccia et al. (eds.), *A Systematic Review of Key Issues in Public Health*,
DOI 10.1007/978-3-319-13620-2_7

lung disorders characterized by a significant burden of disease, but they are discussed in other chapters of this book.

Box 1 Characteristics of Included Studies

A search for reviews on respiratory diseases epidemiology, respiratory diseases burden, and respiratory diseases cost-effective treatments was performed by means of a snowball search on the main scientific databases (Cochrane Database, Pubmed-Medline, SCOPUS, Scholar). The publication date of the retrieved reviews ranges from 1997 to 2013. The most recent data on respiratory diseases were extracted from institutional databases (World Health Organization, WHO). The publication date of the data on respiratory diseases ranges from 2004 to 2013 and was retrieved in the form of excel spreadsheets and analyzed with SPSS 13.0 software for Windows.

Asthma and Respiratory Allergies

Asthma is a chronic inflammatory disorder of the airways characterized by recurrent attacks of breathlessness, wheezing, chest tightness, and cough. Its symptoms vary in severity and frequency from person to person and may occur several times in a day or week in affected individuals. Physical activity, allergens, smoke, air pollutants, and cold air may trigger an asthma attack. Symptoms may get worse at night or in the early morning. During an asthma attack, the hyperresponsiveness of the airways leads to airflow obstruction which is usually reversible (either spontaneously or with treatment). However, despite a low fatality rate, asthma affects more than 200 million people and recurrent asthma symptoms may cause sleeplessness, daytime fatigue, reduced activity levels and school, and work absenteeism [1, 2].

Respiratory allergies are often associated with asthma. They are now estimated to affect about 400 million people all over the world, and although their symptoms are usually mild, their manifestations can be fatal [3].

Epidemiology

WHO estimates that 235 million people currently suffer from asthma, and these estimates may be too conservative. Asthma is the most common chronic disease among children. According to the Centers for Disease Control and Prevention (CDC), its prevalence is higher in the 0–17-year age group (9.5 %) compared to the group of subjects aged 18 or more (7.7 %) and among females (9.2 vs. 7.0 %). Asthma prevalence decreases with income, being 11.2 % in people with incomes less than 100 % of the poverty level, 8.7 % for persons with incomes from 100 % to less than 200 % of the poverty level, and 7.3 % for persons with incomes at least 200 % of the poverty level [4]. Asthma is estimated to affect above 10 % of the populations of North American countries and Australia, while Russia, China, and the Pacific countries report the lowest prevalence (<2.5 %). In Europe, the prevalence of asthma is lower in Poland, Portugal, Switzerland, and the Mediterranean countries (below 5 %); higher in Spain, France, and the Northern countries (5–10 %); and the highest in the UK (above 10 %). Middle Eastern countries usually show asthma prevalence values of 5–7.5 %, while asthma affects 7.5–10 % of the population of the Indian subcontinent. The prevalence of asthma is very high also in South America, where it ranges from 5 to 7.5 % in Argentina and Chile up to above 10 % in Brazil and Peru. Data on African countries is limited and inconsistent. Differences in terms of prevalence among countries are wide and probably they are partly due to different methods of diagnosis [5].

Risk Factors

A number of factors increase the risk of developing asthma. They are:

- Genes predisposing to atopy or to airway hyperresponsiveness
- Overweight
- Firsthand and secondhand tobacco smoke and smoking during pregnancy
- Exposure to air pollutants
- Low birth weight

Asthma attacks are, hence, triggered if a combination of genetic predisposition and environmental factors occur. These factors include:

- Indoor and outdoor allergens
- Tobacco smoke
- Chemical irritants in the workplace
- Air pollution

Other triggers include cold air, physical exercise, nonsteroidal anti-inflammatory drugs (NSAIDs), and beta-blocker drugs [1, 2, 6].

Indoor and outdoor respiratory allergens, also known as aeroallergens, include pollens, house dust mites, molds, and pet fur (or proteins from other biological materials). In allergic subjects, they can cause anaphylaxis, allergic rhinitis, eczema, or urticaria, while in patients suffering from asthma they may trigger attacks.

Burden

Asthma is a public health problem not only for high-income countries, but it occurs in all countries regardless of the level of development. Most asthma-related deaths occur in low- and lower-middle-income countries. Today, asthma is likely to be greatly underdiagnosed and undertreated. It creates substantial burden to individuals and families and often restricts individuals' activities for lifetime. Asthma accounts

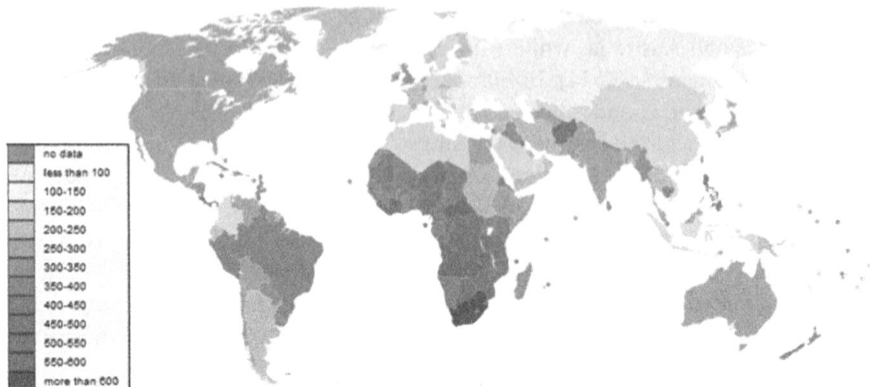

Fig. 7.1 Age-standardized DALY rates from chronic obstructive pulmonary disease by country (per 100,000 inhabitants). *DALY* disability-adjusted life years. (Reproduced from: Death and DALY estimates for 2004 by cause for WHO Member States [6])

for up to 250,000 deaths each year. Most of these deaths are preventable and are due to limited access to both long-term medical care and drugs for the management of the asthma attacks. Mortality is higher in low-income countries, where it exceeds ten cases per 100,000 people suffering from asthma (5–34-year age group, Fig. 7.1) [3, 6–7]. In 2010, asthma was responsible for 13.8 million years lived with disability (YLD) and 22.5 million disability-adjusted life years (DALYs; 201 YLDs and 326 DALYs per 100,000 inhabitants) [8, 9].

The economic burden of asthma is increasing worldwide. A systematic review from Bahadori et al. [10] evaluated and synthesized the current literature regarding the economic burden of asthma. Direct costs of asthma include inpatient care, emergency visits, physician visits, nursing services, ambulance use, drugs and devices, blood and diagnostic tests, research, and education. Indirect costs or morbidity costs include school days lost, traveling, waiting time, and lost productivity for the caretaker of asthmatic children. It is unclear whether the direct costs are higher or lower than the indirect costs, but the total mean annual costs of asthma per person range from US$ 151 to 4158 per person among the different studies [10].

Best Practices

Asthma cannot be cured, but its management allows people to control the disease and have a good quality of life. Adherence to the Global Initiative for Asthma (GINA) guidelines would allow effective management and a reduction of the number of hospitalizations [2, 11]. Diagnosis is based on the clinical signs and symptoms and supported by the data emerged from the spirometry, that is the forced expiratory volume in 1 s (FEV1) and the peak expiratory flow (PEF). Asthma care is based on four components: development of patient/doctor partnership; identification and reduction of exposure to risk factors; assessment, treatment, and monitoring of asthma; management of its exacerbations. Short-term medications relieve symptoms during asthma attacks. These are represented by rapid-acting β_2-agonists. People with persistent symptoms must take long-term medication daily to control the underlying inflammation and prevent the exacerbations. Inhaled corticosteroids are essential for achieving the control of the disease, together with the long-acting β_2-agonists for more severe cases. However, patients are likely to under-use inhaled corticosteroids because, unlike rapid-acting β_2-agonists, they do not provide quick relief from symptoms. Therefore, patients' education is a very important factor in asthma control [2].

In conclusion, asthma is currently underdiagnosed, its treatment is poorly available in many countries (inhaled corticosteroids have high costs), many physicians do not apply guidelines, and patients may be incompliant. However, the application of the recommendations from international guidelines was proven to be cost-effective in many studies (although a high proportion of these were funded by pharmaceutical companies), and their actual use could reduce the burden of the disease [10]. That is why physicians should be provided with the international guidelines and taught to develop a partnership with their patients, the aim of which is the guided self-management of the disease. Patients should learn to avoid the exposure to risk factors, understand the difference between "controller" and "reliever" drugs, take medications correctly and as needed, recognize signs of asthma, and seek medical advice as appropriate [2].

Concerning respiratory allergies, their most effective management is to avoid exposure to allergens known to exacerbate the symptoms. However, this is not always possible, and some patients are forced to deal with the clinical manifestations of the disease. Nowadays, it is possible to treat symptoms with pharmacotherapy (which, among others, includes adrenaline, corticosteroids, and antihistamines), but also with immunotherapy, based on the administration of sublingual or subcutaneous increasing doses of allergen extracts, proved to be effective. The cost-effectiveness of immunotherapy has not yet been definitively proven, even though some studies seem to support it. Little is known on the difference in terms of cost-effectiveness between sublingual and subcutaneous immunotherapy [12].

Key Elements

Asthma is a chronic disease characterized by recurrent attacks of breathlessness and wheezing affecting 235 million people all over the world, mostly children.

Allergic conditions and exposure to tobacco smoke are among the main risk factors and can trigger asthma attacks.

Despite the fact that asthma today is underdiagnosed, it is clear that its burden is increasing worldwide, with most asthma-related deaths occurring in low-income countries. Asthma often restricts individuals' activities for a lifetime.

Education of clinicians and affected people is essential in order to ensure accurate diagnosis, treatment, and follow-up of the disease.

Chronic Obstructive Pulmonary Disease

It is not easy to define the COPD and clearly distinguish it from other conditions such as emphysema, chronic bronchitis, and even asthma. These difficulties come from the fact that the definitions of COPD, emphysema, and chronic bronchitis are not mutually exclusive and are differentially based on clinical, anatomic, or functional conditions [13]. A satisfactory functional definition of COPD is: Disease characterized by airflow limitation that is not fully reversible. The airflow limitation is usually both progressive and associated with an abnormal inflammatory response in the lungs to noxious agents including cigarette smoke, biomass fuels, and occupational agents. The chronic airflow limitation characteristic of COPD is caused by a mixture of small airway disease (obstructive bronchiolitis) and parenchymal destruction (emphysema), the relative contribution of which may vary from person to person. Structural abnormalities, narrowing of the small airways, and loss of lung elastic recoil lead to airflow limitations which are best measured by spirometry [13, 14]. Based on spirometric criteria, COPD is defined by using the post-bronchodilator FEV1 and its ratio to the forced vital capacity (FVC). According to the Global initiative for chronic Obstructive Lung Disease (GOLD) criteria, the main criterion for COPD is a FEV1/FVC ratio <70% (Table 7.1) [14].

Epidemiology

According to WHO estimates, 64 million people suffered from COPD in 2005 [15]. The real prevalence of COPD is probably greatly underestimated because the disease is usually not diagnosed until it is clinically apparent and moderately advanced. Moreover, it varies between studies, increasing the inaccuracy of the estimates, mainly because of different definitions used to assess the disease. In fact, diagnosis in different studies may be spirometry based, symptoms based, or self-reported by patients [16]. Global prevalence of the disease is estimated at 7.6%, but is higher in studies in which diagnoses were based on spirometry (9.2%) and even higher using the GOLD criteria (9.8%) [17]. The prevalence is usually higher in males (9.8%) than females (5.6%), and increases with age, being 3.1% in the population below 40 years of age, 8.2% in the population aged 40–64, and 14.2% in the population above 64 years. Although it is not easy to determine the age of onset of COPD because of its long natural history, this condition is rarely seen

Table 7.1 Global initiative on Obstructive Lung Disease (GOLD) classification of severity of airflow limitations in COPD (patients with FEV1/FVC <70%), based on post-bronchodilator FEV1 [13]

Stage	Characteristics
Mild	FEV1 ≥ 80% predicted
Moderate	50% ≤ FEV1 < 80% predicted
Severe	30% ≤ FEV1 50% predicted
Very severe	FEV1 < 30% predicted

Table 7.2 Prevalence (millions) of symptomatic COPD by WHO Region, 2004 [17]

Africa	10.5
The Americas	13.2
Eastern Mediterranean	30.3
Europe	11.3
Southeast Asia	13.9
Western Pacific	20.2
World	63.6

before the age of 20 [3, 17]. Analyzing the various WHO regions, although the epidemiology of COPD has been poorly studied in many low- and middle-income countries, the prevalence was estimated at 4.6 % in the Americas, 7.4 % in Europe, 11.4 % in Southeast Asia, and 9.0 % in the Western Pacific [17]. The prevalence of symptomatic cases was estimated by WHO and amounts to 63.6 million people all over the world (Table 7.2) [18].

Risk Factors

Cigarette smoke is the main risk factor for COPD. The prevalence of COPD is 15.4 % in smokers and 10.7 % in ex-smokers, while it is only 4.3 % in never smokers. The risk attributable to active smoking in COPD is thought to vary from 40 to 70 % [16, 17]. Active smoking by females during pregnancy alters fetal lung development and is responsible for asthma in predisposed children. The mechanisms of action of smoke are probably multiple and involve the reaction of the immune system to the components of smoke and the subsequent inflammation and progressive destruction and remodeling of the lung tissue [16]. Not all smokers develop COPD in their lifetime, which implies that genetic factors may be involved. At present, only a severe deficit in α1-antitrypsin, caused by having inherited a simple nucleotide polymorphism on both the maternal and paternal SERPINA1 genes (PiZZ phenotype), is considered a proven genetic causal factor [16]. Occupational exposure is a recognized risk factor for COPD, with an attributable risk ranging from 19 % in all workers to 31 % in nonsmokers. Exposure is generally observed in rural environment (vegetable dust; bacterial or fungal toxins), in the textile industry (cotton dust), and in the industrial environment (mining, smelter plants, iron and steel industry, wood industry, building trade) [16]. Domestic pollution particularly affects females and represents an important risk for COPD in developing countries (risk accounting for 35 % of cases). It is usually due to exposure to smoke when cooking or to the method of heating in badly ventilated housing [16]. Infections may play a role in the pathogenesis of the disease, but their importance is mainly due to the fact that they tend to heavily degenerate the clinical situation of the subjects already suffering from COPD [16].

Burden of Disease

Deaths attributable to COPD have increased sharply as data on mortality in the different countries became available. COPD was the fourth leading cause of death in the world in 2011 and was responsible for about three million deaths (5.4 % of all deaths), and there is concern that available data on mortality may underestimate COPD as a cause of death by around 50 % [3, 19]. Mortality greatly increases with age, as more than 2.9 of the 3.2 million deaths estimated in 2008 and caused by COPD were observed in people aged 60 or more. Mortality may be higher in males: 2008 global estimates counted 1.8 million deaths in males and 1.4 million deaths in females [20, 21]. Middle-income countries have the highest mortality due to COPD, where it causes 7.4 % of all deaths. In low- and high-income countries, COPD causes 3.6 and 3.5 % of all deaths, respectively [18].

In 2010, COPD was responsible for 29.4 million YLDs (426 YLDs per 100,000 inhabitants) [8] and 76.7 million DALYs (1114 DALYs per 100,000 inhabitants, Fig. 7.2) [9, 21]. In 2004, COPD was responsible for 17.3 million DALYs in males and 12.8 million DALYs in females. As regards age, COPD caused 14.1 million DALYs in the 15–59 age group and 15.9 million DALYs in people aged 60 or above, minimally affecting the younger age groups [21]. DALYs due to COPD have slightly declined in the past 20 years (there was a 1.5-million-DALY decrease). This may be the result of the reduction of some determinants of COPD such as household air pollution and exposure to particulates from biomass and coal fuels, especially in India and China, despite the increase in cumulative exposure to tobacco [9].

However, according to some projections from Mathers and Loncar, based on the Global Burden of Disease Study, COPD may cause 7.8 % of all deaths and 3.1 % of all DALYs in the world in 2030 [22].

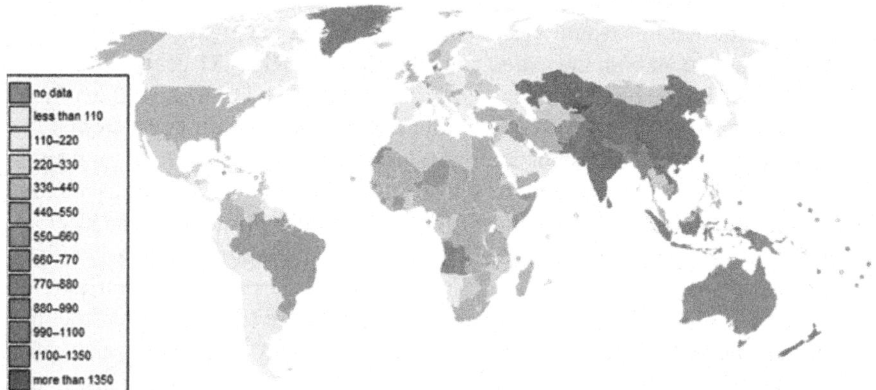

Fig. 7.2 Age-standardized DALY rates from chronic obstructive pulmonary disease by country (per 100,000 inhabitants). (Reproduced from: Death and DALY estimates for 2004 by cause for WHO Member States [6])

Table 7.3 Principal comorbidities associated with COPD by organ/system affected

Cardiovascular	*Endocrine*
Coronary artery disease	Obesity
High blood pressure	Diabetes
Left heart failure	Dyslipidemia
Tachyarrhythmia	Denutrition
Malignant tumors	*Gastroenterology*
Nonsmall cell lung cancer	Gastric ulcer
	Gastroesophageal reflux
Respiratory	*Osteoarticular*
Pneumonia	Fractures
Pulmonary embolism	Osteoporosis
Chronic cor pulmonale	
Asthma	
Rhinitis	
	Psychiatric
	Depression
	Anxiety

Economic costs of COPD are correspondingly high: Patients with COPD tend to get sick frequently, and management of exacerbations of the disease is particularly costly for the health care systems. COPD is the most expensive of the chronic diseases found in elderly patients and direct costs increase with severity. In addition, patients are often smokers or ex-smokers, and approximately two thirds of patients with COPD have one or two comorbidities (Table 7.3) [16, 23]. It has been estimated that the mean management costs for the health systems of COPD are at least twice compared to the management costs of the average patient [24]. According to some estimates, in 2010, the economic costs of COPD were 49.9 billion dollars in the USA, of which 29.5 billion dollars were direct costs. Moreover, COPD annually generates 38.6 billion euros loss in the European Community, 28.5 of which attributable to productivity losses [14, 25, 26]. In developing countries, direct costs may be less relevant, but as a result of a lack in long-term supportive care, COPD would force twice the individuals to leave the workplace: the affected individuals and at least one family member for each case, responsible for the management of the patient [14].

Best Practices

The treatment of COPD is extremely complex and expensive, and requires managing the stable pathology and its exacerbations according to the GOLD guidelines, which are adopted worldwide [14]. The first step for the management of the disease is its diagnosis. COPD should be suspected in each patient above the age of 40 showing at least one sign/symptom among dyspnea, chronic cough, sputum production, or a history of exposure to its risk factors. All these patients should undergo a post-bronchodilator spirometry, an evaluation of the severity of the disease and its comorbidities, and an assessment of the risk of exacerbations and hospitalization. Therapy of the stable COPD includes inhaled (short- and long-acting β2-agonists, glucocorticosteroids, long-acting muscarinic antagonists) and oral drugs (mucolytics, corticosteroids, theophylline, antitussive drugs, antioxidants, antibiotics) and may require surgery and oxygen therapy. Exacerbations may require all these treatments but also hospitalization, intensive care, invasive ventilation, palliative care, social services, rehabilitation, and management of the comorbidities. The triple therapy (a long-acting anticholinergic bronchodilator, a long-acting beta-agonist bronchodilator, and an inhaled corticosteroid) is the most effective but not necessarily the most cost-effective option. Influenza vaccination is considered a cost-effective intervention for reducing mortality and morbidity in patients with COPD. Programs for early detection of COPD have been suggested but their cost-effectiveness have yet to be fully evaluated [14, 27, 28].

In this framework, primary prevention appears to be the wisest choice and the priority objective. Primary COPD prevention requires the reduction or avoidance of personal exposure to common risk factors, to be started during pregnancy and childhood. At the moment, controlling the cigarette smoke consumption is the most sustainable and effective action to be taken. Smoking cessation, pulmonary rehabilitation, and reduction of personal exposure to noxious particles and gases can reduce symptoms, improve quality of life, and increase physical fitness [27–30].

Tobacco Smoking as a Risk Factor and its Control

There are currently about one billion smokers in the world. Manufactured cigarettes represent the major form of smoked tobacco. Tobacco smoke contains more than 4000 chemicals, of which 50 are known to be carcinogenic, and is associated with lung cancer (71 % of all cases), chronic respiratory diseases (42 % of all cases), and cardiovascular disease (10 % of all cases). Moreover, tobacco smoking is an important risk factor for tuberculosis and lower respiratory infections [30–33]. Also, secondhand smoke is harmful for health. Globally, smoke accounts for 6 % of all female and 12 % of all male deaths, so almost 6 million people die from tobacco use and exposure each year, of which 600,000 die because of secondhand smoke [30, 32].

While many interventions for tobacco smoking control may be cost-effective, some are considered "best buys" (actions that should be undertaken immediately to produce accelerated results in terms of lives saved, diseases prevented, and heavy costs avoided). These are: protecting people from tobacco smoke and banning smoking in public places; warning about the dangers of tobacco use; enforcing bans on tobacco advertising, promotion, and sponsorship; and raising taxes on tobacco. In addition to best buys, another cost-effective and low-cost population-wide intervention that can reduce tobacco smoking is offering help to people who want to stop using tobacco through nicotine dependence treatment. All these interventions were included in the WHO 2008–2013 Action Plan for the Global Strategy for the Prevention and Control of Non-communicable Diseases, together with monitoring tobacco use and tobacco-prevention policies [29, 30].

Key Elements

COPD prevalence is estimated at 7.6 % globally, but increases with age, is higher in males, and might be far higher than is recorded.

COPD accounts for 5.4 % of all deaths and is responsible for 76.7 million DALYs.

The management of COPD is extremely complex and expensive; therefore, primary prevention must not be neglected.

Active smoking is the most important risk factor for COPD and its control is the most important intervention for primary prevention (and an essential part of the treatment).

Outdoor and Indoor Air Pollution

As previously described, outdoor and indoor air pollutants are significant risk factors for asthma and COPD. Indoor exposure to air pollutants alone, tobacco and solid fuels smoke excluded, is estimated to account for 20 % of asthma prevalence [34]. Globally, total indoor and outdoor environmental exposures (pollens excluded) account for 44 % of total disease burden from asthma, with occupational exposures being responsible for about 11 % of the total burden from asthma [35, 36]. Regarding COPD, it has been estimated that occupational exposures to airborne particulate and indoor smoke from solid fuels account for 12 and 22 % of its global disease burden, respectively. However, air pollution is also a proven risk factor for numerous diseases, accounting outdoor air pollution alone for 3 % of global cardiopulmonary mortality, about 5 % of trachea, bronchus, and lung cancer mortality and about 1 % of mortality in children from acute respiratory infection in urban areas [35–37].

Outdoor and Urban Air Pollution: Definitions and Problem Framing

Monitoring of outdoor air pollution is currently based on the measurement of the concentrations of particulate matter (PM, either PM10 or PM2.5 if the diameter of the particulate is less than 10 or 2.5 μm in diameter, respectively). PM is a mixture of liquid and solid particles varying in size and composition associated with higher mortality and morbidity, especially in the elderly, the infants, and those suffering from preexisting cardiovascular and respiratory diseases [38]. PM is generally generated by fuel combustion sources, industrial production, and natural sources. Mobile sources (road vehicles) contribute to more than 50% of PM concentrations in urban areas, while biomass burning may be the largest source in rural areas [38].

The presence of PM is commonly associated with a mixture of primary and secondary gaseous air pollutants that are also commonly routinely monitored. Primary air pollutants are emitted directly from combustion sources, while secondary pollutants are formed in the atmosphere from directly emitted pollutants. These pollutants include toxic gases such as sulfur dioxide (SO_2), nitrogen oxides (NOX), carbon monoxide (CO), ozone (O_3), and carcinogens such as benzo(a)pyrene, benzene, and 1,3-butadiene. In many developing countries, fuel still contains lead (Pb), another toxic element which can be found in the pollution mix [36].

Urban air pollution is often referred as "smog," but this term, born from the union of the words "smoke" and "fog," indicates the presence of polluting particles (smoke) mixed with water vapor (fog). There are two main types of smog. Winter smog (or London smog) is a thick, dirty mist that greatly reduces the visibility and is characterized by low temperatures (typically between −1 and 4 °C), high relative humidity, and high concentration of PM and SO_2. It occurs in case of thermal inversion, generally in the early morning in wintertime, when a layer of irradiated warm air settles over a layer of cold air near ground level. On the contrary, summer smog (or photochemical smog) occurs in the presence of a clear sky, a strong solar irradiation, the presence of ultraviolet (UV) rays, and a high concentration of NOX and hydrocarbons. It generally occurs in the summer, during the hottest hours, when the solar rays cause photochemical reactions and generate secondary pollutants such as SO_2 and O_3 from vehicular traffic emissions. It causes reduced visibility and appears as a layer of fog above the polluted cities.

Burden of Outdoor Air Pollution

Outdoor exposure to PM in the air is associated with life-shortening, respiratory, and cardiopulmonary hospital admissions and deaths and lung cancer. The effect on shortening life expectancy has been estimated at 1–2 years, but may be greater in disadvantaged population groups since effects on life expectancy depend on education and antioxidant vitamin status. In children, air pollution is associated with bronchitis and asthma [34, 39, 40].

Worldwide, outdoor air pollution was responsible for more than 1.3 million deaths (13 attributable deaths per 100,000) and more than 30,000 deaths in children under 5 years of age in 2008. This means that outdoor air pollution accounts for 1.4% of all mortality and 0.4% of all DALYs [38, 41]. According to some estimates, this burden may be half as much as that of tobacco. The burden of disease due to urban air pollution occurs predominantly in developing countries (Fig. 7.3) with Asia contributing approximately two thirds of the global burden [37].

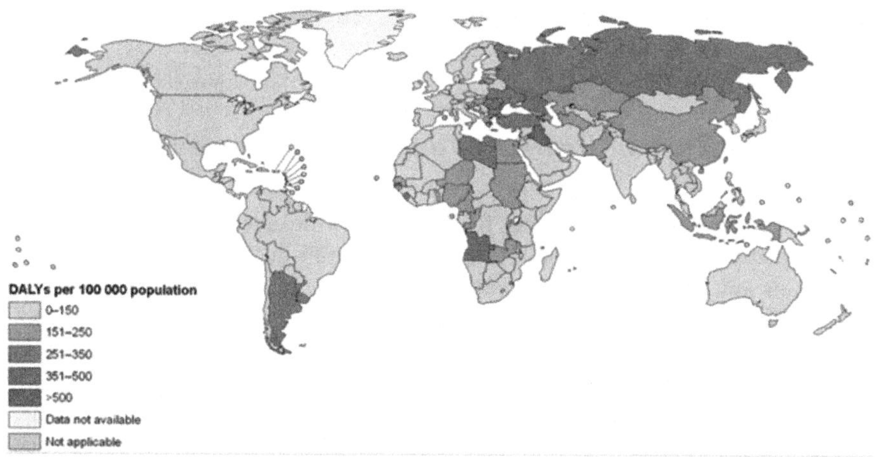

Fig. 7.3 DALY rates from outdoor air pollution by country (per 100,000 inhabitants) in 2011. (Based on WHO Global Health Observatory 2013 data [41])

Table 7.4 Outdoor air pollutants concentration thresholds according to WHO [42]

$PM_{2.5}$[a]	10 μg/m^3 annual mean 25 μg/m^3 24-h mean
PM_{10}[a]	20 μg/m^3 annual mean 50 μg/m^3 24-h mean
O_3[a]	100 μg/m^3 8-h mean
NO_2[a]	40 μg/m^3 annual mean 200 μg/m^3 1-h mean
SO_2[a]	20 μg/m^3 24-h mean 500 μg/m^3 10-min mean

[a]*PM2.5* particulate matter (diameter: 2.5 μm), *PM10* particulate matter (diameter: 10 μm), O_3 ozone, NO_2 nitrogen dioxide, SO_2 sulfur dioxide, *WHO* World Health Organization

Air quality standards are set by each country, but WHO recommends to control four common pollutants in particular: PM, nitrogen dioxide (NO_2), SO_2, and O_3 (Table 7.4), because of their important burden and strong scientific evidence of negative effects on health. Moreover, these pollutants are easier to measure and they often coexist with other toxic substances [42].

Attention must be paid to the measurement methods, as the sampling of ambient air can be more or less representative of the reality on the basis of where they were carried out. In fact, outdoor air should be periodically monitored in different types of microenvironments, such as busy roads, urban areas, human settlements close to productive activities, and rural areas distant from the sources of pollution [42]. Since pollutants and their concentrations widely vary among the different regions of the world, WHO encourages authorities to conduct health impact assessments (HIA) in order to quantitatively link to a given air pollutant the magnitude of the health effects it causes and provide tailored cost-effective improvements in public health for each situation [42].

Indoor Air Pollution: Definitions and Problem Framing

Research on indoor air pollution has focused worldwide on environmental tobacco smoke, volatile organic compounds (VOCs) from furnishings and human activities, radon from soil, and indoor smoke from household use of solid fuels [36]. The significant effects on health of tobacco smoke have already been described. VOCs are associated with the sick building syndrome (SBS) and different degrees of discomfort in the indoor environments [43]. The SBS term is used to describe nonspecific symptoms that may be caused by factors in the indoor environment as headache, fatigue, eye or upper airway discomfort, and skin disorders. [44]. The prevalence of SBS is easily controlled by adjusting (generally reducing) room temperature and with effective cleaning routines of the floors and the other horizontal surfaces. It is more frequent in the presence of carpeting and other textile materials, especially if not properly cleaned, and when personal outdoor air supply rate drops below 10 l/s [44]. Other diseases related to specific indoor environment agents are included among the "building-related illnesses" (BRIs). These include infectious diseases (like Legionnaires' disease and Pontiac fever or flu-like illnesses from respiratory viruses), immunologic and allergic reactions (like dermatitis, rhinitis and asthma from dust mites, plant products, animal allergens, fungi), and other disorders caused by irritant fibers, resins, and combustion products [45]. The BRIs require that the causative agent is removed. When this is not possible (generally in case of some allergens), the employee is kept away from the agent, directing him to another task or microenvironment [45].

Radon is a radioactive gas that emanates from rocks and soils and concentrates in enclosed spaces such as mines or houses. It is the second cause of lung cancer (lung cancers attributable to radon range from 3 to 14%), but it can be effectively controlled on both new and already existing buildings with various different techniques (sealing membranes and barriers, under-floor ventilation, soil pressurization) [46]. These techniques vary in cost, and cost-effectiveness of radon control interventions is strongly influenced by radon concentrations and by the costs of the identification of the affected buildings. However, in areas of high radon concentrations, remediation should still be undertaken [46].

Indoor smoke from household use of solid fuels is the most widespread source of indoor air pollution worldwide and its burden is the most studied among all indoor air pollutants [36]. Main indoor pollutants coming from solid fuels combustion are fine particles, CO, NOX, SO_2, polycyclic aromatic hydrocarbons, arsenic, and fluorine. Indoor air pollution is clearly associated with acute lower respiratory tract infections in children and COPD and lung cancer in adults. However, it is suspected that indoor air pollution is also associated with increased risks of asthma, cataract,

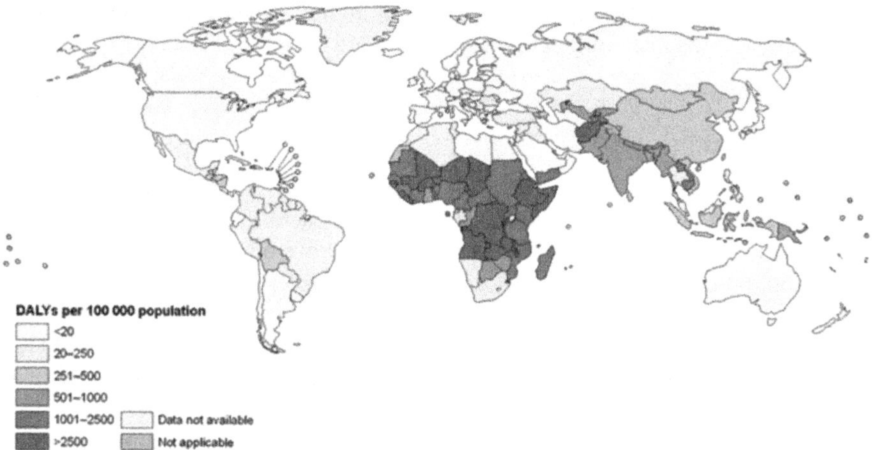

Fig. 7.4 DALY rates from indoor air pollution by country (per 100,000 inhabitants). (Based on WHO Global Health Observatory 2013 data [47])

active tuberculosis and, in case of exposure during pregnancy, intrauterine mortality, low birth weight, prematurity, and early infant death [36].

Burden of Indoor Air Pollution

Lower respiratory tract infections in children account for 59 % of all attributed premature deaths and 78 % of DALYs due to household solid fuels, while COPD accounts for almost all the remainder (lung cancer contributes for less than 1 % of premature deaths and DALYs). Africa and Asia account for almost all deaths and DALYs from household solid fuels [36]. Globally, indoor air pollution was responsible for nearly two million deaths in 2004, of which 872,000 were in children under 5 years of age (24 attributable deaths per 100,000), and about 40 million DALYs (Fig. 7.4) [47].

An extremely cost-effective way to reduce the burden of indoor air pollution is to make cleaner fuels (such as LPG: liquefied petroleum gas) as well as cleaner-burning and more efficient stoves widely available [48]. It was estimated that if the global population without access to LPG was halved, the annual economic benefits from less expenditure on health care, health-related productivity gains, fuel collection, and cooking time savings and environmental impacts would amount from 91 billion dollars at the negative cost of 13 billion. Providing a cheap chimneyless rocket stove in half of the homes not equipped with it would generate 105 billion dollars in economic benefits at a cost of 34 billion. Greater benefits would clearly be observed in regions with higher burden such as the West Pacific and urban areas (net benefits up to US$ 63.7 per person), but these interventions are cost-effective in all developing countries and even cost saving in many regions, as fuel cost savings greatly exceed intervention costs [48].

Key Elements

Outdoor and indoor air pollutants are significant risk factors for asthma and COPD, but they also represent a proven risk factor for numerous other diseases, in particular cardiopulmonary disorders, lung cancer, and acute respiratory infections.

Outdoor air pollution kills 1.3 million people each year. It can be visible, as occurring in the presence of smog, but it should be monitored nonetheless. WHO suggests to measure at least the concentration in the outdoor air of PM (PM10 and PM2.5), NO_2, SO_2, and O_3, and encourages authorities to conduct HIA in order to plan public health interventions that are consistent with the local situations.

Tobacco smoke, VOCs, radon, and smoke from solid fuels are among the main components of indoor air pollution, which kills each year about two million people (of which 872,000 are children under 5 years of age). Africa and Asia account for almost all the burden of indoor air pollution, which is mainly due to the use of solid fuels for cooking and heating. Providing these populations with cleaner fuels and stoves would be an extremely cost-effective way to reduce the burden of indoor air pollution.

Obstructive Sleep Apnea Syndrome

OSAS was first clearly documented in 1966 and its clinical importance is now widely recognized. Patients suffering from OSAS have frequent pauses in breathing during sleep, usually accompanied by snoring, gasps, and chokes. This causes frequent awakenings (micro-arousals) that may be unrecognized by the patients, thus leading to undiagnosed cases. Impaired sleep quality causes disabling daytime symptoms such as fatigue, sleepiness, morning headaches, and difficulty in concentrating. The typical patient is above the age of 40 (the prevalence of the disease has a peak between the ages of 55 and 60 years), obese, may suffer from retrognathia (a retro-positioning of the chin), and have a large neck circumference. Most patients are unaware of their disease and show no respiratory abnormality while awake. These patients usually suffer from hypertension, which can be both a risk factor and a result of OSAS. Other risk factors are alcohol consumption, chronically swollen or enlarged tongue, tonsils or adenoids, and a family history of OSAS (that is generally related to the shape of the craniofacial structures). Typically, the syndrome is associated with an increased risk of traffic accidents (three- to sevenfold) and depression, but a correlation with myocardial infarction and stroke was also observed [3, 49–51].

A diagnosis of OSAS requires daytime sleepiness and evidence of more than five episodes per hour of apnea (breathing cessation above 10 s) or hypopnea (a reduction of the airflow) during sleeping despite the chest wall showing ventilatory efforts. The disease is diagnosed by means of full polysomnography. Between 30 and 70 years of age, 9 % of women and 24 % of men show signs of OSAS at the polysomnography with no daytime sleepiness, but only 2 % of women and 4 % of men of the overall population show both sleepiness and night signs of OSAS. However, according to the scientific literature, the prevalence of the disease may be as high as 6 % of the population. Moreover, OSAS being strongly associated with severe overweight, its prevalence is likely to increase in parallel with the current epidemic of obesity seen in many countries [3].

The exact costs of the disease are difficult to gauge, but they are mainly due to the work limitation (a substantial proportion of patients suffering from OSAS are of working age), the occupational injuries, and the traffic accidents. It was estimated that the medical costs of OSAS prior to diagnosis are US$ 2720 (compared to US$ 1384 in a matched population) and that the annual excess total direct and indirect costs for patients with obstructive sleep apnea are 3860 €, but can be three times higher among the obese subjects [52, 53]. Once the disease is identified, it can be effectively treated. Obese patients should be first treated with weight loss. Other effective treatments are the nocturnal continuous positive air pressure (CPAP) and surgery in patients for whom the anatomy of the upper airways is a determining factor [50].

While surgery may be an expensive solution, there is evidence that nocturnal CPAP is a cost-effective intervention that improves hypertension and quality of life, reduces traffic accidents and depression, and has an incremental cost-effectiveness ratio (ICER) that ranges from 4000 £ and US$ 3,354 to CND$ 3626 in the various studies [50, 52, 53].

References

1. World Health Organization (2013) Asthma fact sheet. http://www.who.int/mediacentre/factsheets/fs307/en/. Accessed date Jul 2013
2. Global Initiative for Asthma (2012) Global strategy for asthma management and prevention. Updated 2012. http://www.ginasthma.org/local/uploads/files/GINA_Report_March13.pdf. Accessed 15 Jul 2013
3. World Health Organization (2010) Chronic respiratory diseases. http://www.who.int/gard/publications/chronic_respiratory_diseases.pdf. Accessed 15 Jul 2013
4. Akinbami LJ, Moorman JE, Bailey C et al (2012) Trends in asthma prevalence, health care use, and mortality in the United States, 2001–2010. NCHS data brief, no 94. National Center for Health Statistics, Hyattsville
5. Global Initiative for Asthma (2013) Global burden of asthma. http://www.ginasthma.org/Global-Burden-of-Asthma. Accessed 15 Jul 2013
6. World Health Organization (2004) Death and DALY estimates for 2004 by cause for WHO Member States. http://www.who.int/healthinfo/global_burden_disease/estimates_country/en/. Accessed 15 Jul 2013

7. Subbarao P, Mandhane PJ, Sears MR (2009) Asthma: epidemiology, etiology and risk factors. CMAJ 181(9):E181–E190
8. Vos T, Flaxman AD, Naghavi M et al (2012) Years lived with disability (YLDs) for 1160 sequelae of 289 diseases and injuries 1990–2010: a systematic analysis for the Global Burden of Disease Study 2010. Lancet 380(9859):2163–2196
9. Murray CJ, Vos T, Lozano R et al (2012) Disability-adjusted life years (DALYs) for 291 diseases and injuries in 21 regions, 1990–2010: a systematic analysis for the Global Burden of Disease Study 2010. Lancet 380(9859):2197–2223
10. Bahadori K, Doyle-Waters MM, Marra C et al (2009) Economic burden of asthma: a systematic review. BMC Pulm Med 9:24
11. Fitzgerald JM, Quon BS (2010) The impact of asthma guidelines. Lancet 376(9743):751–753
12. Simoens S (2012) The cost-effectiveness of immunotherapy for respiratory allergy: a review. Allergy 67(9):1087–1105
13. Guerra S (2005) Overlap of asthma and chronic obstructive pulmonary disease. Curr Opin Allergy Clin Immunol 11(1):7–13
14. Global Initiative for Chronic Obstructive Lung Disease (2013) Global strategy for the diagnosis, management, and prevention of chronic obstructive pulmonary disease. Updated 2013. http://www.goldcopd.org/uploads/users/files/GOLD_Report_2013_Feb20.pdf. Accessed 15 Jul 2013
15. World Health Organization (2012) COPD. Fact Sheet No. 315. http://www.who.int/mediacentre/factsheets/fs315/en/index.html. Accessed 15 Jul 2013
16. Raherison C, Girodet PO (2009) Epidemiology of COPD. Eur Respir Rev 18(114):213–221
17. Halbert RJ, Natoli JL, Gano A et al (2006) Global burden of COPD: systematic review and meta-analysis. Eur Respir J 28(3):523–532
18. World Health Organization (2004) The Global Burden of Disease 2004 Update. http://www.who.int/healthinfo/global_burden_disease/GBD_report_2004update_full.pdf. Accessed 15 Jul 2013
19. World Health Organization (2013) COPD. Fact Sheet No. 310. http://www.who.int/mediacentre/factsheets/fs310/en/index.html. Accessed Jul 2013
20. World Health Organization (2011) Data elaborations. http://www.who.int/gho/mortality_burden_disease/global_burden_disease_death_estimates_sex_2008.xls. Accessed 15 Jul 2013
21. World Health Organization (2011) Data elaborations. http://www.who.int/gho/mortality_burden_disease/global_burden_disease_death_estimates_sex_age_2008.xls. Accessed 15 Jul 2013
22. Mathers CD, Loncar D (2006) Projections of global mortality and burden of disease from 2002 to 2030. PLoS Med 3(11):e442
23. Mapel DW, McMillan GP, Frost FJ et al (2005) Predicting the costs of managing patients with chronic obstructive pulmonary disease. Respir Med 99(10):1325–1333
24. Chapman KR, Mannino DM, Soriano JB et al (2006) Epidemiology and costs of chronic obstructive pulmonary disease. Eur Respir J 27(1):188–207
25. European Respiratory Society (2003) European lung white book. European Respiratory Society Journals Ltd, Huddersfield
26. National Heart, Lung, and Blood Institute (2009) Morbidity and mortality chartbook on cardiovascular, lung and blood diseases. US Deparment of Health and Human Services, Public Health Service, National Institutes of Health, Bethesda. http://www.nhlbi.nih.gov/resources/docs/2009_ChartBook.pdf. Accessed 15 Jul 2013
27. National Clinical Guideline Centre (2010) Chronic obstructive pulmonary disease: management of chronic obstructive pulmonary disease in adults in primary and secondary care. National Clinical Guideline Centre, London
28. World Health Organization (2002) WHO strategy for prevention and control of chronic respiratory diseases. http://whqlibdoc.who.int/hq/2002/WHO_MNC_CRA_02.1.pdf. Accessed 15 Jul 2013
29. World Health Organization (2013) 2008–2013 Action plan for the global strategy for the prevention and control of noncommunicable diseases. http://whqlibdoc.who.int/publications/2009/9789241597418_eng.pdf. Accessed 15 Jul 2013

30. World Health Organization (2010) Global status report on noncommunicable diseases 2010. http://whqlibdoc.who.int/publications/2011/9789240686458_eng.pdf. Accessed 15 Jul 2013
31. World Health Organization (2009) Global health risks: mortality and burden of disease attributable to selected major risks. World Health Organization, Geneva.
32. Oberg M, Jaakkola MS, Woodward A, Peruga A, Prüss-Ustün A (2011) Worldwide burden of disease from exposure to second-hand smoke: a retrospective analysis of data from 192 countries. Lancet 377(9760):139–146
33. Lin HH, Ezzati M, Murray M (2007) Tobacco smoke, indoor air pollution and tuberculosis: a systematic review and meta-analysis. PLoS Med 4(1):e20
34. Melse JM, de Hollander AEM (2001) Environment and health within the OECD region: lost health, lost money. Background document to the OECD Environmental Outlook. RIVM (Dutch National Institute of Public Health and the Environment), Bilthoven. http://www.rivm.nl/bibliotheek/rapporten/402101001.pdf. Accessed 1 Aug 2013
35. Prüss-Üstün A, Corvalán C (2006) Preventing disease through healthy environments: towards an estimate of the environmental burden of disease. World Health Organization, Geneva
36. Ezzati M, Lopez AD, Rodgers A, Murray CJL (2004) Comparative quantification of health risks: global and regional burden of disease attributable to selected major risk factors, vol. 2. World Health Organization, Geneva
37. Cohen AJ, Ross Anderson H, Ostro B et al (2005) The global burden of disease due to outdoor air pollution. J Toxicol Environ Health A 68(13–14):1301–1307
38. Ostro B (2004) Outdoor air pollution: assessing the environmental burden of disease at national and local levels. World Health Organization, Geneva
39. Brunekreef B, Holgate ST (2002) Air pollution and health. Lancet 360:1233–1242
40. Curtis L, Rea W, Smith-Willis P, Fenyves E, Pan Y (2006) Adverse health effects of outdoor air pollutants. Environ Int 32(6):815–830
41. World Health Organization (2013) Data elaborations. http://apps.who.int/gho/data/node.main.156. Accessed 1 Aug 2013
42. World Health Organization (2005) WHO air quality guidelines for particulate matter, ozone, nitrogen dioxide and sulfur dioxide. Global update 2005. http://www.euro.who.int/__data/assets/pdf_file/0005/78638/E90038.pdf. Accessed 1 Aug 2013
43. Wang, S, Ang, HM, Tade MO (2007) Volatile organic compounds in indoor environment and photocatalytic oxidation: state of the art. Environ Int 33(5):694–705
44. Norbäck D (2009) An update on sick building syndrome. Curr Opin Allergy Clin Immunol 9(1):55–59
45. Menzies D, Bourbeau J (1997) Building-related illnesses. N Engl J Med 337(21):1524–1531
46. World Health Organization (2009) WHO handbook on indoor radon: a public health perspective. http://whqlibdoc.who.int/publications/2009/9789241547673_eng.pdf. Accessed 1 Aug 2013
47. World Health Organization (2013) Data elaborations. http://apps.who.int/gho/data/node.main.140. Accessed 1 Aug 2013
48. Hutton G, Rehfuess E, Tediosi F (2007) Evaluation of the costs and benefits of interventions to reduce indoor air pollution. Energy Sustain Dev 11(4):34–43
49. Gibson GJ (2005) Obstructive sleep apnoea syndrome: underestimated and undertreated. Br Med Bull 72:49–65
50. Myers KA, Mrkobrada M, Simel DL (2013) Does this patient have obstructive sleep apnea?: The rational clinical examination systematic review. J Am Med Assoc 310(7):731–741
51. Durán J, Esnaola S, Rubio R, Iztueta A (2001) Obstructive sleep apnea-hypopnea and related clinical features in a population based sample of subjects aged 30 to 70 year. Am J Respir Crit Care Med 163:685–689
52. AlGhanim N, Comondore VR, Fleetham J, Marra CA, Ayas NT (2008) The economic impact of obstructive sleep apnea. Lung 186(1):7–12
53. Leger D, Bayon V, Laaban JP, Philip P (2012) Impact of sleep apnea on economics. Sleep Med Rev 16(5):455–462

Chapter 8
Public Health Gerontology and Active Aging

Andrea Poscia, Francesco Landi and Agnese Collamati

Definition

What is Aging and Who is "Old"?

Aging is the natural process of growing old. It is a biological process which involves physical, psychological, and social changes. Besides any objective definition, aging implies a deeper subjective dimension quite difficult to be defined. In fact, the age at which an individual is considered and considers himself/herself "old" varies worldwide depending on several complex factors. The age of 60 or 65, roughly equivalent to retirement ages, is said to be the beginning of old age [1] in most developed countries and many World Health Organization (WHO) documents often define "older people" as those over 60 years of age [2].

However, extended life expectancy and improved quality of life have led to the identification of other two new categories: on the one hand with the term "oldest old" (also called "fourth age" [3]) we usually refer to over 80/85, a new exploding population group, on the other hand we have the "youngest old," defined as 50–60+ (also called "third age"), a group of people who would not define themselves as "old," but which represent a fundamental target population to be addressed in order to take preventive measures to stave off health-related problems in the coming decades [4].

A. Poscia (✉)
Institute of Public Health, Section of Hygiene, Università Cattolica del Sacro Cuore, L.go F. Vito 1, 00168 Rome, Italy
e-mail: andrea.poscia@edu.rm.unicatt.it

F. Landi · A. Collamati
Institute of Gerontology, Università Cattolica del Sacro Cuore, L.go F. Vito 1, 00168 Rome, Italy
e-mail: francesco.landi@rm.unicatt.it, agnese.collamati@gmail.com

A. Collamati
e-mail: agnese.collamati@gmail.com

S. Boccia et al. (eds.), *A Systematic Review of Key Issues in Public Health*,
DOI 10.1007/978-3-319-13620-2_8

Many factors contribute to the dynamic process of aging: genetic characteristics, gender, behavior, socioeconomic class, culture (instruction), and environment. As a consequence, we will have a diversity in health profiles among older people with an assorted range of health needs. However, aging does not always mean getting ill. Many of the disabilities and diseases suffered by older people, although more common at this age, are not a natural or an inevitable part of growing older. Health decline in later life is the result of the combined effect of intrinsic and extrinsic causes: While the human body undergoes a natural functional decline, there is a cumulative effect of a lifetime exposure to lifestyle and environmental factors that contribute to the pathogenesis of a disease [5].

This consideration brings a fundamental consequence: If some disease conditions are preventable, or at least treatable, health programs should go in that direction. For this reason, there is a growing interest in how to promote a healthier old age and how to carry out effective interventions to reduce disability and health risks in later life [6]. In 1999, the director general of WHO stated,

> there is much the individual can do to remain active and healthy in later life. The right lifestyle, involvement in family and society and a supportive environment for older age all preserve well being. Policies that reduce social inequalities and poverty are essential to complement individual efforts towards Active Ageing. [7]

Active Aging

The WHO defined active and healthy aging as the process of optimizing opportunities for health, participation, and security in order to enhance the quality of life as people age. [8] According to the *European Commission's* contribution to the Second World Assembly on Active Ageing, it is seen as "an orientation towards policies and practices (…) including life-long learning, working longer, retiring later and more gradually, and engaging in capacity-enhancing and health sustaining activities. Such practices aim to raise the average quality of individual lives and, at the same time, at a societal level, contribute to higher growth, lower dependency burdens and substantial cost savings in pensions and health. They therefore represent win-win strategies for people of all ages." [9] The European Union, after that various Presidencies of the Council have prioritized the theme of healthy aging, has identified 2012 as the "European Year for Active Ageing and Solidarity between Generations" and many countries are developing national programs to improve and preserve health and physical, social, and mental wellness.

Usually, the term "healthy" refers to physical, mental, and social well-being [10]. "Active" refers to continuing participation in social, economic, cultural, spiritual, and civic affairs. "*Successful aging,*" commonly used in gerontology and geriatrics, refers to the optimization of life expectancy while minimizing physical and mental deterioration and disability. It focuses on the absence or avoidance of disease and risk factors for disease, maintenance of physical and cognitive functioning, and active engagement with life (including maintenance of autonomy and social support). Some investigators have broadened the model to include more psychosocial elements [11], such as life satisfaction, social participation, and functioning, and psychological resources, including personal growth, resolution and fortitude, happiness, relationships between desired and achieved goals, self concept, mood, and overall wellbeing. Successful aging is seen as a dynamic process, as the outcome of one's development over the life course [12], and as the ability to grow and learn by using past experiences to cope with present circumstances.

A structured literature review was conducted using PubMed with the following keywords [(healthy or active or positive or successful or productive or optimal) *and* (aging or ageing)]. To be included in this review, papers had to be published in peer-reviewed journals or by international scientific society/agencies, had to be written in English, Italian, or Spanish, and had to be about humans aged 65+ years. No publication date restrictions were set a priori. The initial search was done in February 2013 and repeated in August 2013 independently by two researchers: It highlighted 52,180 articles (6764 reviews), with 17,434 (2,369 reviews) in the past 5 years. Using the inclusion criteria, the selection was reduced to 22,074 articles (2187 reviews). Considering the high number of articles published on this topic, the authors limited the research strategy to the reviews. Authors excluded 2058 reviews looking at their title or abstract. In addition, authors assessed articles listed in the "Related articles" section and in the bibliography of the remaining 129 reviews to identify and include additional relevant articles. In parallel, an investigation of websites through Google using the same keywords was done to include also important articles from gray literature and acknowledged international institutions (such as WHO, Organisation for Economic Co-operation and Development (OECD), Centers for Disease Control and Prevention (CDC), etc.). At the end of the process, authors selected and reviewed 124 references: 82 reviews, 14 articles, 22 documents from international agencies, and 6 books.

Burden

Population is Aging and Changing: the Modern Challenge

Europe and many other countries in the world are currently facing increasingly complex and systemic societal challenges. Due to health care advances, increased wealth, improved well-being, and living standards, life expectancy has dramatically increased during these past decades [13]. The world will have more people who live to see their 80s or 90s than ever before, even because we are witnessing (attending) the baby boomer generation growing and becoming older.

It is projected that between 2010 and 2060, the number of Europeans aged over 65 will double, from 88 to 153 million (about 30% of the EU population will be aged 65+ [14]). The rise of the "oldest old" is the fastest growing part of the total population, since those over 80 will nearly triple, from 24 to 62 million (Fig. 8.1).

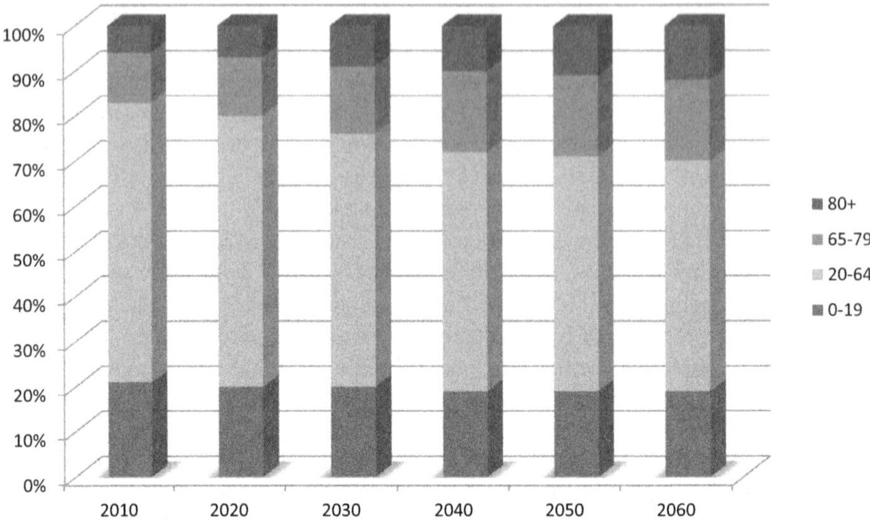

Fig. 8.1 Changes in the EU structure of population, by main age group (Reproduced from [15])

What happens in Europe is the counterpart of a global situation: The world's population aged 65 and over is projected to grow from 524 million to nearly 1.5 billion between the years 2010 and 2050. The number of people aged 65 or older will outnumber children under age 5 and this population aging is not only going to continue but also accelerate.

In early nonindustrial societies, the risk of death was high at every age, with a high perinatal and neonatal mortality so that only a small proportion of people reached oldness. In the early part of the twentieth century, most of the increase in life expectancy was due to improvements in infant and childhood mortality; after 1960 began a progressive increase in survival among those over 60. As a result in modern societies, most people live past middle age, and deaths are highly concentrated at older ages. Furthermore, a significant decline of death rates among people above age 100 have led to an increasing number of centenarians [16, 17].

This transition implies a broad set of changes in the characteristics of the society; first of all, it implies a decline from high to low fertility. As a matter of fact, fertility rate has declined substantially and in most countries is much below the mortality ratio and what it is considered the replacement rate of 2.1 children per woman [18, 19]

As a consequence, we assist at a change in what is called the potential support ratio, that is the number of persons aged 15–64 years per one older person aged 65 years and over (an expression of the ratio of working age people to people of nonworking age [20]). In 1950, the OECD average potential support ratio was 7.21, but by 2000 it had fallen to 4.17 and is predicted to fall to 3.34 by 2020 and 2.08 by 2050 [21] with the obvious implications for social security schemes. Together, the parent support ratio (the number of persons aged 85 years or over in relation to those between 50 and 64 years) is quickly shooting up as the demands on families to provide support for their oldest-old members.

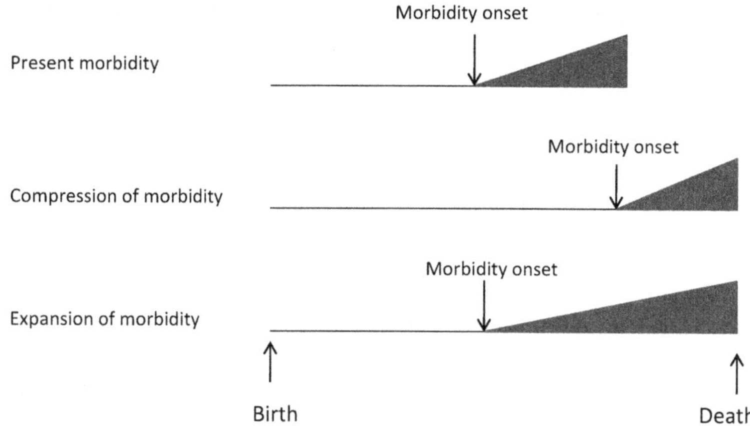

Fig. 8.2 Graphical exemplification of the three theories about mortality and morbidity in different scenarios. (Reproduced from [24])

The population is not only aging but also changing its characteristics. The transition from high to low mortality and fertility that accompanied socioeconomic development has also meant a shift in the leading causes of disease and death. Demographers and epidemiologists describe this shift as part of an "epidemiologic transition" characterized by the waning of infectious and acute diseases (commonly associated with poverty, poor diets, and limited infrastructure as it happens in developing countries) and the emerging importance of chronic and degenerative diseases including cardiovascular disease, cancer, dementia, and diabetes. [22]

Consequently, a question arises: Has the increased longevity generally occurred in parallel with improved health and quality of life? We live longer, this is pretty much a given, but is it a life worth living? Are we living healthier as well as longer lives, or are our additional years spent in poor health?

In this sense, there has been much debate in the past 50 years between opposite theories: the compression versus the expansion of morbidity, with a third option that sounds like something in between, the so called dynamic equilibrium scenario [23] (Fig. 8.2).

From Burden to Opportunity

If increased longevity is a great achievement, it is also a formidable challenge for both public and private budgets, for public services and for older people and their families. In a recent publication, Ahtonen spurs policymakers to realize that the "silver economy" represents a huge potential market and encourages to turning the aging challenge into a "golden opportunity" [25].

The issue of demographic change due to population aging has obviously taken an increasing importance in both national and international agenda over the past 20 years since it is going to have a deep impact on economic growth, investments and consumption, labor markets, pension reforms, and taxation. For health care systems, this situation creates two potentially major pressures: increased utilization of health services and decreased revenues (as a declining share of the population is economically active).

In 2011, the total health expenditure in the USA was about US$ 2.8 trillion—17.9 % of the gross domestic product (GDP) [26]—and it has been reported that only 5 % of Medicare beneficiaries, presumably many with chronic diseases, accounted for almost half (47 %) of total spending, while a much larger segment of the population (40 %), those in relatively good health, accounted for only 1 % of the total [27]. Older people typically account for about half of the hospital workload, when measured in terms of bed days [28], per capita consumption of health services by elderly people is three to five times higher than for younger people [29] and a study in eight OECD countries found that they between one third and one half of total health expenditure was spent for them [30].

The recent work about economic and budgetary projections for the 27 EU member states reports that strictly age-related spending (unemployment benefits excluded) was 25 % of GDP and unemployment benefit spending was 1.1 % of GDP in 2010 (health care expenditures account for 7.1 % of GDP in EU27 and 7.3 in the euro area) [31]. It considers for the period 2010–2060 an increase in strictly age-related public expenditure on average by 4.1 percentage points of GDP (4.5 p.p. in the euro area). Most of this increase will be on pensions (+ 1.5 p.p. of GDP), long-term care (+ 1.5 p.p. of GDP), and health care (+ 1.1 p.p. of GDP). Through two hypothetical scenarios, the authors reported that between 2010 and 2060 the health care spending will increase between 0.5 and 2.8 % of GDP, ranging between 0.4p.p. of Belgium and Cyprus and 2.9p.p. of GDP of Malta. This is considered reasonable, as increasing economic wealth puts governments at pressure to provide more health services and to improve the quality of care, while growing living standards change people's attitude toward their own health, raising their expectations on living a longer and healthier life.

However, the greater impact of an aging population will be expected on public spending for long-term care that is projected to double, increasing from 1.8 % of GDP in 2010 to 3.4 % of GDP in 2060 in the EU as a whole (to 3.4 % of GDP in the EA).

Nevertheless, while expenditure on long-term care is certain to increase with the aging of the population, the effects on health care expenditure are disputed [32] and other factors can magnify (especially the increasing complexity of technology) or mitigate (successful promotion of healthy aging) the impact on it [33]. Rechel et al. highlight that elderly people are not just recipients of pensions or health and long-term care but they also provide a large proportion of care for other elderly people (including spouses). Given that the overwhelming majority of care received by older people is informal and usually provided without financial compensation, improvements in their health status may effectively enlarge the pool of potential carers. Additionally, a significant number of older people in many countries engage in volunteer work or help to look after their grandchildren, providing an important input into society that would otherwise have to be purchased in the marketplace.

These considerations incite a growing consensus about the idea that population aging does not have to be an inevitable drain on health care resources and a negative effect on health and social care systems is not inevitable if appropriate measures are

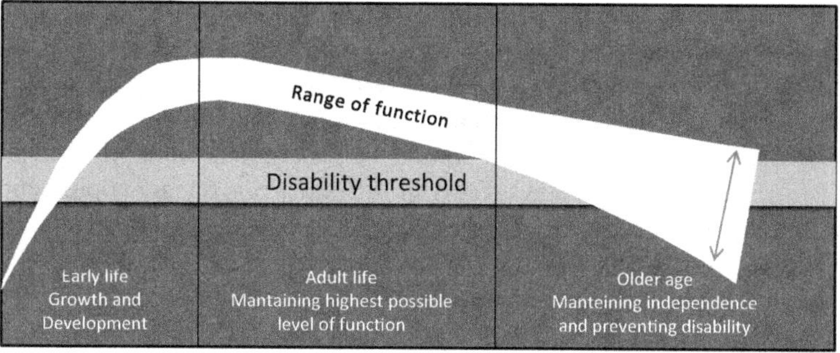

Fig. 8.3 A life course approach to active aging. (Reproduced from [34])

implemented in time. Even if promoting active aging seems one of the most promising ways, ensuring an adequate response from health systems, building adequate systems of long-term care, and supporting economic and social integration will also help to make sure that health systems are properly equipped to accommodate population aging.

Best Practices

How well we age depends on many factors. The functional capacity of an individual's biological system increases during the first years of life, reaches its peak in early adulthood, and naturally declines thereafter (Fig. 8.3).

The rate of decline is determined, at least in part, by behaviors and environmental exposures across the whole life course. These include what we eat, how physically active we are, and our exposure to smoke, alcohol consumption, or toxic substances. Other possible modifiable factors aroused in different studies *are diet, disability, aptitude toward prevention (screening and vaccination), oral health, stress, sleep, and social participation*. The more factors on which positive tendencies were reported, the greater the likelihood of having good health [35–38].

This paragraph provides an update review of the evidence about the most important determinants of healthy aging, including international programs and policies, especially if they are cost-effective.

Stop Smoking and Reduce Alcohol Use

Smoking is considered a proved risk factor for morbidity and mortality throughout all life span. Although tobacco consumption often starts at a young age, the lag between smoking and negative health effects is long. The impact of continued smoking tends to be larger at older ages and the risks of illness and death increase as people age and continue smoking. Smokers lose on average 13 years of healthy life expectancy and smoking is associated with increased risks (sometimes as much as 10 to 20 times) of contracting 40 or more different diseases. Peel et al. found that nonsmoking—along with moderate alcohol consumption—are correlated with healthy aging. Ex-smokers and never smokers with a high level of physical activity were 2.5 times more likely to age successfully. Studies on younger populations also suggest that this is the case. Effect sizes for the association of healthy aging with current nonsmoking or low tobacco consumption ranged from 1.2 [39] to 4.5 [40]. Even though stopping smoking when aged 65–70 halves the excess risk of premature death, some studies show that older smokers are less likely to try to stop than younger smokers (but are more successful when they do). In summary, smoking cessation has very high payoffs in terms of healthy aging and remains one of the key policy levers in improving health in old age.

There is some inconclusive evidence of the positive effects of moderate alcohol consumption (particularly of red wine) on heart disease and other medical problems. Alcohol consumption has been touted as beneficial for health [41], and while it may be true for moderate consumption in younger persons, there is considerable risk associated with increased alcohol intake in older adults. This increase is partially due to age-related physiological changes, comorbidity, and polipharmacotherapy. Specifically, regarding sedative-hypnotic drugs use, older persons may be more susceptible to addictive central nervous system effects than younger persons because of physiologic changes in psychotropic drug and alcohol metabolism [42] so it should be important to consider patients' alcohol consumption patterns before prescribing potential interfering drugs. High alcohol consumption is linked to liver disease [43] and produces detrimental effects on executive function (for example, the ability to form concepts, organize thoughts and activities, prioritize tasks, and think abstractly).

Nonetheless, alcohol misuse disorders are common among older people, often ignored, or under-assessed. A recent report titled "Working with Older Drinkers" by Alcohol Research UK showed that older people consume more alcohol in recent years, with an estimated 20 % of men and 10 % of women exceeding their drinking limit and this trend is projected to be particularly evident in the baby boomer cohort [44].

A systematic review by Reid et al. [45] examined potential association with alcohol consumption: 20 % of the 84 studies demonstrated harm associated with increased alcohol exposure, 70 % found no association with any of the selected outcomes, and 10 % reported benefit from greater alcohol use. Hence, the magnitude of risk posed by alcohol use for falls or fall injuries, functional impairment, cognitive impairment, and all-cause mortality among older adults remains uncertain.

Panza et al. [46] investigated current evidence about the potential alcohol protective effect. The authors found that the studies are limited by cross-sectional design, restriction by age or sex, or incomplete ascertainment. Different outcomes, beverages, drinking patterns, or follow-up periods, or possible interactions with other lifestyle-related (i.e., smoking status, regular exercise or healthy diet) or genetic factors (apolipoprotein E (APOE) genotyping) may be sources of great variability.

In conclusion, in line with what was said in a previous review of Peters et al. [47], they come out that light to moderate alcohol use may be associated with a reduced risk of unspecified incident dementia and Alzheimer's disease, while for vascular dementia, cognitive decline, and predementia syndromes, the current evidence is only suggestive of a protective effect. The protective effects are more likely with wine consumption and the absence of an APOE e4 allele. At present, there is no indication that light to moderate alcohol drinking would be harmful to cognition and dementia, and it is not possible to define a specific beneficial level of alcohol intake (see also below cognitive impairment).

A systematic review of 78 papers conducted as part of the European project VINTAGE confirms the paucity of data on this topic but suggests, even if with scarce evidence, that the elderly seems to respond equally well to alcohol policy, screening instruments, and brief interventions as do younger adults [48]. However, until specific recommendations for alcohol intake will not be established for the 65 year and older population, the best way to act is through a common sense approach of a moderate alcohol use in a more complex frame of healthy lifestyle.

Healthy Eating

Nutrition is emerging as a key element for health throughout life and in particular in the elderly, since both obesity (and behavior related) and malnutrition (especially when associated to hospitalization) constitute risk factors for morbidity and disability. There is also evidence that important aspects of adult health status are determined even before birth (during intrauterine life) and across infancy [49, 50], strengthening the idea that promoting healthy diets throughout all life and since its very beginning results in substantial health benefits.

Sarcopenia [51], defined as the age-related loss of skeletal muscle mass and function, is associated with serious health consequences in terms of frailty, disability, and morbidity and it predicts future mortality in middle-aged as well as older adults [52]. Sarcopenia is strictly connected with the concept of frailty and correlates with both musculoskeletal aging and their many causes: age-related changes in body composition, inflammation, and hormonal imbalance. Its negative impact on disability, disease incidence and dependency, affects healthcare services deeply: for example, in the USA, direct costs for sarcopenia were estimated in $18.5 billion[53], about 1.5% of total healthcare expenditures for that year. [53].

Older people's energy requirements decline with age but the need for nutrients remains the same. Food intake falls by 25 % between 40 and 70 years of age, putting older people at risk of having inadequate nutrient supply. A great number of factors can affect the intake of food in the elderly population and bring to the so-called anorexia of aging. There could be physiological, psychological, and social factors that influence appetite and food consumption, such as loss of taste and olfaction, increased satiation effects of meals, chewing and swallowing difficulties, and impaired gut function [54, 55]. Lack of exercise can diminish appetite and, more generally, interest in food may be affected by dementia and depression. Secondary effects of medicines may also negatively affect the desire to eat.

There is a growing literature suggesting that diet could have an important modifiable influence on sarcopenia [56], with the most consistent evidence pointing to roles for protein, vitamin D, and antioxidant nutrients. There is good observational evidence that links low protein intake to declining muscle mass [57], and supplementation with protein and/or amino acids should therefore have the potential to slow sarcopenic muscle loss. However, the results from trials have been inconsistent. A Cochrane review [58] found that the use of protein and energy supplements in older people at risk of malnutrition produced a small but consistent weight gain and mortality appeared to be reduced in those who were undernourished. However, there was no evidence of functional benefit and further work is needed to establish protein and specific amino acid requirements to support optimal physical function in older people.

On the contrary, *obesity* remains a major public health problem in the general population but also in the geriatric one. Like malnutrition and sarcopenia, obesity starts early in life: The development of childhood obesity is predictive of future obesity in adulthood [59, 60] and increased risk of premature morbidity (hypertension, type II diabetes, hyperlipemia) and mortality for cardiovascular diseases with consequent impact on health care cost [61]. A special attention must reserve the so-called "baby boomer generation" since a recent study documented among them a poorer health status and an increased rate of obesity, hypertension, diabetes, and hypercholesterolemia, with consequent health-care costs, so that this situation deserves a special effort at prevention and healthy lifestyle promotion in this specific generation.

In this sense, starting on the right path is critical to achieving a long life spent in good health [62]. There is some evidence that "healthy" diets, characterized by greater fruit and vegetable consumption and whole meal cereals, are associated with greater muscle strength in older adults [63] Also, the close connection between correct diet and physical exercise is largely proved in the literature. A recent study demonstrated that a modest increase in fruit and vegetable intake, or leisure time physical activity could have a marked effect on the self-related health in older adults [64]. Despite the challenges of changing dietary behavior, nutrition interventions in older community-dwelling adults have been shown to be effective [65]. This goal can be reached through a nutritional education aimed to establish good alimentary habits since adolescents and childhood, coupled with a clear message discouraging a sedentary lifestyle. There is a need to educate health-care professionals as to what constitutes a healthy diet for the elderly population, and to give practical guidance to prevent both malnutrition and obesity within this age group.

Enjoy Physical Activity

Physical activity is very important for maintaining health and physical functioning as people age; it increases strength and, more importantly, it is a strong predictor of healthy aging. A systematic review and meta-analysis published on *BMJ* by Cooper et al. [66] demonstrated that objective measures of physical capability are predictors of all-cause mortality in older community-dwelling populations. The four measures of physical capability investigated were grip strength, walking speed, chair rising, and standing balance. Those people who performed less well in these tests were found to be at a higher risk of all-cause mortality.

Physical activity reduces many major mortality risk factors and improves many diseases and conditions including arterial hypertension [67], diabetes mellitus type 2 [68], dyslipidemia [69], coronary heart disease, chronic heart failure [70], chronic obstructive pulmonary disease, stroke [71, 72], and cancer (colon [73] and breast [74] while possibly endometrial, lung, and pancreatic are reduced). It is associated with a lower incidence of cardiovascular disease, osteoporosis, and bone loss. It can also reduce the risk of falls. On the other side, physical inactivity represents a major independent risk factor for mortality accounting for up to 10 % of all deaths in the European region. Hence, because a 40 % lower mortality rate corresponds to an approximately 5-year higher life expectancy, one would expect an approximately 3.5- to 4.0-year higher life expectancy in physically active persons compared to that in inactive persons [75].

Interestingly, the years gained with physical activity are not spent in frailty and depending on assistance: Nusselder et al. [76] reported a gain of disability-free years of life with a higher life expectancy. However, studies have shown that older adults are insufficiently active. One of the reported barriers to physical activity is fear of injuries [77].

Exercise may reduce the risk of depression and may decrease the chances of developing dementia [78], although it is difficult to isolate exercise from other factors that are often associated with other health-aging policies such as social networks. Better physical condition reduces the risk of dependency [79].

A review by Landi et al. [80] address the role of physical activity on frailty, a specific geriatric syndrome as very common in the elderly, defined as a state of high vulnerability for adverse health outcomes, such as disability, falls, hospitalization, institutionalization, and mortality. Regular physical activity has been shown to protect against different components of the frailty syndrome, in the specific against sarcopenia, functional impairment, cognitive performance, and depression.

There is evidence that aerobic physical activities which improve cardiorespiratory fitness are beneficial for cognitive function in healthy older adults, with effects observed for motor function, cognitive speed, delayed memory functions, and auditory and visual attention [81]. Furthermore, through improving social participation, it enhances the quality of life [82].

However, there is still no agreement regarding what intensity and what kind of exercise is required. A Cochrane review [83] provides evidence that progressive resistance strength training is an effective intervention for improving physical functioning in older people, including improving strength and the performance of some simple and complex activities. However, some caution is needed with transferring these exercises for use with clinical populations because adverse events are not adequately reported. According to the results of the meta-analysis on all-cause mortality in relation to physical activity performed by Samitz et al. [84], reduction in mortality risk was greatest for vigorous exercise and sports and smaller for moderate-intensity activities of daily living. Relative mortality reductions corresponding to 150 and 300 min of moderate to vigorous physical activity per week were 14 and 26 %, respectively, supporting the "some is good; more is better" message.

Promoting physical activity can be an example to prove that programs for older people can be very cost-effective. Munro et al. estimate the likely costs, health benefits, and consequences for the National Health Service which might result from a publicly funded program of regular exercise made available to a population of 10,000 people over the age of 65. With a cost of approximately 854,700 pounds per year, the program would prevent 76 deaths and 230 in-patient episodes and would cost about 330 pounds per life-year saved (ranging from 100 pounds to 1500 pounds) [85]. In another trial, Munro et al. demonstrated that, despite a low level of adherence to the exercise program, there were significant gains in health-related quality of life (quality-adjusted life year (QALY) gain of 0.011 per person). Furthermore the program, resulted in an incremental cost per QALY ratio of € 17,174 (95 % confidence interval (CI) = € 8300 to € 87,120), was more cost-effective than many existing medical interventions [86].

In sum, it is clear from the literature that sedentary behaviors, which are linked to complex sociodemographic and health factors [87], are related with poor health in old people as in young people [88]. On the contrary, exercise is the "best preventive medicine for old age" since it reduces significantly the risk of dependency. In this sense, the motto "It's never too late" sounds incredibly true.

Preventing Falls

Preventing falls is also a fundamental target in a prospective of healthy aging, since approximately 30 % of people over 65 years living in the community fall each year, with even higher cases in institutions. Falls increase in frequency with advancing age and increasing frailty; although less than one fall in ten results in a fracture, a fifth of fall incidents require medical attention [89]. The main and dreaded consequence of falls is disability and dependency in daily living, expensive hospital stays, and long-term residency in institutions: In the year 2000, the cost of treating fall-related injuries was estimated to be US$ 19 billion in the USA [90]. The fear of falling can also lead to reduced physical exercise, increasing further the risk of falls. Women are particularly vulnerable to injury as they may be physically weaker and suffer from osteoporosis, particularly later in life. The major modifiable risk factors for falls include impaired mobility, reduced muscle strength and balance, low levels of physical activity, low body mass index, fear of falling, environmental hazards both indoor and outdoor, such as obstacles, poor lighting, and irregular floor.

A recent Cochrane meta-analysis [91] analyzed randomized trials of intervention to reduce the incidence of falls in older people living in the community. Multiple-component group exercise reduced rate of falls and risk of falling, as did Tai Chi and individually prescribed multiple-component home-based exercise. Multifactorial intervention programs have also been found to be most effective. Vitamins did reduce falls but only in people with lower vitamin D levels before treatment. Home safety interventions were effective, especially in people with severe visual impairment and in others at higher risk of falling. Gradual withdrawal of psychotropic medication and medication reviews reduced rate of falls, but not risk of falling. Pacemakers reduced rate of falls in people with carotid sinus hypersensitivity and cataract surgery did the same if applied to the first eye. Globally, there is evidence that fall prevention strategies can be cost saving.

Moving to the care facilities and hospitals, another revision of the same authors [92] confirmed that, despite the large number of trials, there is limited evidence to support any kind of intervention. The systematic review by Neyens et al. [93] focused on the effectiveness and implementation aspects of interventions aimed at reducing falls in elderly residents in long-term care facilities, supports the conclusions of Gillespie et al.: Multifactorial interventions seem more likely to be beneficial, even if single interventions (i.e., targeting vitamin D insufficiency) can be effective. McClure et al. reviewed 23 population-based studies and, despite some methodological limitations, suggest that the consistency of reported reductions in fall-related injuries across all programs supports the preliminary claim that the population-based approach to the prevention of fall-related injury is effective and can form the basis of public health practice [94]. Several fall prevention programs have shown to be also cost-effective: For example, the Stay on Your Feet [95] resulted in benefit to cost ratio of 20.6:1.21 [96]. Robertson et al. show that a home exercise program cost £441 per fall prevented [97], while Wilson reports that Yang-style Tai Chi classes given twice a week to nursing home residents comports a net cost savings of US$ 8.04 per participant per year (US$ 1274.43 per person per year when direct plus indirect benefits were considered) [98].

Coordinated, effective falls prevention strategies are needed in order to fight the emotional, physical, personal, and health resource costs associated with the increasing number of falls among the elderly.

Contrast Cognitive Impairment

There are currently 5.5 million people with dementia in Europe and 36 million worldwide. Alzheimer's disease, the most common form of dementia, affects 4% of people over the age of 65 and this figure is set to double within 50 years. For this reason, it has been called the "plague of the twenty-first century." The prevalence rises from around 2% among 65–69-year-olds to 22% among 85–89-year-olds. The number of people with cognitive impairment is expected to rise by more than 60% over the next 30 years. On the other hand, new reassuring evidences come from the literature challenging the alarming predictions about the future global burden of dementia. Christensen and colleagues' findings seem to identify an important plateau in dementia incidence after age 90 years, already suggested by the Rotterdam study investigators [99]. According to them, medical factors such as increased use of antithrombotics and lipid-lowering agents have brought to cognitive improvement over time.

The financial costs of managing dementia are enormous in terms of both public and private resources. The WHO estimates that the total cost of treating and caring for people with dementia is currently more than US$ 604 billion a year worldwide [100]. In several high-income countries, between a third and one half of people with dementia live in resource- and cost-intensive residential or nursing homes [101].

Much of the financial burden for caring for Alzheimer patients lies on the shoulders of family members, often with considerable financial strain, because home care and residential care services are lacking. Even when community services do exist, they are often not covered by state health insurance and thus remain the full financial responsibility of individuals and their families.

There is no definite cure for dementia, except when dementia is caused by drugs or vitamin imbalances, nor is there a standard course of development and death often occurs for pneumonia or other complications. For this reason, in the past decades the research has been focused not only on potential cures for the disease but also on possible determinants, with the aim of identifying possible preventive strategies. In 2008, the WHO launched the Mental Health Gap Action Programme which included dementia as a priority condition. This was then followed by a major report in 2012.

Epidemiological evidence has been accumulating that hypertension, hypercholesterolemia, and obesity are potential modifiable risk factors of Alzheimer's disease [102]. On the other hand, physical and social activity [103], a healthy diet [104], minimizing exposure to toxins (such as lead and mercury), and not smoking or abusing alcohol may all help reduce the risk of cognitive decline. Diabetes also increases the risk of dementia, and vascular dementia in particular, especially when it occurs together with severe systolic hypertension or heart disease [105].

Vaccination

Vaccines are a very powerful arm against infectious diseases with unquestioned benefits in terms of both individual and herd protection. Infectious diseases are the fifth leading cause of death [106] among older adults and approximately 90 % of influenza-related deaths occur among adults ages 65 years or more [107]. Since immunization is one of the most effective means of preventing disease and consequent disability and death, a fundamental opportunity for healthy aging consists in a correct use of vaccination programs in order to minimize the burden of preventable disease such as pneumococcal pneumonia [108, 109]. However, it is important to keep in mind that in the older adults the benefits of vaccination are limited, mainly because of the adaptive immune system's inability to generate protective immunity. The age-dependent decrease in immunological competence, often referred to as "immunosenescence" [110], results from the progressive deterioration of innate and adaptive immune responses (antibody titers are generally lower in the elderly and—particularly for inactivated vaccines—decline fast). It has been proved by Goodwin et al. [111] that rather than the estimated 70–90 % clinical vaccine efficacy in younger adults, the clinical efficacy in the elderly is 17–53 %, depending which

Table 8.1 Routinely recommended vaccines for the elderly (Reproduced from [115])

Vaccine	Inactivated influenza	Pneumococcal polysaccharide	Varicella-Zoster	Tetanus and diphtheria
Type of vaccine	Killed or inactivated virus	23 valent purified bacterial capsular polysaccharides	Live attenuated virus	Bacterial toxoids
Indications for vaccination	All adults equal or greater than 50	All adults equal or greater than 65	All adults equal or greater than 60	All previously unvaccinated adults. Patients with contaminated wound if 5 years have elapsed since last done
Contraindication for vaccination	Severe hypersensitivity reaction to the vaccine or eggs	Severe allergic reaction to the vaccine	Immunocompromised adults*. Persons with and without anaphylactic reaction to neomycin or gelatin	Severe allergic reaction to the vaccine
Revaccination schedule	Annually	One-time revaccination after 5 years if first dose before age 65	None	Every 10 years
Route of administration	Intramuscular injection	Intramuscular injection	Subcutaneous injection	–

* such as those with leukemia, lymphoma, or generalized malignancy and in patients receiving chemotherapy, radiation, and large doses of corticosteroids.

viruses were prevalent that year. This highlights the need for more immunogenic vaccine formulations for the elderly. Novel approaches, such as viral vectors for antigen delivery, DNA-based vaccines, and innovative adjuvants, particularly toll-like receptor agonists, will help to achieve optimal protection against infectious diseases also in old age [112, 113]. The current indications, in line with CDC recommended schedule for those over 65, are reported in Table 8.1 [114].

Screening

Unlike the relative consensus for immunization recommendations, there is considerable controversy regarding screening for specific disease states in older adults since the guidelines for the early diagnosis present more blurred boundaries than those defined for the adult population. Here follows an overlook of the role of early diagnosis to ensure a "healthy aging" protected by the chronic degenerative diseases.

Nicholas and Hall [116] pointed out how, with advancing age, the days of life lost when stopping the different screening programs progressively decrease. However, more and more studies show the importance of not relying on age alone, but to a more complex approach when referring to the older patient [117] since healthy elderly people seem to benefit from continuing cancer screening in respect of frail older individuals [118].

There is no doubt that the early diagnosis, when performed in accordance with the guidelines shared by the scientific community, provides a great benefit in many asymptomatic patients in terms of increased survival and quality of life. However, frail older people do not always profit from such maneuvers.

Considering the long latency in the onset of many chronic diseases, the relatively invasivity (or poor acceptability) of some of the screening procedures and consequent interventions in the event of a positive test, the reduced life expectancy, and the highest frequencies of comorbidities in the old population, it is very hard to establish a shared definition of a standard practice. The real goal should remain the warranty of a quality-of-life improvement after screening tests rather than simply a promise of "more years of life."

In addition, the cultural level and the cognitive status could compromise the ability of the subject to provide a truly informed consent, requiring a new definition of an individualized approach to screening procedures that should be adjusted to comorbidity, life expectancy, and patient preference [119]

This problem is particularly pressing when considering the neoplastic diseases. Hoffe and Balducci [120] in their review underline that also the natural history of cancer, the patient tolerance to treatment, the caregiver opinion, and the financial considerations are important in assessing treatment benefits and risks. They conclude that cooperation between geriatricians and oncologists can improve the decision making in the cancer of older patients. Eckstrom et al. [121] stress the need of additional research to fulfill the lack of evidence for older adults about the harms of screening tests in terms of overdiagnosis, effects of inaccurate test results, and possible complication of disease treatment. Globally, strong evidences lend support to the recommendation that clinicians should prioritize counseling about healthy lifestyle over cancer screening.

The guidelines are clear about the starting age for all the screening programs, but the evidence rating is lower on how long to continue cancer screening in older patients. Albert and Clark [122] in their review summarize that cervical, breast, colon, and prostate cancer screening can be discontinued, respectively, at the age of 65 years (Pap smear), approximately 75–80 years (mammography), 75 years (men)/80 years (women) (fecal occult blood test, barium enema, sigmoidoscopy/colonoscopy) and 75 years (prostate-specific antigen (PSA) testing and digital rectal examination). However, there is no shared consensus and different scientific societies expressing different opinions.

Until it will not be possible to decide on the basis of new screening guidelines based on individual life expectancy adjusted for comorbidities, poli pharmacotherapy and a variety of concurrent interventions/outcomes rather than for age only, the actual suggestion is to decide whether to continue or stop cancer screening after a careful two-way dialogue, combining evidence-based guidelines with individual patient preferences, better if with a "comprehensive geriatric assessment," as recommended by Terret et al.

In addition to the neoplastic diseases, an increasing awareness is growing in the scientific community about the need for more precise indications for early diagnosis also concerning other pathologies such as cardiovascular diseases, but also osteoporosis, diabetes, visual and hearing impairment. A recent review by Nicholas JA et al. about recommendations from various American agencies for "conventional" screening and prevention for the "young old" (>65 years), and for older adults (>80) has come after the increased emphasis that Medicare put over preventive care services for older adults after the Obama Reform (Affordable Care Act). In the same direction also the newly revised (2011–2012) guidelines for screening and preventive services by the US Preventive Services Task Force (USPSTF) and the CDC, even if all these recommendations are limited by the paucity of effectiveness studies in geriatric populations.

Key Elements for Decisions Makers

- Increasing life expectancy has led to higher expectations among people in the EU not only to live longer but also to live better lives with morbidity and disability compressed in fewer years and with a relatively high quality of life.
- As mortality rates between countries in the EU and also among different groups within the EU countries vary considerably, the age at which an individual is considered and considers himself/herself "older" also varies. The spectrum of aging has become rich with the definition of the "young old" (those aged 55–65) and the "oldest old" (those over 85). Subpopulations of nonagenarians and centenarians represent growing parts/slices of the society.
- Increased longevity is a great achievement, but also a formidable challenge for both public and private budgets, for the health system, and for the consequent impact on the future labor force and on economic growth. It the need to consider aging as an opportunity rather than a burden, valorizing older people, and their contribution to society is emerging.
- Healthy aging is therefore much more than increasing the number of healthy life-years without any activity limitation or disease. It has been defined as the process of optimizing opportunities for health to enable older people to take an active part in society and to enjoy an independent and positive life.
- Healthy aging should ideally start in childhood and take a lifelong perspective. A particular stress should be given to encourage/foster a healthy lifestyle also among the elderly, since it has been proved that "it is never too late." It should regard stopping harmful habits (smoke and alcohol), encouraging safe behavior such as physical exercise, correct diet, social relations, and participation in meaningful activities. For most of them the message should be: "some is good; more is better."

- Investing in prevention can have important benefits for the individuals involved but also for the whole society, since it has been demonstrated that it is cost-effective.
- Vaccination programs should be proposed to the geriatric population as they represent an effective strategy to prevent infectious diseases and related complications and death. New research must be focused on the creation of more powerful vaccines in order to avoid the well-known problem of immunosenescence.
- Screening programs in older people must be carried out with a more personalized and patient-tailored approach. New guidelines which take into consideration polimorbidity and polipharmacotheraly should be created in order to help clinicians in routine management of health promotion.
- Active aging should not remain only an isolated program. Healthy aging policies and practice, including life-long learning, working longer, retiring more gradually, and living actively after retirement, should be encouraged and supported at the international, national, and local level and should be integrated in all policy areas such as economy, housing, transport, and the environment.

References

1. Gorman M (1999) Development and the rights of older people. In: Randel J et al (Eds) The ageing and development report: poverty, independence and the world's older people. Earthscan Publications Ltd, London, p 3–21
2. WHO (2013) Definition of an older or elderly person. http://www.who.int/healthinfo/survey/ageingdefnolder/en/index.html. Accessed 20 Aug 2013
3. Baltes PB, Smith J (2003) New frontiers in the future of aging: from successful aging of the young old to the dilemmas of the fourth age. Gerontology 49(2):123–135
4. WHO (2013) Global health and aging. http://www.who.int/ageing/publications/global_health.pdf. Accessed 20 Aug 2013
5. WHO Regional Office for the Western Pacific (2013) Ageing and health a health promotion approach for developing countries. http://www.wpro.who.int/publications/pub_9290610662/en/index.html. Accessed 20 Aug 2013
6. Bowling A, Dieppe P (2005) What is successful ageing and who should define it? Br Med J 331:1548–1551
7. WHO (2001) Active ageing makes the difference. http://www.who.int/ageing/publications/alc_embrace2001_en.pdf. Accessed 22 Aug 2013
8. WHO (2002) Active ageing: a policy frame work. http://whqlibdoc.who.int/hq/2002/WHO_NMH_NPH_02.8.pdf. Accessed 21 Aug 2013
9. Europe's response to world ageing—Promoting economic and social progress in an ageing world. A contribution of the European Commission to the 2nd World Assembly on Ageing. COM (2002) 143 Final. Brussels
10. Oxley H (2009) Policies for healthy ageing: an overview. OECD health working papers. no 42. DELSA/HEA/WD/HWP (2009) 1
11. Vaillant GE (2002) Aging well: surprising guideposts to a happier life from the Landmark Harvard study of adult development. Little Brown, Boston
12. Ryff CD (1989) Beyond Ponce de Leon and life satisfaction: new directions in quest of successful aging. Int J Behav Dev 12:35–55
13. Leon DA (2011) Trends in European life expectancy: a salutary view. Int J Epidemiol 40:271–277

14. European Commission (2011) The 2012 ageing report: underlying assumptions and projection methodologies. Brussels: Joint Report prepared by the European Commission (DG ECFIN) and the Economic Policy Committee (AWG). European Economy 4/2011 37–45, 113–114
15. European Commission—Directorate-General for Economic and Financial Affairs (2012) The 2012 Ageing Report: economic and budgetary projections for the EU27 Member States (2010–2060). Joint Report prepared by the European Commission (DG ECFIN) and the Economic Policy Committee (AWG). EUROPEAN ECONOMY 2/2012 +
16. Kannisto V (2001) Development of oldest-old mortality, 1950–1990: evidence from 28 developed countries. Odense University Press, Odense
17. Robine JM, Saito Y, Jagger C (2003) The emergence of extremely old people: the case of Japan. Exp Gerontol 38:735–739
18. OECD (2011) Ageing, health and innovation: policy reforms to facilitate healthy and active ageing in OECD countries. OECD:delsa/hea (2011) 14
19. Stauner G (2008) The future of social security systems and demographic change. Eur View 7:203–208
20. Bloom DE, Canning D (2008) Global demographic change: dimensions and economic significance. Popul Dev Rev 34:17–51
21. United Nations (2008) World population prospects, 2008 revision
22. Centers for Disease Prevention and Control (2003) Public health and aging: trends in ageing—United States and worldwide. MMWR Weekly 52(6):101–106
23. Lagiewka K (2012) European innovation partnership on active and healthy ageing: triggers of setting the headline target of 2 additional healthy life years at birth at EU average by 2020. Arch Public Health 70(1):23
24. Fries JF, Bruce B, Chakravarty E (2011) Compression of morbidity 1980–2011: a focused review of paradigms and progress. J Aging Res 2011: 261702. doi:10.4061/2011/261702
25. Ahtonen A (2012). Healthy and active ageing: turning the 'silver' economy into gold. European Policy Centre. POLICY BRIEF
26. World Bank data. http://data.worldbank.org/country/united-states. Accessed 21 Aug 2013
27. Liberman SM, Lee J, Anderson T et al. (2003) Reducing the growth of medicare spending: geographic versus patient-based strategies. Health Aff (Millwood) (Suppl Web Exclusives) W3-603-13.
28. McKee M, Healy J (2002) Pressures for change. In: McKee M, Healy J (Eds) Hospitals in a changing Europe. Open University Press, Buckingham, p 36–58
29. Casey B et al (2003) Policies for an ageing society: recent measures and areas for further reform. OECD, Paris
30. Anderson G, Hussey P (2001) Comparing health system performance in OECD countries. Health Affairs 20:219–232
31. The European Union (2012) The council endorses the 2012 ageing report: economic and budgetary projections for the 27 EU Member States (2010–2060). European Economy 2012(2)
32. Rechel B et al (2009) Investing in hospitals of the future. WHO Regional Office for Europe, Copenhagen
33. Rechel B, Doyle Y, Grundy E, McKee M (2009) How can health systems respond to population ageing? Health Systems and Policy Analysis
34. The Swedish National Institute of Public Health (2007) Healthy ageing: a challenge for Europe. Huskvarna
35. Ramage-Morin PL, Shields M, Martel L (2010) Health-promoting factors and good health among Canadians in mid- to late life. Health Rep 21(3):45–53
36. Centers for Disease Control and Prevention and The Merck Company Foundation (2007) The state of aging and health in America 2007. The Merck Company Foundation, Whitehouse Station
37. Ljubuncic P, Globerson A, Reznick AZ (2008) Evidence-based roads to the promotion of health in old age. J Nutr Health Aging 12(2):139–143

38. Peel NM, McClure RJ, Bartlett HP (2005) Behavioral determinants of healthy aging. Am J Prev Med 28(3):298–304
39. Newman AB, Arnold AM, Naydeck BL et al (2003) Successful aging: effect of subclinical cardiovascular disease. Arch Intern Med 163:2315–2322
40. Vaillant GE, Mukamal K (2011) Successful aging. Am J Psychiatry 158:839–847
41. Rimm EB, Klatsky A, Grobbee D, Stampfer MJ (1996) Review of moderate alcohol consumption and reduced risk of coronary heart disease: is the effect due to beer, wine, or spirits. BMJ 312(7033):731–736
42. Ilomäki J, Paljärvi T, Korhonen MJ et al (2013) Prevalence of concomitant use of alcohol and sedative-hypnotic drugs in middle and older aged persons: a systematic review. Ann Pharmacother 47(2):257–268
43. Meier P, Seitz HK (2008) Age, alcohol metabolism and liver disease. Curr Opin Clin Nutr Metab Care 11:21–26
44. Alcohol Research UK (2011) Working with older drinkers. Alcohol Research, London
45. Reid MC, Boutros NN, O'Connor PG, Cadariu A, Concato J (2002) The health-related effects of alcohol use in older persons: a systematic review. Subst Abus 23(3):149–164
46. Panza F, Capurso C, D'Introno A et al (2009) Alcohol drinking, cognitive functions in older age, predementia, and dementia syndromes. J Alzheimers Dis 17(1):7–31
47. Peters R, Peters J, Warner J, Beckett N, Bulpitt C (2008) Alcohol, dementia and cognitive decline in the elderly: a systematic review. Age Ageing 37(5):505–512
48. Anderson P, Scafato E, Galluzzo L, VINTAGE project Working Group (2012) Alcohol and older people from a public health perspective. Ann Ist Super Sanita 48(3):232–247
49. Sayer AA, Syddall HE, Gilbody HJ, Dennison EM, Cooper C (2004) Does sarcopenia originate in early life? Findings from the Hertfordshire Cohort Study. J Gerontol 59A:930–934
50. Robinson SM, Simmonds SJ, Jameson KA et al (2012) Muscle strength in older community-dwelling men is related to type of milk feeding in infancy. J Geront A Biol Sci Med Sci 67:990–996
51. Sayer AA, Robinson SM, Patel HP, Shavlakadze T, Cooper C, Grounds MD (2013) New horizons in the pathogenesis, diagnosis and management of sarcopenia. Age Ageing 42(2):145–150. doi:10.1093/ageing/afs191
52. Cooper R, Kuh D, Hardy R (2010) Objectively measured physical capability levels and mortality: systematic review and meta-analysis. Br Med J 341:c4467
53. Janssen I, Shepard DS, Katzmarzyk PT, Roubenoff R (2004) The healthcare costs of sarcopenia in the United States. J Am Geriatr Soc 52:80–85
54. Nieuwenhuizen WF, Weenen H, Rigby P, Hetherington MM (2010) Older adults and patients in need of nutritional support: review of current treatment options and factors influencing nutritional intake. Clin Nutr 29(2):160–169. doi:10.1016/j.clnu.2009.09.003
55. Murphy C (2008) The chemical senses and nutrition in older adults. J Nutr Elder 27(3–4):247–265
56. Robinson S, Cooper C, Aihie SA (2012) Nutrition and sarcopenia: a review of the evidence and implications for preventive strategies. J Aging Res 2012:510801
57. Houston DK, Nicklas BJ, Ding J et al (2008) Dietary protein intake is associated with lean mass change in older, community-dwelling adults: the Health, Aging, and Body Composition (Health ABC) Study. Am J Clin Nutr 87:150–155
58. Milne AC, Potter J, Vivanti A, Avenell A (2009) Protein and energy supplementation in elderly people at risk from malnutrition. Cochrane Database Syst Rev 15(2):CD003288. doi:10.1002/14651858.CD003288.pub3
59. Guo SS, Wu W, Chumlea WC, Roche AF (2002) Predicting overweight and obesity in adulthood from body mass index values in childhood and adolescence. Am J Clin Nutr 76:653–658
60. Guo SS, Roche AF, Chumlea WC, Gardner JD, Siervogel RM (1994) The predictive value of childhood body mass index values for overweight at age 35 y. Am J Clin Nutr 59:810–819

61. McNaughton SA, Crawford D, Ball K, Salmon J (2012) Understanding determinants of nutrition, physical activity and quality of life among older adults: the Wellbeing, Eating and Exercise for a Long Life (WELL) study. Health Qual Life Outcomes 10:109
62. Shepherd A (2009) Nutrition through the life span. Part 3: adults aged 65 years and over. Br J Nur 18(5):301–307
63. Robinson SM, Jameson KA, Batelaan SF et al (2008) Diet and its relationship with grip strength in community-dwelling older men and women: the Hertfordshire cohort study, J Am Geriatr Soc 56(1):84–90
64. Södergren M, McNaughton SA, Salmon J, Ball K, Crawford DA (2012) Associations between fruit and vegetable intake, leisure-time physical activity, sitting time and self-rated health among older adults: cross-sectional data from the WELL study. BMC Public Health 12:551
65. Bandayrel K, Wong S (2011) Systematic literature review of randomized control trials assessing the effectiveness of nutrition interventions in community-dwelling older adults. J Nutr Educ Behav 43:251–262
66. Cooper R, Kuh D, Hardy R, Mortality Review Group, FALCon and HALCyon Study Teams (2010) Objectively measured physical capability levels and mortality: systematic review and meta-analysis. Br Med J 341:c4467
67. Pedersen BK, Saltin B (2006) Evidence for prescribing exercise as therapy in chronic disease. Scand J Med Sci Sports 16(S1):3–63
68. Walker KZ, O'Dea K, Gomez M, Girgis S, Colagiuri R (2010) Diet and exercise in the prevention of diabetes. J Hum Nutr Diet 23(4):344–352
69. Kelley GA, Kelley KS (2006) Aerobic exercise and HDL2-C: a meta-analysis of randomized controlled trials. Atherosclerosis 184(1): 207–215
70. Adami PE, Negro A, Lala N, Martelletti P (2010) The role of physical activity in the prevention and treatment of chronic diseases. Clinica Clin Ter 161(6):537–541
71. Warburton DE, Charlesworth S, Ivey A, Nettlefold L, Bredin SS (2010) A systematic review of the evidence for Canada's Physical Activity Guidelines for Adults. Int J Behav Nutr Phys Act 7:39
72. Lee CD, Folsom AR, Blair SN (2003) Physical activity and stroke risk. A meta-analysis. Stroke 34:2475–2482
73. Halle M, Schoenberg MH (2009) Physical activity in the prevention and treatment of colorectal carcinoma. Dtsch Arztebl Int 106(44):722–727
74. Monninkhof EM, Elias SG, Vlems FA et al (2007) Physical activity and breast cancer: a systematic review. Epidemiology 18(1):137–157
75. Reimers CD, Knapp G, Reimers AK (2012) Does physical activity increase life expectancy? A review of the literature. J Aging Res 2012:243958
76. Nusselder WJ, Looman CW, Franco OH, Peeters A, Slingerland AS, Mackenbach JP (2008) The relation between non-occupational physical activity and years lived with and without disability. Epidemiol Community Health 62(9):823–828
77. Dunsky A, Netz Y (2012) Physical activity and sport in advanced age: is it risky? A summary of data from articles published between 2000–2009. Curr Aging Sci 5(1):66–71
78. Paillard-Borg S, Fratiglioni L, Xu W, Winblad B, Wang HX (2012) An active lifestyle postpones dementia onset by more than one year in very old adults. J Alzheimers Dis 31(4):835–842
79. Callaghan P (2004) Exercise: a neglected intervention in mental health care? J Psychiatr Ment Health Nurs 11(4):476–483
80. Landi F, Abbatecola AM, Provinciali M (2010) Moving against frailty: does physical activity matter? Biogerontology 11(5):537–545
81. Angevaren M, Aufdemkampe G, Verhaar HJ, Aleman A, Vanhees L (2008) Physical activity and enhanced fitness to improve cognitive function in older people without known cognitive impairment. Cochrane Database Syst Rev (3):CD005381

82. Figueira HA, Figueira AA, Cader SA et al (2012) Effects of a physical activity governmental health programme on the quality of life of elderly people. Scand J Public Health 40(5):418–422
83. Liu CJ, Latham NK (2009) Progressive resistance strength training for improving physical function in older adults. Cochrane Database Syst Rev (3):CD002759
84. Samitz G, Egger M, Zwahlen M (2011) Domains of physical activity and all-cause mortality: systematic review and doseresponse meta-analysis of cohort studies. Int J Epidemiol 40(5):1382–1400
85. Munro J, Brazier J, Davey R, Nicholl J (1997) Physical activity for the over-65s: could it be a cost-effective exercise for the NHS? J Public Health Med 19(4):397–402
86. Munro JF, Nicholl JP, Brazier JE, Davey R, Cochrane T (2003) Cost effectiveness of a community based exercise programme in over 65 year olds: cluster randomised trial. J Epidemiol Community Health 58(12):1004–1010
87. Rhodes RE, Mark RS, Temmel CP (2012) Adult sedentary behavior: a systematic review. Am J Prev Med 42(3):e3–e28
88. Inoue S, Sugiyama T, Takamiya T, Oka K, Owen N, Shimomitsu T (2012) Television viewing time is associated with overweight/obesity among older adults, independent of meeting physical activity and health guidelines. J Epidemiol 22(1):50–56
89. Hill K et al (2004) An analysis of research on preventing falls and falls injury in older people: community, residential care and hospital settings (2004 update). National Ageing Research Institute and Centre for Applied Gerontology, report to the Australian Government, Department of Health and Ageing, Injury Prevention Section: Melbourne.
90. Stevens JA, Corso PS, Finkelstein EA, Miller TR (2006) The cost of fatal and non-fatal falls among older adults. Injury Prevention 12:290–295
91. Gillespie LD, Robertson MC, Gillespie WJ, Gates S, Clemson LM, Lamb SE (2012) Interventions for preventing falls in elderly people. Cochrane Database Syst Rev 9:CD007146
92. Cameron ID, Gillespie LD, Robertson MC et al (2012) Interventions for preventing falls in older people in care facilities and hospitals. Cochrane Database Syst Rev 12:CD005465
93. Neyens JC, van Haastregt JC, Dijcks BP et al (2011) Effectiveness and implementation aspects of interventions for preventing falls in elderly people in long-term care facilities: a systematic review of RCTs. J Am Med Dir Assoc 12(6):410–425
94. McClure R, Turner C, Peel N, Spinks A, Eakin E, Hughes K (2005) Population-based interventions for the prevention of fall-related injuries in older people. Cochrane Database Syst Rev (1):CD004441
95. http://www.health.wa.gov.au/stayonyourfeet/home/. Accessed 23 Aug 2013
96. Kempton A et al (2000) Older people can stay on their feet: final results of a community-based falls prevention programme. Health Promot Int 15(1):27–33
97. Robertson MC, Gardner MM, Devlin N, McGee R, Campbell AJ (2001) Effectiveness and economic evaluation of a nurse delivered home exercise programme to prevent falls. Controlled trial in multiple centres. Br Med J 322(7288):701–704
98. Wilson C, Datta K (2001) Tai Chi for prevention of fractures in a nursing home population: an economic analysis. J Clin Outcomes Manag 8:19–27
99. Schrijvers EM, Verhaaren BF, Koudstaal PJ, Hofman A, Ikram MA, Breteler MM (2012) Is dementia incidence declining? Trends in dementia incidence since 1990 in the Rotterdam Study. Neurology 78:1456–1463
100. WHO (2012) Mental Health Gap Action Programme (mhGAP). http://www.who.int/mental_health/mhGAP_nl_June_2012.pdf. Accessed 17 Aug 2013
101. WHO (2012) Dementia: a public health priority. WHO, Geneva. http://whqlibdoc.who.int/publications/2012/9789241564458_eng.pdf. Accessed 17 Aug 2013
102. Solomon A, Sippola R, Soininen H et al (2010) Lipid-lowering treatment is related to decreased risk of dementia: a population-based study (FINRISK). Neurodegener Dis 7(1–3):180–182. doi:10.1159/000295659
103. Rovio S, Kåreholt I, Helkala EL et al (2005) Leisure-time physical activity at midlife and the risk of dementia and Alzheimer's disease. Lancet Neurol 4(11):705–711

104. Frisardi V, Panza F, Seripa D et al (2010) Nutraceutical properties of Mediterranean diet and cognitive decline: possible underlying mechanisms. J Alzheimers Dis 22(3):715–740. doi:10.3233/JAD-2010-100942
105. Xu WL, Qiu CX, Wahlin A, Winblad B, Fratiglioni L (2004) Diabetes mellitus and risk of dementia in the Kungsholmen project: a 6-year follow-up study. Neurology 63(7):1181–1186
106. National Center for Health Statistics (2007) Trends in health and aging. Trends in causes of death among older persons in the United States. http://www.cdc.gov/nchs/agingact.htm. Accessed 16 Aug 2007
107. Thompson WW, Matthew R et al (2009) Estimating influenza-associated deaths in the United States. Am J Public Health 99(2):S225–S230. doi:10.2105/AJPH.2008.151944
108. Ludwig E, Unal S, Bogdan M et al (2012) Opportunity for healthy ageing: lessening the burden of adult pneumococcal disease in Central and Eastern Europe, and Israel. Cent Eur J Public Health 20(2):121–125
109. Assaad U, El-Masri I, Porhomayon J, El-Solh AA (2012) Pneumonia immunization in older adults: review of vaccine effectiveness and strategies. Clin Interv Aging 7:453–461
110. Goronzy JJ, Weyand CM (2013) Understanding immunosenescence to improve responses to vaccines. Nat Immunol 14(5):428–436
111. Goodwin K, Viboud C, Simonsen L (2006) Antibody response to influenza vaccination in the elderly: a quantitative review. Vaccine 24(8):1159–1169
112. Weinberger B, Grubeck-Loebenstein B (2012) Vaccines for the elderly. Clin Microbiol Infect. 18(5):100–108. doi:10.1111/j.1469-0691.2012.03944.x
113. Derhovanessian E, Pawelec G (2012) Vaccination in the elderly. Microb Biotechnol 5(2):226–232
114. Centers for Disease Control and Prevention (CDC) (2006) Recommended adult immunization schedule: United States, October 2006-September 2007. MMWR Morb Mortal Wkly Rep 55:Q1–Q4
115. Bader M.S (2007) Immunization for the elderly. Am J Med Sci 334(6):481–486
116. Nicholas JA, Hall WJ (2011) Screening and preventive services for older adults. Mt Sinai J Med 78(4):498–508
117. Flaherty JH (2008) Cancer screening in older patients: life expectancy, prioritization, and health literacy. Am Fam Physician 78(12):1336–1338
118. Terret C, Castel-Kremer E, Albrand G, Droz JP (2009) Effects of comorbidity on screening and early diagnosis of cancer in elderly people. Lancet Oncol 10(1):80–87. doi:10.1016/S1470-2045(08)70336-X
119. Clarfield AM (2010). Screening in frail older people: an ounce of prevention or a pound of trouble? J Am Geriatr Soc 58(10):2016–2021
120. Hoffe S, Balducci L (2012) Cancer and age: general considerations. Clin Geriatr Med 28(1):1–18
121. Eckstrom E, Feeny DH, Walter LC, Perdue LA, Whitlock EP (2013) Individualizing cancer screening in older adults: a narrative review and framework for future research. J Gen Int Med 28(2):292–298
122. Albert RH, Clark MM (2008) Cancer screening in the older patient. Am Fam Physician 78(12):1369–1374, 1376

Chapter 9
Some Ethical Reflections in Public Health

Maria Luisa Di Pietro

The Field of Investigation

Before commencing an ethical reflection in public health, it is necessary to define the field of investigation. This is not an easy task since the concepts of both "public health" and "health" have largely evolved in time.

The different interpretations of the concept of "health" are the symptom of the difficulty to define "health" if not by referring to its opposite: "disease." In *The Conflict of the Faculties (Third section),* Kant argues that the definition of health is problematic, because we can only perceive disease [1]. In [2] other words, we are not able to "measure" well-being but only to distinguish disease from a state of normal health. Furthermore, in the *Letter on the deaf and dumb for the use of those who hear and speak,* Diderot writes: "When we are well, we are unconscious of any part of our body; and if any part draws attention to itself by pain, we are certainly not well; and if it is by a pleasurable sensation, it is by no means certain that we are the better for it" [3].

The definition of "health" represents, therefore, a philosophical issue to the same degree as its reflection on public health: "The first decision—MacKee and Raine write—to make when developing a public-health strategy must be to decide the philosophical basis on which it is to stand" [4]."Health" could be interpreted according to three paradigms: the reductionist paradigm, the static paradigm, and the dynamic paradigm.

The reductionist paradigm refers exclusively to the human body. The concept of "health" does not consider the psychological, affective, social, and moral dimensions of the human being, but only the physical efficiency and absence of disease.

M. L. Di Pietro (✉)
Institute of Public Health, Section of Hygiene, Università Cattolica del Sacro Cuore,
L.go F. Vito 1, 00168 Rome, Italy
e-mail: mldipietro@rm.unicatt.it

S. Boccia et al. (eds.), *A Systematic Review of Key Issues in Public Health,*
DOI 10.1007/978-3-319-13620-2_9

The diagnosis and the cure of a disease, which is considered an incidental event in life, is the aim of medical intervention in order to eliminate the symptoms and to reestablish physical efficiency.

In 1946, the World Health Organization (WHO) defined health as "a state of complete physical, mental and social well-being and not merely the absence of disease or infirmity." This definition, which includes both the words "state" and "complete," gives space to two interpretations: the static interpretation and the dynamic interpretation.

According to the static interpretation, the abovementioned state of complete health is in realty rather impossible to reach and all conditions of discomfort are to be considered illness with the consequent risk of a "medicalization" of life. In this interpretation, for example, even some physiological conditions (dissatisfaction during adolescence, symptoms of menopause, the lack of energy in old age) become "disease."

According to the dynamic interpretation, on the other hand, health becomes an equilibrium within the dynamics of everyday experience. An alteration of this equilibrium can cause disease, which in this case does not assume the characteristics of a mere accident but represents, instead, the necessity to seek a new equilibrium, through a growth process in one's self-awareness and responsibility. The human being, therefore, is to be considered "healthy" when he/she is capable to carry out his/her intentions in a conscious and free way within the various situations of life. On the contrary, the human being is to be considered "sick" when he/she is unable to manage life and to enhance his/her skills. As a consequence, in addition to "perfect" health, there is also a condition of "relative" health: it is possible to find one's own equilibrium even in a condition of lifelong disability. Therefore, it is evident that the search for health is part of a search for the meaning of life and that "health" is a duty, a lifestyle, which includes not only the physical, mental, and social dimensions but also the ethical dimension. In other words, health is directly related to one's individual choices and behaviors. In this perspective, the aim of medicine is not only diagnosis, treatment, and rehabilitation (such as in the static interpretation) but also health promotion, and disease prevention.

Within this context, the determinants of health (medical, environmental, educational, economic, etc.) and the possibilities of intervention in public health increase. And the areas of public health are not simply hygiene and the prevention of communicable diseases but also the health condition of the population, the health promotion, the prevention of noncommunicable diseases, the availability and administration of health services, and the management of economic resources.

In public health, you can, therefore, identify two fields of intervention, which differ in extension: (1) a narrower field, which includes only interventions designed to identify (monitoring) and reduce the risk factors of disease (prevention); (2) a wider field, which also addresses the socioeconomic factors (organization of health services and social health services, assistance management, resource allocation, etc.). In this chapter, we refer to the narrower field of intervention in public health organization, whose mission is: the promotion of physical and psychosocial health and the prevention of disease, accidents, and disability. We also mention, as regards to justice, the issue of priorities in health interventions.

Health Promotion and Prevention of Disease: The Difference Between Public Health and Clinics

Health promotion and disease prevention are two areas of intervention that often get overlapped, although their objectives and approach are different [5].

Health promotion is based, in fact, on a positive and holistic interpretation which encompasses physical, psychological, social, and moral dimensions. The Ottawa Charter, presented in 1986, states that health promotion must be conceived as a process that enables people to increase control over, and to improve, their health, to identify and to realize their aspirations, to satisfy needs, and to change or cope with the environment [6]. Therefore, the real protagonist of health is the person, not the institution. In fact, the institution must put the person in a position to have the power (empowerment) and the knowledge to make choices, while ensuring conditions of complete physical, mental, and relational well-being. This involves responsibilities on both a social (health, social, and environmental policies) and personal level (of the individual, of the group, of the community). Health promotion should, in fact, accommodate the needs of each person and try to eliminate the differences and conditions of inequity [7].

In order to obtain this objective, it is necessary that there be a sense of justice and an educational project and—sometimes—normative interventions (coercive or noncoercive). However, the necessity for normative interventions is an evident signal that the educational project was not implemented or that it was not adequate for the obtainment of the desired objective (for example, to promote and overcome the resistance toward a healthy lifestyle).

When the cultural and educational dimensions are absent in health, health may not even have a public dimension. In fact, if healthy individuals adapt to their tasks in silence and live their lives in the relative freedom of their choices, the society could also ignore them and perceive their presence only when they become sick. Health promotion, however, precedes the "noise" of disease and works not only for the "silence" of the organs but also for the discretion of social relations.

It is then evident that the promotion of health also moves from dynamics that are outside of the world of health care but that are instead cultural, educational, social, economic, and environmental. Promoting health means, in fact, also taking care of, for example, the environment, food and drug safety, urban planning, and occupational health. In this context, health education transcends the objective of "remedy" and becomes a space for the acquisitions of skills: to acquire the capability to distinguish needs from desires; to become aware of one's own actions, responsibility, critical thought, evaluation criteria, and motivations; and to take actions according to freedom and responsibility.

Health education thus becomes: "the art of maieutics" that brings forth (*e-ducere*) the positive elements that can be found in each person; "the pedagogy of freedom" that indicates what can improve our health so as to be able to make choices that ameliorate our life. Society's commitment is, therefore, not only to give an education that indicates "what to do" but also that helps each person acquire the ability of obtaining their own good.

Health is not affected, of course, only by individual behavior but also by the environment and the context in which the given behavior takes place. For this reason, individual and social responsibilities are closely intertwined. This indicates the necessity that there be a balance between responsibility on a personal and public health level in order to prevent forms of "health fascism" or "preventive fanaticism."

Unlike the promotion of health, the prevention of disease derives from the negative interpretation of health, in other words, its opposite: disease. "Prevention" means, in fact, to act against something that could cause harm. The strategies that promote health (salutogenesis), therefore, become replaced by defensive strategies toward what may determine the loss of health (pathogenesis).

Prevention is, without doubt, an asset since its objectives are: the improvement of the quality and expectancy of life; the acquisition of knowledge about risk factors and diseases, allowing the reduction of morbidity and mortality in the population. It is sufficient to say that prevention has: a universal dimension (diminishing inequalities); an anticipatory value (prediction of a future harm/ disease); and a good cost–benefit ratio (reduction of pain and suffering).

Prevention, however, presents some critical aspects. For example, prevention: targets subjects who are "healthy" or in a preclinical stage of disease; it is sometimes only a "promise" of prevention; in some cases it determines a benefit to society but not to the individual; it may reduce personal freedom and cause a "stigmatization" of the individual; it may cause a "medicalization" of life and expose the individual to the risk of side effects and at times even reduce their quality of life. According to some, it is from this point of view that preventive medicine reveals its impersonal and presumptuous character.

In fact, we cannot deny that disease prevention tends to focus on the needs of society and not on those of the individual. This idea of prevention is evident in those intervention policies that simply favor forms of "risk reduction." These interventions, in fact, invite the individual to sponsor certain remedies in order to obtain a reduction of risk within risk behaviors, but they do not help the individual to abandon these behaviors.

Respect for human life and health requires that the application of preventive measures in the population must always be preceded by sufficient research, the minimization of associated risks, and the adequate information of the population on any possible damage, burdens, and side effects. Prevention should also be guaranteed to the greatest number of people possible, assuring also in the case of diagnosis the necessary assistance. Information decisively plays a central role in prevention, because, while respecting the individual's autonomy, it is what makes him/her understand and desire to adhere to the proposed program. It is, in addition, an important element in not creating a false sense of security. For example, the positive result of a screening (i.e., the absence of risk factors) should not determine in the individual a reduction in the importance given to certain lifestyles (nor, on the other hand, should the screening generate anxiety regarding their health).

From the analysis of these two areas of intervention (health promotion and disease prevention), it is already possible to identify the profound differences between public health and clinical activity.

Clinical activity is focused on diagnosis, treatment, care, and rehabilitation based on the request of the patient, who seeks the doctor because of a specific need. An interpersonal relationship is therefore established in which the doctor declares his/her knowledge and skills and promises to help the patient. Medicine is, therefore, not only clinical interaction but also:

- A relationship between that specific doctor and that specific patient
- An interaction that focuses on the human body and its main objective (though not exclusive) is the restoration of a condition of health
- An unbalanced relationship in which the physician possesses the necessary knowledge and expertise to respond to the patient's request for health

Public health programs do not respond, however, to a request expressed by the "patient" (in fact, the absence of symptoms makes this definition inapplicable) but are targeted to the general population rather than the individual. As regards to the population, public health is interested in: measuring the health status through epidemiological and biostatistic methods; identifying health risks and developing health policies to contrast them; and providing certain health services.

On the other hand, in public health some elements are lacking compared to clinical activity, and they are, above all, the interpersonal relationship (doctor–patient) and the attention to the specific characteristics of the single individuals. For example, the sensitivity of mass communication toward the individual is often inadequate and there is also a tendency to overlook the individual when analyzing the effectiveness of an intervention.

The needs of the community may, as a consequence, be in conflict with the needs of the individual. Some examples are: quarantine in the case of an infectious disease, the allocation of resources in areas of public intervention that subtract funds for individual needs, or the determination of risk acceptance criteria only on the basis of cost–benefit assessment.

How can we avoid slipping toward a paternalistic approach in public health? Does the individual have a responsibility in promoting public health and participating in the protection of the community? And most importantly, what is public health? Is it "health of the population" or "health in the population"?

According to the first definition ("health of the population"), public health is to be understood as the knowledge of the health conditions of the population (incidence of morbidity and mortality) or as the sum of the states of health of all the members of society (aggregational dimension) and the distribution of the level of health within the population (distributional dimension). In the second definition ("health in the population"), public health includes all the collective public interventions which favor the population's health without taking into account the actions of individuals [8].

Ethics in Public Health

The ethical debate (or rather, the "bioethical debate") has given little attention to the problems in public health. On the other hand, the field of bioethics developed in the 1970s mostly in response to other necessities: the repetitive abuses in research on human beings, the birth of movements in support of human rights, and the risks due to a medicine enriched by constantly more powerful technology [9].

Public health, however, falls inside the areas of bioethical reflection. The definition of 1978 ("the systematic study of human behavior in the context of the study of life, health and conduct examined in the light of values and moral principles") and the definition of 1995 ("systematic study of the moral dimensions—including the moral view, decisions, conduct and policies in the sciences and health—using a variety of ethical methodologies with an interdisciplinary approach") of the Encyclopedia of Bioethics include, in fact, much broader areas of intervention, than simply clinical activity [10]. The peculiar nature of public health interventions makes it also necessary to make some specific reflections.

For this reason, bioethics started taking interest in public health starting from the mid-1990s. It became evident, in fact, that the health of the population is also affected by actions of good health governance and by adequate socioeconomic conditions, and not just by medical dynamics. This, of course, does not mean to say that public health does not depend also on medical knowledge. It is sufficient to think, for example, of screening programs and of the use of biomedical techniques.

Being the result of human choices, public health interventions can be assessed by an ethical point of view, just like any other human action that is the fruit of individual freedom and will. What are the ethical issues in public health?

In time, the already evident public health issues (health promotion, disease prevention, risk reduction, epidemiology, and other forms of research in public health, structural, and socioeconomic disparities in health interventions) have been enriched by other important challenges such as the increase of chronic diseases, conditions of disability, and the health risks caused by environmental pollution. And it is in this context that further questions arise: what degree of risk may be considered acceptable for individuals and society? Is it justified to put in act interventions that may violate the autonomy (i.e., by not following the rules of informed consent) and the privacy of the individual in order to reduce the risk for society? How to avoid socioeconomic inequality and enable equal access to health care? These decisions are not always simple, often due to the lack of precise data and because besides the biological, epidemiological, and clinical aspects, we must also take into account the social and behavioral aspects [11].

That having been said, it becomes necessary not only to reflect on the individual ethical issues but, above all, also to define our ethical basis. We can identify four ethical approaches (subjectivism, intersubjectivism, descriptivism, objectivism), which differ in their parameter of reference (freedom, utility, behavior of the majority, and person).

Freedom Freedom is the first reference value in subjectivist ethics to which other philosophical currents such as emotionalism, decisionism, and liberalism refer. "Good" is exclusively that which is freely desired, without taking into account the action's consequences on oneself or on others. It is a freedom without constraints, a freedom without responsibility, yet a limited freedom, since it cannot be exercised by all but only by those who are able to express and assert it; a freedom that can exist only in a context of tolerance toward one another.

Usefulness The intersubjectivist philosophy tries to overcome the social weakness of subjectivism and considers usefulness as the ethical parameter of reference. Utility is measured by the calculation of the cost–benefit ratio. Benefit is evaluated in economical terms or in pleasure obtained. Something is considered "useful" if it is economically profitable or if it is able to maximize the well-being and minimize the pain for the greatest number of people.

Social Behavior In descriptivism, the moral norm is determined by the behavior of the majority of the people within a particular historical and social context. If the social and historical contexts change, even the moral judgment can change and ethics therefore adapts to the situation that is in continuous evolution.

The Person For objectivism, the measure of lecitness or illecitness of an act is the person, conceived in a holistic sense. Freedom considered as the capability to plan, be aware, choose, etc., is a characteristic that depends on the nature of the human being. In this context, autonomy is based on the integration of freedom and responsibility. Autonomous agents can adopt moral constraints, willingly submitting to norms to which they have given their consent. Autonomy is equated with positive freedom, with self-mastery, and with being in charge of oneself. Being a person imposes then—as Kant would write—the categorical imperative to act so as to treat oneself and others always as an end and never as mere means. In this sense, the *bonum,* the ultimate value that measures any moral action is the promotion of the human being and of its great value as a person.

Given the complexity of public health and within a context of ethical pluralism, how can we overcome certain issues and conflicts? For example, how can we solve the conflict between the paternalistic approach of public health and the respect of autonomy in the case of vaccinations?

From Obligation to Responsibility: The Case of Vaccinations

The debate whether some vaccinations should be mandatory or recommended is an example of a conflict between the paternalistic approach of some interventions in public health and the right to exercise autonomy [12]. As we know, the attitude toward vaccinations is ambivalent. Though some reject mandatory vaccinations for religious reasons or because they consider them to be an abuse of individual freedom, on the other hand, others draw attention to their undeniable advantages. In fact, from a scientific point of view, it has been demonstrated that vaccinations have:

- A positive efficacy–safety ratio. The health risks are, in fact, modest, especially with the use of the newer preparations, which are subjected to randomized control trials (RCTs) that ensure their safety and effectiveness. In addition, while the number of deaths prevented by vaccinations is constantly increasing, a large number of people still are dying because they were not vaccinated.
- A positive cost–effectiveness ratio. We must compare the cost of the administration of the vaccine with the costs that arises in case the corresponding disease is contracted: direct costs (i.e., health care, therapeutic treatments, possible hospitalization, suffering, pain, dependency) and indirect costs (i.e., loss of work days or school).

It is also necessary to emphasize the social value of vaccinations. In fact, through the mechanism of herd immunity, it is possible to obtain a dual effect: by safeguarding those who undergo the vaccination we also obtain a "protection" of the remaining part of the population.

Vaccinations are, therefore, beneficial at both a personal and social level: Should they, however, be considered mandatory? Although mandatory vaccinations have allowed us to achieve results that would not have been obtained in any other way, there is an attempt to find alternative models in order to switch from mandatory administration to a responsible choice. In fact, it could not be otherwise in a time in which medical practice is characterized by the patient's exercise of autonomy and by the necessity of an informed consent.

Exercising autonomy, however, requires that the subject take responsibility for his/her own choices. This underlines the moral dimension of the transition from a compulsory administration to a free choice. There would no longer be the imposition on the subject of a behavior that has been established by others (the so-called ethics of the third person), but an attempt to help the subject to understand the motivations and to freely make a choice that is good for their own and others' lives (the so-called ethics of the first person).

That the logic behind vaccinations is connected to the ethics of the third person is evident from the two reasons used in its support [13]:

- The first reason is that a contagious disease can also cause unintentional damage to others and this risk can be reduced by a vaccine. Since there is a moral obligation not to cause harm to others through acts or omissions, there is also subsequently the obligation to reduce the risk of causing harm to others by accepting a vaccination. Some objections could be: (1) since many people contract the disease, it cannot depend on one person's responsibility and (2) there are also diseases (i.e., tetanus) in which, even if the subject is not vaccinated, they can only harm themselves and not others.
- The second reason derives from Kant's third categorical imperative—"Act so that your will may establish a universal law"—each person must, therefore, contribute to the good of the society to which they belong also through the use of vaccinations and the immunization of the population. Those who object to this

motivation point out that the introduction of an obligation is detrimental to the autonomy of the subject and that if a person refused to participate in a vaccination program, it would then be necessary to provide a sanction, which would limit even more the freedom of choice.

A conscious choice must instead refer, as already mentioned, to the "ethics of the first person" or to the "virtue ethics," and to the search for the global well-being of the person (the well-being of human life in its entirety and complexity). This ethic derives from Aristotle, according to which the virtuous man "judges righteously everything, and in everything to him appears the truth (…) perhaps the good man is distinguished by the fact that he sees the truth in everything, in that he is the rule and measure of it" (*Nicomachean Ethics,* III, 4, 1113 at 28–32) [14]. Ethics would therefore be a form of "discussion" on the different lifestyles and on the different ways of living, and only secondly would it deal with the individual actions to be taken.

An appropriate method to pass from the ethics of the third person to the ethics of the first person is through a new interpretation of Jonas' ethics of responsibility [15]. According to the ethics of responsibility, the "fathers" have a duty to intervene to save the succeeding generations ("the children") from the catastrophe of the uncontrolled use of technology. The responsibility "of the fathers toward the children" is the most evident example of a responsibility and a duty that is not mutual and is recognized and practiced spontaneously. For Jonas, in fact, the origin of responsibility is not in the relationship between independent adults but rather in the relationship with those who are in conditions of greater fragility (the "children") and who are in need of protection. The parental attention toward one's children is therefore the archetype of the responsible action which does not derive from the compliance to rules or principles, but that is rooted in the nature of every human being.

The same could, in fact, be said for any other situation in which an "adult" has a responsibility toward a person who is in a situation of fragility. In other words, according to Jonas, also the administration of public matters by those who govern must be directed according to their responsibility toward each member of society, since their role in society was spontaneously taken. The fundamental difference between the two situations is given by the natural origin of the parental condition, on one hand, and by the artificial origin of the responsibility to govern, on the other. The responsibilities of parents toward their children, and of those who govern toward the citizens, according to Jonas, have five characteristics in common:

- *Totality*. The responsibility toward others is "global." One should take care of all the needs of those (children/citizens) for whom they are responsible: ranging from the simple existence to higher aspirations, from security to the fullness of life, and from good behavior to happiness.
- *The object*. Parental responsibility also includes the education of children in society and the state helps the parents in the education of their children.
- *The "sentiment*." The reason behind the sense of responsibility is for parents the love for the child and for those who govern the affective relationship with the community/country (of which they are not fathers but 'sons').

- *The historicity*. The exercise of responsibility has a temporal continuity and character of historicity. The responsibility of parents and governors also includes the duty to pass on traditions and prepare for the future.
- *The perspective view*. In the parental responsibility and in that of those who govern, there is the concern for the future. In the context of a global responsibility, every action is evaluated on the basis of the future consequences on the life of the child/population. This is the so-called diachronic ethics which measures (unlike "synchronic ethics") the ethics of an action not based on the intentions, means, goals, or circumstances with which it is done, but on the anticipation of the future consequences.

In public health interventions, it is possible to see a real convergence between the responsibility of parents toward their children and of those who govern toward their citizens: the case of vaccinations is an interesting illustration of this. In the case of the vaccination of children, the abovementioned aspects of the responsibility of the parents and of those who govern (the totality, the object, the sentiment, the historicity, and the perspective view) seem to be more united than ever. In fact, the ethics of responsibility can reinforce the motivations behind the decisions regarding vaccinations.

And so, while the "ethics of the third person" tends to transform preventive medicine (including vaccinations) in a combination of obligations and prohibitions, the "ethics of the first person" recalls first of all to the responsibility toward what in Descartes' words is our "largest" asset: health. When reasoning from this perspective, to make vaccinations mandatory would be superfluous. In fact, considering their high medical, scientific, and social value, vaccinations would have to be considered "a moral duty" (or responsibility) since they are useful instruments in the path toward the asset "health."

In order to favor parents in their responsible search for "health" seen as an asset, it would be necessary to implement certain interventions and guarantees, which are in fact promoted (among other things) by those who are in favor of the abandonment of compulsory vaccinations. For example, it is the health authorities' duty to: (1) give parents complete information about the benefits and risks of preventive immunization, (2) train health personnel on health education, (3) offer free vaccines, and (4) organize an effective service of control of communicable diseases and of the adverse reactions to vaccinations. When a government implements these interventions, it is in fact, on the one hand, exercising its responsibility and, on the other hand, favoring the exercise of responsibility by part of the parents.

In conclusion, even though the positive value of vaccinations is supported by a series of medical–scientific and social considerations, today's conception of human rights make compulsory measures of administration very problematic. In addition, adequate education on a responsible attitude toward one's health would eliminate the need for compulsory methods. The desirable transition from compulsory to recommended must be, however, accompanied by the understanding that vaccinations call into question a double moral responsibility: that of parents toward their children, and that of those who govern toward the community. Second, in order for the free adherence to vaccinations to be effective (not taking in consideration cases of emergencies), some measures become necessary, such as education, information, and training. These measures guarantee the protection of community and allow parents to exercise their responsibility toward their children.

Individual Responsibility and Collective Responsibility: The Centrality of Communication

When dealing with the responsibility toward one's own health, another element to take into consideration is the fact that the majority of diseases is at least in part the result of unhealthy lifestyles. It is sufficient to consider the contribution to the global burden of disease given by high blood pressure, consumption of alcohol, tobacco smoking, elevated levels of cholesterol, and obesity. We thus witness a rise in health care costs, which could be limited by more appropriate lifestyles.

This statement, for however obvious it may seem, raises some objections:

- To consider the individual accountable for his/her own health would be in conflict with the function of medicine, which is to take care of the sick, and the obligation of the society to take care of the more vulnerable individuals.
- It is unfair to consider people responsible for their own health when, for example, they are not able to make the correct choices because of ignorance, incompetence, addiction to drugs, or the presence of cultural pressures.
- Conditions of illness or disability do not depend only on the responsibilities of the individual, but are the result of complex interactions also with genetic and environmental factors.

Having said that when disease is already in act, the presence or absence of individual responsibilities is irrelevant as regards to the right to receive care, society is co-responsible for promoting health and preventing disease through careful and effective informative campaigns.

The difficulty of communicating is, however, exactly the major obstacle in this communion of responsibility. In this regard, we shall analyze the dynamics of interpersonal communication based on the scheme proposed by Slama-Cazacu [16]. According to this model the elements of a communicative act are: (1) the transmitter, who produces the message, (2) the message conveyed according to the rules provided by code; (3) the code according to which the message is produced; (4) the transmission channel; (5) the context in which the message is found and to which it refers; and (6) the receiver.

In health communication, the transmitter is usually an agency that tries to reach the receiver through forms of mass communication.

The content of a message holds in itself two levels of meaning: denotative and cognitive. The denotative meaning indicates what the words mean in themselves; the cognitive meaning refers to the emotions that the words can evoke. A message is also characterized by explicit and implicit elements, which affect both the reception and the emission. In other words, the content of a message can be decoded in a different way by each receiver and this must condition—through a system of feedback—the method of communication used by the transmitter. Furthermore, every communication takes place within a specific sociocultural and organizational context, which may also influence the result that is achieved.

In communication on issues regarding healthy lifestyles, the receiver's reaction is characterized by three consecutive stages: (1) the perception of the risk (cognitive moment), (2) the representation of the risk (affective moment), (3) the acceptance of the risk (operative moment). Stage 3, however, is not necessarily always present after stages 1 and 2. Some will recognize how risky a certain behavior is and will decide not to adopt it, while others will consciously accept the risk.

In some cases, there can be a discrepancy between the cognitive and the affective moment, which can instead exert an attraction toward the effects of a certain behavior and is therefore also responsible for the acceptance of the consequences. Furthermore, there might be a discrepancy between the risk's perception and representation, that is, between the knowledge of the frequency with which a negative event occurs and the subjective perception of the frequency. This is a very important element for preventive purposes: a preventive measure, which is based only on information and that does not take into consideration the propensity of individuals toward risky behavior, would be incorrect and insufficient.

The question "why are you willing to take the risks of certain behaviors?" receives different answers and there are countless studies that have linked risky behaviors with a series of "predisposing" factors. These are not "etiological factors," in other words, that are responsible for the behavior at risk, but are "risk factors." This means that these factors, although detectable, are not always isolable and easily removable and can also be responsible for a greater vulnerability of the subject. The concept of "vulnerability factors" has in fact replaced that of "risk factors," in the fear that by talking about risk factors there could be a stigmatization of certain groups of people and also a consequent diminishment of their responsibility. Some argue that the group at risk could even be genetically determined to take that risk. However, even assuming there be a genetic predisposition, does this means that one can necessarily act only in one way? And how much does the environmental factor interact with the possible genetic factor?

While the genetic factor is still the object of research, it should be emphasized that the environmental factor has instead been the most studied factor in the analysis of the etiology of risk behavior. This refers to the so-called ecological theory, which analyzes the influence of the economic, cultural, and social contexts on the choice of behaviors.

Each environment is created by four systems: microsystem, mesosystem, exosystem, and macrosystem. The microsystem is composed by the environment which is closest to the subject: some microsystems are the family, friends, school, or workplace. The interaction between the different microsystems forms the mesosystem. The community and the mass media, from which the subject can be influenced, but with which he cannot interact directly, create the exosystem; the cultural, social, and political context determine the macrosystem.

Finally, there is another aspect in the management of lifestyles that needs to be considered: the moral dimension, in other words the influence that is exerted on our choices by our perception of lecitness/illecitness of each behavior. Alongside with the other interpretations we must, therefore, also remember the "moral theory" according to which any activity, which is considered ethically unacceptable, should be also considered at risk. Even though there are undoubtedly many situations of vulnerability/weakness that influence a choice, in order for a choice to be responsible, it is first of all fundamental to acquire a sense of limit of what is bad or good. And, therefore, it becomes again necessary to underline how much knowledge is one of the fundamental dimensions in the exercise of responsibility.

Public Health as a "Common Good": A Matter of Justice

Public health's focus on the population must never cause us to forget the needs of the individuals. There are two methods of analyzing the population's and individuals' coexisting interests: in the first, the focus is on the individual, and the community is considered as the sum of the actions, motivations, and characteristics of the single individuals; in the second, the attention is focused on the community, of which the individuals are parts.

Whether you choose an approach that privileges the individual or the population, it is a fact that the limited resources available in health care often make choices difficult [17]. This is true not only for the economical resources. For example, how can we solve problems such as the shortage of organs and the long waiting lists for transplants? Although we may think about allocating a greater amount of resources in health care (which at the moment is in itself difficult because of the current economic crisis) and finding alternatives to organ donation (stem cells, xenotransplantation), it is a fact that these are currently insuperable limits. What criteria can be used to ensure just treatment for all?

In these cases, it is usual to refer to the criterion of justice. It is, however, not sufficient to announce justice: we must also give it a basis and a content. While in classical thought it was usual to distinguish between commutative justice (it regulates and controls the relationships between individuals, i.e., exchanges, transitions, and contracts) and distributive justice (distributes the available resources), in bioethical debate we can identify four models of justice:

Liberal Individualism The liberal individualist model focuses on the search of the maximum freedom of the individual. As a consequence, the state cannot interfere with personal choices, but must merely put the individual in a position to exercise its autonomy through appropriate laws and promotion of a market economy. Choices regarding one's health are subject to the will and economic availability of the individual, and those who govern do not have any moral obligation to protect health. It is obvious that this type of justice excludes all those who are not capable of exercising their autonomy.

Utilitarianism According to the utilitarian vision, every choice is to be judged according to the sum of all the forms of utility that it generates. The main goal is to obtain the maximum benefit for the greatest number of people at the lowest cost. Therefore, even though this model apparently takes into account everyone's interest, the benefit of society prevails over that of the individual. The state, in this case, has the role of promoting what is useful for society, and not that of responding to individual needs. For example, in the field of microallocative decisions, treatment would be given in preference to acute situations, as opposed to conditions that are not curable or that cause permanent disabilities.

Egalitarianism Social egalitarianism favors the needs of society over individual freedom. Egalitarian health care is based on the right to health, of which the state is responsibile: in this case, the areas of public intervention increase, leaving less space for individual choices. It is necessary to give equally to everyone, and the poor must receive that of which they are in need: only this way is it possible to correct the inequalities created by the "lottery" present in nature and society. And if the institution of a health care system that is universal (for all) and based on solidarity is in itself positive, one should not underestimate the critical issues. The equality promoted in egalitarianism does not, in fact, take into account individual differences and by treating everyone the same way; it creates the possibility of developing new forms of inequalities and discrimination.

Substantialism It refers to the human person in its concrete reality; the objective is to put each person in the position of achieving the maximum potential health according to their situation. Ensuring justice, therefore, means not only respecting the equality of human beings but also responding to the different needs of each person, in relation to their state of health/disease. In this case, the individual becomes the unit of measurement in public health; the protection of health and life is the supreme value; justice is the instrument used to obtain that value.

In this case, both commutative justice and distributive justice are fully achieved. According to distributive justice it is necessary to give everyone what they deserve objectively and concretely on the basis of their individual need; commutative justice intersects with the concept of community, according to which the individual develops at his best within the search of common good. In the context of public health, this translates into a particular attention to the needs of each person. In each decision, it is necessary to make reference to the criteria of urgency, therapeutic proportionality and subsidiarity, yet without forgetting that the pursuit of health is always influenced by the meaning that is given to life.

References

1. Kant I (1979) The conflict of the faculties. Abaris, New York
2. Canguilhem G (1991) The normal and the pathological. Zone Books, New York
3. Jourdain M (ed) (1916) Diderot's early philosophical works. The Open Court Publishing Company, Chicago, p. 185

4. McKee M, Raine R (2005) Choosing health? First choose your philosophy. Lancet 29:369–371
5. MacDonald T (1998) Rethinking health promotion: a global approach. Routledge, London
6. World Health Organization (1986) The Ottawa Charter for Health Promotion. http://www.who.int/healthpromotion/conferences/previous/ottawa/en/. Accessed 22 Dec 2013
7. Allotey P, Verghis S, Alvarez-Castillo F, Reidpath DD (2012) Vulnerability, equity and universal coverage—a concept note. BMC Public Health 12(Suppl 1):S2
8. Dawson A, Verweij M (eds) (2007) Ethics, prevention and public health. Clarendon Press, Oxford
9. Beauchamp TL, Childress JF (1978) Principles of biomedical ethics. Oxford University Press, New York
10. Reich WT (ed) (1995) Encyclopedia of bioethics. Simon & Schuster Macmillan, New York
11. Buchanan DR (2008) Autonomy, paternalism, and justice: ethical priorities in public health. Am J Pub Health 98:15–21
12. Di Pietro ML, Refolo P, Gonzales-Melado FJ (2012) About "responsibility" of vaccination. Cuadernos de Bioetica 23:323–336
13. Dawson A (2007). Herd Protection as a Public Good: Vaccination and Our Obligations to Others. In: Dawson A, Verweij M (eds) Ethics, prevention and public health. Clarendon Press, Oxford, pp. 160–178
14. Aristotle (2007) Nicomachean ethics. Cosimo Inc., New York
15. Jonas H (1985) Technik, Medizin und Ethik. Zur Praxis des Prinzips Verantwortung. Insel, Frankfurt
16. Slama-Cazacu T (1973) Introduction to psycho-linguistics. Mouton, The Hague
17. Pellegrino ED (2002). Rationing health care: Inherent conflicts within the concept of justice. In: Bondeson WD, Jones JW (eds) The ethical ethics of managed care: professional integrity and patient rights. Kluver Academy Publishers, Dordrecht, pp. 1–18

Chapter 10
Injury Prevention and Safety Promotion

Johan Lund, Paolo Di Giannantonio and Alice Mannocci

Introduction

Injuries (outcomes of accidents, assaults, and intentional self-harm) place heavy burdens on societies worldwide in terms of human suffering, health expenses, and compensation costs. In 1990, injuries were responsible for 10 % of world mortality, and this rate is predicted to increase to 12 % by 2020 [1]. It is also estimated that injuries account for 14 % of global life years lost when using the measure years of life lost [2].

There is an increasing global effort to control the injury problem and to establish prevention strategies [3]. A prerequisite for planning, implementation, and evaluation of injury prevention strategies is an understanding of the *epidemiology of injuries,* i.e. the occurrence of injuries in terms of time, place, person, and factors contributing to injuries in the population [4]. Here, we focus on the epidemiology and prevention of *accidental injuries* (also called unintentional injuries), as outcomes of traffic, occupational, home, and leisure accidents. *Assault* (interpersonal violence) and *intentional self-harm* (self-inflicted violence) are viewed as separate phenomena in terms of the preventive strategies that are employed. As aspects of the general injury problem, however, they are included in discussions of treatment and registration in the medical sector.

J. Lund (✉)
Institute of Health and Society, Section for Social Medicine, University of Oslo, 0318 Oslo, Norway
e-mail: Johan.lund@medisin.uio.no

P. Di Giannantonio
Institute of Public Health, Section of Hygiene, Università Cattolica del Sacro Cuore, L.go F. Vito 1, 00168 Rome, Italy
e-mail: paolo.di.giannantonio@gmail.com

A. Mannocci
Department of Public Health and Infectious Diseases, Sapienza University of Rome, Ple Aldo Moro 5, 00185 Rome, Italy
e-mail: alice.mannocci@uniroma1.it

S. Boccia et al. (eds.), *A Systematic Review of Key Issues in Public Health,*
DOI 10.1007/978-3-319-13620-2_10

Definitions and Concepts

Some important concepts in accident analysis and prevention and a model of the relations between them are given in Fig. 10.1 [5].

Dangers Are the Origins of Accidents and Injuries

Accidents might happen wherever humans are present, and at all hours. Each day, we are exposed to, or expose ourselves to, dangers: external sources of energy, or something that causes or is likely to cause harm [6]. The dangers are mostly "normal" and are coped with in the daily life (Fig. 10.1). However, when a person loses control over the situation, or observes a danger too late, an accident occurs (Fig. 10.1). An accident is defined as an unintentional event, characterised by the sudden release of an external force or impact which can manifest itself as a body injury [7], if the threshold of the human tolerance is exceeded [6, 8]. Humans with low mastering abilities, e.g. children and the elderly, have more accidents than humans with high mastering abilities.

There are two main strategies for avoiding accidents and injuries:

1. Remove or modify/diminish the dangers, mostly connected to injury prevention: environmental changes, hindrances, lack of freedom, rules, and regulations. Examples are: drain swimming pools of season, do not permit elderly people to use stairs, enforce speed limits on roads, make bathtubs less slippery, place guards on dangerous machines, enforce safety regulation on playground equipment, etc. Availability and use of safety equipment might influence the outcome of the accident (Fig. 10.1).
2. Master the dangers, mostly connected to safety promotion. Examples are: train to master dangers (very relevant in child development), traffic training (bicycling, etc.), but only when the child is able/ripe to fulfil the requirements, physical and mental training, exercises in all ages, tai chi, dancing for the elderly, etc.

To master dangers is an essential part of building self-esteem. Not all dangers should be eliminated. The child needs risk-taking, adventures, and challenges. It is essential to find the balance between development and protection. If a child is falling from a high climbing frame, she/he should fall on a soft surface. When voluntary risks are coped with, the risk-taker might be rewarded with joy, happiness, and realisation of their potentialities. The downside of risk-taking, however, is injury, death, and tragedy. This ambiguity in risk-taking is a challenge to planning and implementing injury prevention strategies [9].

Injury Prevention

A model for accident prevention is proposed, the two lower shaded boxes in Fig. 10.1 [10]. The measures used for prevention of accidents and injuries directly

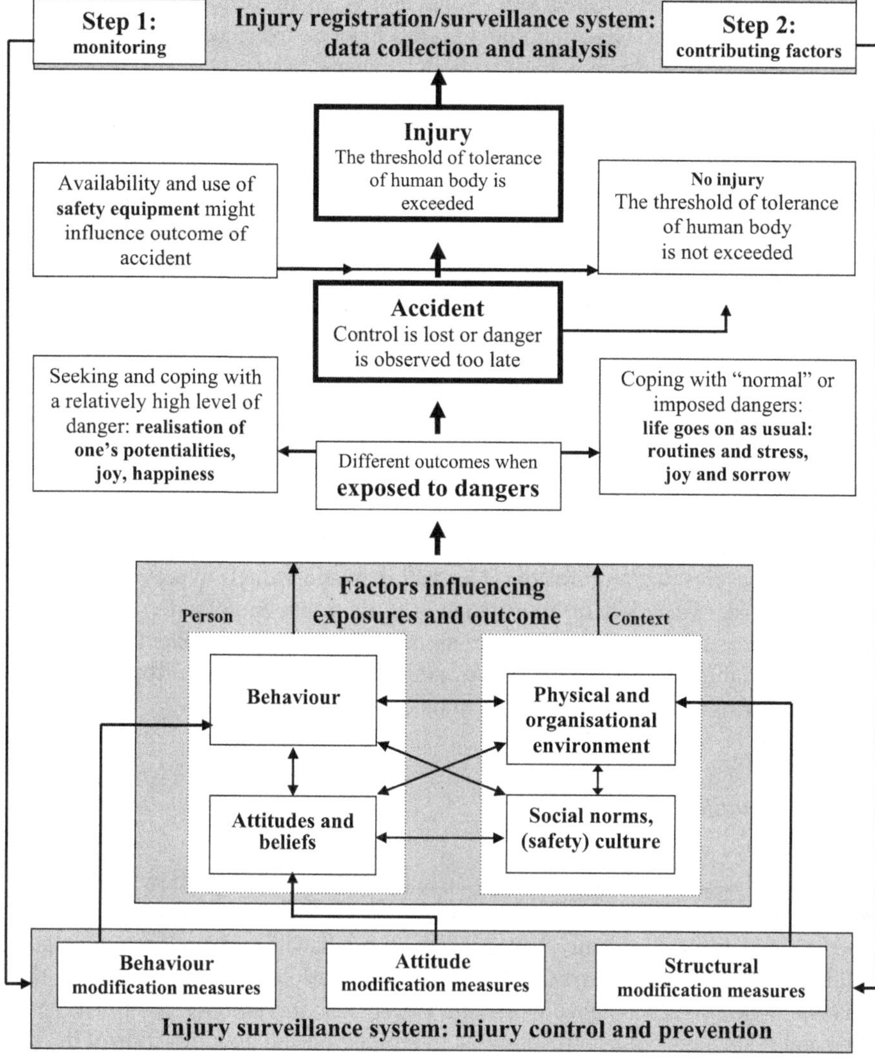

Fig. 10.1 Important concepts in accident analysis and prevention, and a model of the relations between them [5]

and indirectly influence the personal and contextual factors. Here, they are divided into three main categories:

1. *Attitude modification measures:* attitudes are changed by means of persuasive messages in mass media campaigns, leaflets, booklets, films, posters, or direct mail. Also included in this category are one-way counselling schemes, such as counselling on car safety to mothers of newborn children. Health education normally utilises measures from this category.

2. *Behaviour modification measures:* behaviour is changed through more direct approaches, without assuming that attitudes have an intermediary function, for instance by skills training with or without a rewards system.
3. *Structural modification measures:* contextual factors are changed through legislation, regulation, enforcement, organisation, and economy. This also refers to changes in the physical environment and to modification and the availability of products.

The model shows connections between these three types of preventive measures and two risk factors: behaviour and physical/organisational environment, and two process factors: attitudes/beliefs and social norms/(safety) culture.

A classic model for injury prevention has three different phases [11]:

- Primary prevention: preventing new accidents and injuries
- Secondary prevention: reducing the severity of injuries
- Tertiary prevention: decreasing the frequency and severity of disability after injury

Important distinctions between prevention measures are made between:

- Active measures that require conscious action by individuals to prevent or minimize the risk of accident or injury, such as using safety equipment.
- Passive measures that do not require an individual to act to prevent injury, and are often more effective than active measures. Examples are airbags in cars, smoke alarms in homes, and dumps in roads.

Injury Surveillance

A medically based injury registration system is a tool for gaining knowledge of the epidemiology of the injuries that are referred to the medical care system (Fig. 10.1, upper shaded box). Medically based injury surveillance systems have emerged around the world from the early 1970s. The forerunners were computerised trauma registers in the USA established in the late 1960s [12]. *Surveillance* comprises "ongoing and systematic collection, analysis, interpretation and dissemination of health information" [13]. The term "register" is used synonymously with the related term surveillance system. According to Frerichs (p. 265) [14], "a surveillance system goes one step further than a monitoring system by including a 'controller' who is a person or agency with some ability to take corrective actions"(Fig. 10.1, lower shaded box). A controller can be found at national, regional, and local levels. After receiving input from the monitoring system, the controller compares the registered data with established standards or goals. Information on factors contributing to accidents and injuries might lead to proposals for preventive actions. Action follows only "if the administration has the will and political power to act" (p. 265) [14].

The first medically based injury surveillance systems were designed by product safety authorities to identify unsafe products [5]. They are data sources additional to occupational and traffic accident registers that are generally incomplete and fragmented [15, 16]. They are also a valuable data source on home and leisure accidents, the largest accident group in most countries. More current systems are based on reports of all types of injuries: accidental, assaults, and intentional self-harm. All systems collect information on injuries treated in a more or less representative sample of hospitals and/or accident and emergency departments (AED) in the country/region to be surveyed.

The use of the medical care system for acquiring statistics on injuries and injury control has necessitated development of new multiaxial classifications [7, 17]. Minimum data sets (MDSs) are developed for settings where registration resources are scarce [13, 18]. In such settings, the possibilities to identify the contributing factors leading to injuries are restricted because few details on each accident/injury can be collected. For such purposes, expanded data sets (EDSs) are collected in specially designed and funded in-depth investigations, or in accident commissions.

The most important aim of an injury surveillance system is to provide information useful for the prevention of injuries. To fulfil this aim, three different types of data need to be recorded:

1. Data enabling estimation of injury incidence rates (for the purpose of guiding programme priorities and resource allocation)
2. Data for establishing trends (for the purpose of evaluating the effectiveness of prevention programmes
3. Data on factors contributing to injuries (for the purpose of developing prevention measures, strategies, and programmes)

In order to record all three types of data simultaneously, many details from each accident/injury have to be collected in a sufficiently large sample to provide high representativeness of the population to be surveyed. Such an ideal system requires large registration resources, hardly to be found anywhere in the world. As an alternative, a two-step injury surveillance system is suggested (Fig. 10.1, upper shaded box). In the first step, limited data (an MDS) on all or a representative sample of all injuries are recorded within the medical care system using routine collection procedures. This data collection includes injuries sustained by both residents and nonresidents within a defined geographical area and fulfils the need for data types 1 and 2. The second step involves periodic sampling of specific injuries, injured persons, or places for in-depth investigations from the database established in the first step, or selecting relevant injured persons seeking treatment in the medical system, in order to collect many data on a limited number of injuries. This step might provide data for developing prevention measures, strategies, and programmes (data type 3).

Such a two-step injury surveillance system was implemented in Oslo, the capital of Norway, with a population of about 500,000 [19]. During 1 year, 48,283 persons were registered using an MDS. They were treated by 17 general practitioners (GPs) in one city district, at the city's main AED, as inpatients in four hospitals, and deceased persons were registered on death certificates (step 1). Two in-depth investigations of each of a total of 273 serious occupational injuries treated at the AED were carried out. Detailed interviews as well as on-site studies were undertaken (step 2). This two-step injury register showed potential for providing valid monitoring data and revealing factors contributing to accidents and injury.

In the European region, a lot of efforts have been made in order to establish injury surveillance systems. Both the World Health Organization (WHO) European Region (Resolution EUR/RC55/R9) and the European Council (Recommendation 2007/C164/01) have urged member states to develop injury surveillance systems, so that programmes for prevention, care, and rehabilitation can be better targeted, monitored, and evaluated. The WHO European Region evaluation of these actions shows that there has been some progress, but calls for "improved access to reliable and comparable injury surveillance information to make the extent, causes and circumstances of the problem more visible across the Region" p. 34 [20].

A Joint Action on Monitoring Injuries in the EU (JAMIE) has led to an updated methodology and format for collecting basic information in a large number of emergency departments at hospitals at almost no additional costs. At present, a substantial number of hospitals across 26 countries in the European Union (EU) are collecting data in their emergency departments in line with the harmonised methodology and classification. During these years, injury statistics in the EU has been produced based on this system, the last for the years 2008–2010 [21].

These data are currently being used for a wide range of safety promotion purposes including in helping to design better and safer consumer products. That is one of the reasons why a broad coalition of European organisations called earlier this year (2013) on the European Commission to set up a *Pan European Accident and Injury Data System*. These EU-level umbrella organisations in commerce, standardisation, consumer, and health and safety are convinced that such a system would contribute to fewer accidents and injuries.

Current Burden of Injuries in Europe

Injuries due to accidents, assaults, and intentional self-harm are a major health problem, killing more than 230,000 persons in the EU-27 each year (annual average 2008–2010). An estimated one million persons will be permanently disabled [22]. Injuries are the third most common cause of death, after cardiovascular diseases and cancer. Below 45 years of age, it is the number one cause of death [21]. Across the European countries, there is a great variation of injury incidences, from rather high in Russia and the previous Soviet Republics, to rather low in the western countries of Europe. The most recent data show a variation from less than 25 per 100,000 to more than 180 per 100,000, a sevenfold disparity (Fig. 10.2).

Every 2 min., one EU citizen dies of an injury. For each fatal injury case, 25 people across the EU are admitted to a hospital, 145 are treated as hospital outpatients, and many more seek treatment elsewhere, e.g. by family doctors. This means that each year a staggering 5.7 million people are admitted to a hospital and 33.9 million people are treated as hospital outpatients as a result of an accident or violence-related injury [21] (Fig. 10.3).

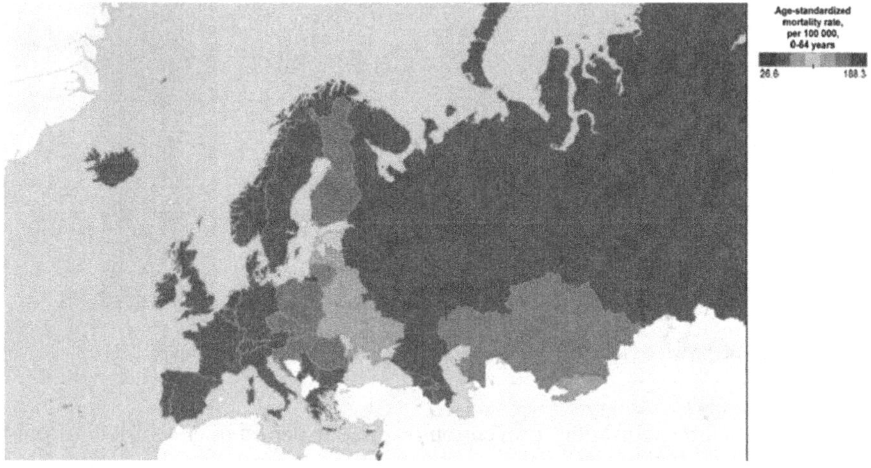

Fig. 10.2 Mortality from all causes of injury incidences in the European Region [21]

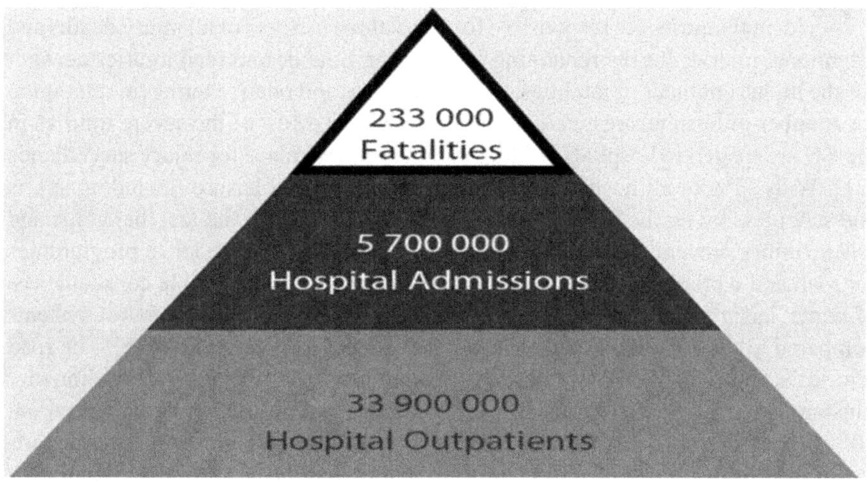

Fig. 10.3 The injury pyramid for the European Union (EU-27) [21]

In addition to hospital treatments, many injuries are treated by GPs and paramedical staff without being referred to a hospital. In the Netherlands for instance, about one third of all injury patients are treated in hospitals and two thirds are seeking consultation in the office of a GP [23]. In Norway in the years 2009–2011, 80 % of the injured patients sought consultation at a GP/municipality AED, Quite many of these are transferred to hospitals, with the result that in the end about 50 % of all medically treated injury patients are finally treated by GPs and 50 % at the hospitals (both as in- and outpatients) [24]. This relation will of course vary across countries depending on the organisation of the health system.

	Road traffic	Work place	School	Sports	Home, leasure	Total of unintentional injuries	Homicide, assault	Suicide, self-harm	Total of all injuries
Fatalites	[illegible] 10%	[illegible] 2%	1 250 1%	7 000 3%	98 891 42%	150 221 65%	4 704 2%	57 514 25%	232 869 100%
Hospital admissions	[illegible] 12%	152 000 4%	32 000 1%	419 000 7%	3 914 000 69%	5 285 000 93%	202 000 4%	219 000 4%	5 700 000 100%
Hospital outpatients	3 524 000 10%	[illegible] [illegible]	792 000 2%	5 644 000 17%	18 951 000 56%	32 465 000 96%	1 231 000 4%	[illegible] 1%	33 900 000 100%
All hospital patients	4 192 000 11%	[illegible] [illegible]	824 000 2%	6 063 000 14%	22 985 000 59%	37 750 000 95%	1 433 000 4%	[illegible] 1%	39 600 000 100%

Fig. 10.4 Comprehensive view on injuries in EU-27 by injury prevention domain [21]

The responsibility for injury prevention is quite dispersed over a variety of policy sectors depending on the setting in which they occur and the circumstances. Figure 10.4 depicts the key figures of the main unintentional and intentional injury categories according to place of occurrence and injury outcomes in terms of severity (death, hospital admission, or outpatient treatment).

Accidental injuries are responsible for about three quarters of all injury deaths and intentional injuries for the remaining one quarter. Suicide and road injuries account for the highest number of fatalities, in both absolute and relative terms (in relation to the number of hospital-treated injuries, i.e. lethality). Most of the severe injuries in the EU are treated in hospitals making them the proper place for injury surveillance [21]. With 73 % of all hospital-treated injuries, home and leisure (including sports and school) is by far the biggest share, which is in contrast to the fact that home and leisure injury prevention programmes appear as far less resourced than programmes for road and workplace safety. In general, the tangible and intangible consequences of home, leisure, and sport injuries are also less well covered by insurance systems compared to the compensation schemes for road and work accidents [25]. The road injuries account for 10 % of all hospital-treated injuries or a total of 4.2 million victims annually. Compared to just 1.7 million injuries reported by the police (about 40 % of the hospital-treated traffic injuries), this indicates a significant underreporting of the problem in official road traffic statistics and the need for complementary information on road injuries treated in health facilities [26]. This level of underreporting in eight European countries varied between 21 and 57 % [27].

Costs of Injuries

Costs of accidents can be measured in human, social, economic, and organisational costs [28]:

- Human
  - The injured person being unable to return to usual work tasks, temporarily or permanently

Table 10.1 Costs per capita, incidence, and mean costs per patient for admitted injury patients (all causes) per country [30]

Country	Cost per capita (€)	Incidence (per 1,000)	Cost per patient (€)	Mean length of stay (days)
Austria	75	22.9	3,242	6.9
Denmark	51	18.1	2,745	6.1
Greece	30	13.4	2,166	7.6
Ireland	26	15.2	1,690	4.2
Italy	25	16.6	1,506	4.2
Netherlands	19	6.5	2,954	8.4
Norway	42	14.7	2,819	5.0
Spain	14	4.8	2,771	9.3
England	18	11.8	1,418	5.9
Wales	23	15.6	1,399	6.5
EUROCOST	24	12.2	1,965	6.4

  - Poor quality of life, due to constant pain measured in QALY (quality-adjusted life years) [29]
  - Emotional physical trauma
  - Financial hardship
- Social
  - Financial burden may fall onto other family members
  - Fellow workers and family may need counselling
  - Economic
  - Medical expenses, compensation, and rehabilitation costs to family, company, and taxpayers
- Organisational
  - Costs of hiring and training of replacement staff
  - Loss of production while staff respond to accident or equipment needs to be shut down to be replaced or repaired
  - Some workers may not wish to return to the usual job due to the severity of accident

Recently (2001–2004), within the framework of a project named EUROCOST, a uniform injury-based method to calculate medical costs of injury was developed and applied to ten EU countries. This method allowed the calculation of medical costs of injury by sex, age, external cause, and type of injury at the country level and EU level.

Home and leisure, sport, and occupational accidents combined make a major contribution (86 %) of the total hospital costs of injury in Europe. Table 10.1 shows the costs of admitted injury patients for each participating EUROCOST country.

In addition, the study shows that the elderly patients aged 65 years and older, especially women, consume a disproportionate share of hospital resources for trauma care, mainly caused by hip fractures and fractures of the knee/lower leg, which indicates the importance of prevention and investing in trauma care for this specific patient group (Fig. 10.5).

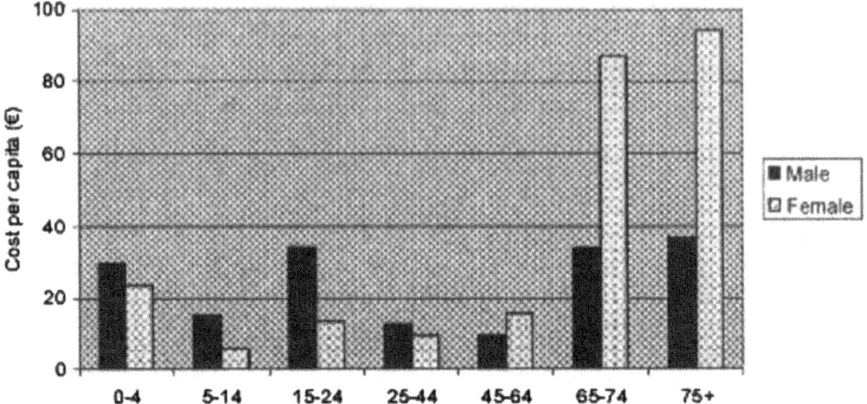

Fig. 10.5 Hospital cost per capita (€) for admitted injury patients by age and sex for the EURO-COST countries [30]

Prevention of Accidental Injuries: Best Practices and Evidence-Based Strategies

What Works Well and What Does Not Work So Well?

According to the model presented in Fig. 10.1 (lower part), accident prevention measures are divided into three main categories: modification of (1) attitudes, (2) behaviour, and (3) structural conditions. Prevention measures from two or three categories might be utilised in the same programme (orchestration), creating a new category of measures across categories. Through a literature review, the pathways and impacts on the incidences of accidental injuries of the various accident prevention measures in Fig. 10.1 were examined [10]. An attempt was made to identify the most effective accident prevention measures. A total of 249 interventions (166 in meta-analysis and systematic reviews and 83 separate interventions) of relatively high quality were identified in the literature. They were divided into the following main and subcategories with regard to which prevention measures they utilised:

1. Attitude modification programmes (N=27):
   a. Information measures: mass media campaigns, leaflets, booklets, films, posters, and direct mail (N=17)
   b. Counselling and education in classrooms, small groups, or individually (N=10)
2. Behaviour modification programmes (N=32):
   a. Instruction, skills training, and feedback, focus on behavioural change (N=24)
   b. Rewards for desired behaviour (N=8)

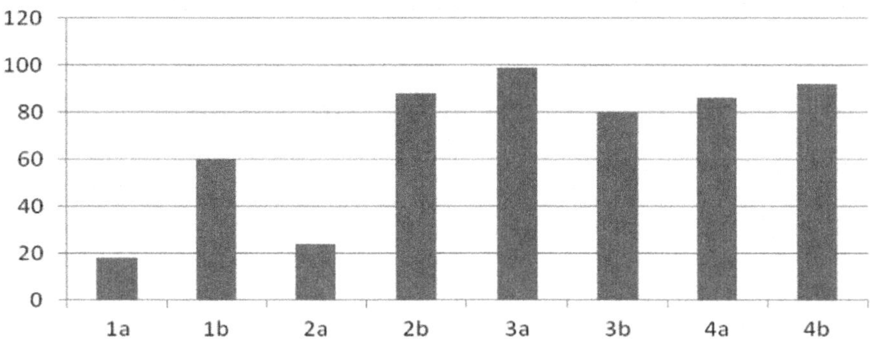

Fig. 10.6 Percentages of all accident prevention interventions in each subcategory with significant positive effect on the incidence rates of accidental injuries, or on changes in behaviours [10]

3. Structural modification programmes (N=156):
   a. Legislation (N=86)
   b. Environmental and product modification (N=70)
4. Programmes combining measures across categories (orchestration; N=34):
   a. Combined prevention measures (N=22)
   b. Community-based interventions (N=12)

All interventions were analysed with regard to the results of the interventions. Some of them had significant positive effects on reductions in accidents or injury incidence rates, or on changes in behaviours that might have an impact on injury rates, e.g. use of bicycle helmets. Others did not have any effects, or sometimes have negative effects. The percentages of interventions in each subcategory with positive results are shown in Fig. 10.6.

Based on Fig. 10.6, some of the hypothesised paths in the model (Fig. 10.1, lower part) seem to be weak: Attitude modification measures (information) → attitude → behaviour → accidents and injuries (the traditional KAP model: knowledge → attitude → practice; subcategory 1a). Others seem strong: Structural modification measures → physical and organisational environment → behaviour → accidents and injuries (subcategory 3a, b). Behaviour modification measures in workplaces have shown positive effects, while there are mixed experiences with educational and skills training programmes for children and adolescents. Such training might create unrealistic beliefs in one's own abilities, and parents might overestimate their children's abilities, so they may be exposed to situations more dangerous than they can master. Behaviour modification measures that concentrate on a single behaviour usually seemed to be more effective than a more general effort directed at a range of hazards [31]. The use of rewards (subcategory 2b) has consistently shown positive effects on children's and adults' use of safety equipment in cars and in workplaces. When attitude, behaviour, and structural modification measures were used in combination (subcategory 4a, b), the interconnections and mutual influences taking place among the personal and contextual factors in the model mostly seemed to produce stronger effects than if one category of preventive measures was used alone. The overview of community-based interventions showed significant positive preventive effects in all but one study reviewed.

Injury prevention, with its broad range of injury types and possible countermeasures, lends itself to community-based approaches. The use of multiple interventions, repeated in different forms and contexts, can lead to a culture of safety being developed within a community [11]. There is evidence that the WHO Safe Community model is effective in reducing injuries in whole populations [32].

Information measures *alone* (such as mass media campaigns or leaflets, Fig. 10.6, subcategory 1a) seemed to produce very little, if any, effect on safety behaviour and on the incidence of accidents and injuries, except when the target groups were highly motivated. The effects were stronger when the message was repeated, was more tailor made, and was delivered face to face in counselling schemes, or even better when this information on accident prevention was based on two-way information in small groups (subcategory 1b). Structural measures, such as regulation and enforcement, environmental and product modifications generally seemed to have a strong positive effect. Environmental changes with negative effects were marked pedestrian road crossings, which probably introduced some sort of false safety.

All 166 interventions in the meta-analyses and systematic reviews dealt with traffic accidents, as well as 51 of the 83 other interventions. The rest dealt with home (17), occupational (6), sport/leisure (5), and all accidents (4). About 80 % of the 249 interventions took place in Anglo-American cultures. Very few of the interventions took place in Africa ($N=4$) and in Asia ($N=2$). This bias restricts any generalisation of results to the Western World. The bias towards traffic accidents reflects the fact that evaluations of traffic accidents have a longer and broader tradition in the English-speaking world compared with evaluation research into home, occupational, and sport/leisure accidents. The bias towards traffic accident interventions, however, should not influence general conclusions, as risk and process factors are not supposed to react differently when other accident types are involved.

Although attitude change measures used alone seem to have little direct impact on behaviour, they may still have an important role in accident prevention. The model presented in Fig. 10.1 (lower part) suggests that by influencing attitudes, other factors can also be influenced, which in turn will reduce accidents and subsequent injuries. Through attitude-changing measures, we might:

- Persuade more people to take both *precautionary actions* and to *initiate passive measures* that in turn will reduce the prevalence of accidents and injuries.
- Contribute to the *shaping of public opinion* that is favourable towards the use of passive measures and legislation. If one does not have convincing support from public opinion, it is more difficult for politicians, union representatives, and others to make the decisions that are necessary to introduce various structural measures.

- *Mobilise social support* for kinds of behaviour that will reduce the risk of accidents and subsequent injuries; for example, support for not driving under the influence of alcohol.
- Contribute to changing *social norms*. Although individuals' private attitudes may have limited impact on their own actions, the attitudes of others often carry more weight.
- Accident-relevant aspects of culture may be influenced through a long-term use of informational and educational approaches, preferably in combination with other measures. Hence, attitude-changing measures also represent an important contribution to the *development of a more safety-minded culture*.

After this more general view on which preventative measures work well, and which not so well, we refer to examples of interventions which have given positive effects in some of the main accident types. We refer to handbooks, overviews of best practices, and other systematic reviews which give information about prevention of accidental injuries. One systematic review describes preventative measures in various settings and includes cost–benefit analyses (CBAs) of the measures [33]. The results of CBA depend strongly on the context to which they refer. Monetary valuations of impacts, which are a key element of CBA, vary substantially between countries. As a rule, one would therefore not expect the results of CBAs made in one country to apply directly to another country.

These CBAs are referred to in the following chapters. The country where and the year when the analysis is made are given in parentheses.

Prevention of Traffic Accidents and Injuries

Evaluations of traffic accidents have a longer and broader tradition than evaluations of other accident types. Traffic safety has been highly prioritised, probably because the field is public, there are many fatalities, and it is a high-energy and dramatic area.

The WHO has published a world report with a lot of information about road traffic injury prevention and how to tackle the situation [34]. The *Handbook of Road Safety Measures* [27] gives a systematic overview of current knowledge about the effects of road safety measures. This is a book of about 1000 pages. Hundreds of scientific papers and reports have been studied and analysed; 110 specific road safety measures are described with the effect on accidents, mobility, environment, costs, and also CBA for many of them.

The road safety measures in this handbook are divided in eight chapters:

- Road design and road equipment: 20 measures, e.g. tracks for walking and cycling, roundabouts, black spot treatment, cross-section improvements, and road lighting
- Road maintenance: nine measures, e.g. improving evenness of the road surface, bright road surface, winter maintenance, correcting erroneous traffic signs

- Traffic control: 21 measures, e.g. speed limits, speed-reducing devices, pedestrian streets, yield signs at junctions
- Vehicle design and protective devices: 28 measures, e.g. studded tyres, ABS and disc brakes, daytime running lights for cars, cycle helmets, and seatbelts in light vehicles
- Vehicle inspections: Four measures: e.g. periodic motor vehicle inspection
- Requirements for drivers, driver training, and professional driving: 13 measures, e.g. driving licence age limits, the driving test, and graduated driving licence
- Road user education and information: four measures, e.g. education of preschool children, education in schools, and road user information and campaign
- Enforcement and sanctions: 11 measures, e.g. stationary speed enforcement, seatbelt enforcement, speed cameras, fines and imprisonments, and warning letters

In addition, there is a chapter on general-purpose policy instruments: 14 measures. These measures are general in nature and are used in many sectors of public policy. Thus, they are not always regarded as road safety measures. Examples of these are: safe community programmes, road pricing, motor vehicle taxation, and road traffic legislation.

Some examples from the review of Elke and Elvik [33] with benefit–cost (BC) ratio:

- Alcohol-control and media campaign (NZ 2004), BC ratio 14–26
- Road lighting (NO 2007), BC ratio: 1.9
- Alco-lock for previous drunken drivers (NO 2007), BC ratio: 8.8
- Roundabouts (NO 2007), BC ratio: 1.9–2.6
- Seatbelt reminder (NO 2007), BC ratio: 16.2
- Speed control (NO 2007), BC ratio 1.5

Prevention of Occupational Accidents and Injuries

In a recently published systematic review of safety intervention for the prevention of accidents at work [35], 318 relevant studies were identified. The screening process started with about 22,000 titles from the international literature from 1966 and up to now. About 6500 abstracts were assessed to be relevant. After studying them, about 600 articles were left to be read. Of the 318 articles, 162 were assessed to be of too low quality, leaving 156 studies to be studied for assessing the effectiveness of safety interventions in preventing accidents and injuries at work.

About 50 % of these studies were from the health and social sector, 10 % from industry, 10 % from construction, 5 % from agriculture, and the rest (25 %) from other sectors. The studies were divided into the same four main groups as with the study of Lund and Aaro [10] (Fig. 10.6). And the same general results were found: Group 1 and 2 had less studies with positive significant results as groups 3 and 4. In the following, some examples of these studies are listed (+: positive effect, –: negative effect, s.: significant, ns.: not significant).

Attitude modification programmes

- Transport, professional driving, and group discussions (SE 1996): +44 %, s.
- Agriculture, one-way communication, and group discussions (DK 2003): +3 %, ns.

Behaviour modification programmes

- Transport, professional driving, and training programmes (SE 1996): +37 %, s.
- Transport, professional driving, and rewards (SE 1996): +26 %, s.
- Supermarkets, cut injuries, knives, and training programmes (USA 1997): +9 %, ns.
- Post workers, back injuries, and educational programmes (USA 1998): – 11 %, s.

Structural modification programmes

- Forestry, technical changes in machinery (USA 2002): +64 %, s.
- Hospital, regulation against violence (USA 2009): +48 %, s.
- Hospital, technical change of syringe (USA 2001): +46 %, s.
- Mining, change of regulation (USA 2002): +45 %, s.

Programmes combining measures across categories (orchestration)

- Hospital, muscle-skeletal injuries (USA 2011): +61 %, s.
- Hospital, needle sticks (AUS 2008): +51 %, s.
- Construction, nail-gun injuries (USA 2008): +37 %, s.
- Construction, all injuries (DK 2002): +25 %, s.

In conclusion, the authors recommend to develop and build strategies based on integrated measures and structural measures (p. 19) [10]. "It is therefore not a viable option for focusing exclusively on attitudinal measures through campaigns and the like, as they cannot stand alone in prevention efforts nor provide the expected pay-off when they do."

Some examples from the review of Elke and Elvik [33] with BC ratio:

- Programme against drugs at the working place (USA 2007): BC ratio: 4–26
- Hospitals, programme for ergonomic lifting of patients (USA 2007), BC ratio: 1.4
- Regulation towards dangerous chemicals (NO 2000): BC ratio: 15
- Active management against muscle-skeletal injuries (UK 2006): BC ratio: 1.4–5.8

Prevention of Accidents and Injuries in the Home

About one third of all medically treated injuries are due to accidents in the home [19]. Because the accidents happen behind closed doors in isolated incidents, they rarely attract public and media attention, in contrast to traffic and occupational injuries. Children and the elderly have the highest incidences of home injuries, but it is also a very common accident type for adolescents and adults.

In an overview of the Swiss home and leisure accident scene, key accident factors are identified [36]. For the accident segments: falls, broken glass/sheet metal, animals, equipment/tools/appliances/machinery, burns/chemical burns, poisonings, and electrocution risk factor profiles are created. Prevention methods for these segments are developed and evaluated.

Some examples from the review of Elke and Elvik [33] with BC ratio:

- Universal design of residences (SE 2006): BC ratio: B>C
- Sprinklers in residences (UK 2004): BC ratio: 1.1–4.5

Prevention of Sports Accidents and Injuries

Based on the Eurostat and WHO mortality databases, the number of fatal sports injuries in the EU can be estimated at 7000 fatalities per year. Based on the European Injury Database (IDB), it is estimated that annually almost six million persons need treatment in a hospital due to an accident related to sport activities, of whom 10% require hospitalization for 1 day or more [37].

There are many possibilities to prevent sports injuries. Approaches that have been shown to be successful include: (1) using equipment designed to reduce injury risk, (2) adopting the rules of play, and (3) specific exercise programmes developed to reduce injury risk. Sports organisations should adopt available injury prevention strategies as part of their policies [38]. See also www.stopsportsinjuries.org/ and www.eurosafe.eu.com/csi/eurosafe2006.nsf/wwwVwContent/l2sportssafety.htm [21].

Some examples from the review of Elke and Elvik [33] with BC ratio:

- Campaigns for the use of ski helmets (CH 2006), BC ratio: B>C
- Use of ski helmets (CH 2006), BC ratio: B>C

Prevention of Child Accident and Injuries

The WHO has published a report on child injury prevention with a lot of information about the situation and about prevention [11]. Important chapters in the report describe main child injury types and how to prevent them: road traffic injuries, drowning, burns, falls, and poisonings. It is referred to a CBA from the USA (2000), showing the following BC ratios: smoke alarms 65, child restraints 29, bicycle helmets 29, prevention counselling by paediatricians 10, poison control centres 7, and road safety improvements 3.

European Child Safety Alliance (ECSA) has since 2000 worked on promoting child safety in the European countries (http://www.childsafetyeurope.org/) [21]. Today, more than 30 countries across Europe are working together to reduce injuries, which are the leading cause of death, disability, and inequity to children in all countries in Europe. A “Good Practice Guide” has been published [39]. The purpose of this guide is to enable countries in Europe to examine strategy options for unintentional child injury prevention that are evidence based and offer guidance on how such strategies can be transferred into action and policy. The guide is divided into four sections and includes at-a-glance tables of evidence-based strategies, as well as European case studies to help injury stakeholders working in European countries to promote good practice in planning and implementing strategies to address child injury. About 20 good practice case studies from various countries in Europe are referred to, and divided into safety areas as: car passenger, pedestrian, cyclist, drownings, falls, poisonings, home, and community safety.

Some examples from the review of Elke and Elvik [33] with BC ratio:

- Regulation towards walking chair for infants (USA 2007), BC ratio: >43.
- Poison control centres (USA 1997), BC ratio: 5.5.

Prevention of Accidents and Injuries in the Elderly

Each year, approximately 10% of the elderly population (65+) will be treated for by medical doctors for an injury. Falls are the dominant cause of injuries, followed by traffic accidents, burns, and fires. In a European project EUNESE (EUropean NEtwork for Safety among Elderly), a manual on elderly safety was published, focusing on accidental injuries [40]. It was referred to quite a few interventions with documented positive effects, mostly with fall injuries.

Some examples from the review of Elke and Elvik [33] with BC ratio:

- Rehabilitation after hip fracture operations (USA 2001), BC ratio: 4.5–5.3
- Programme to reduce fall injuries (Australia 2006), BC ratio: 6.3–20.6
- Hip protectors on nursing homes (USA 2006): BC ratio: 1–2.8

The elderly population in Europe will increase substantially towards 2050. The need to prevent hip fractures and other injuries will increase in importance. It is recommended that each country in Europe should establish a national action plan for the prevention of injuries in the elderly [40].

The Prevention of Falls Network for Dissemination (ProFouND) is a new EC-funded initiative dedicated to bring about the dissemination and implementation of best practice in falls prevention across Europe. Among other activities, they are aiming at promoting the dissemination and adoption of evidence-based best practice in falls prevention throughout Europe and beyond (http://profound.eu.com/).

Key Elements for Decision-Makers

Injury prevention is a good case for public health. It gives rapid and positive results. We have a lot of experiences on best practices and evidence-based strategies on prevention of traffic, occupational, home, sports, child, and elderly accidents and injuries. Many injury interventions have been documented that they give profit to the society.

The challenge with accident prevention is the fragmentation of the field: traffic, occupational, home, sport, and leisure. There is a need for an effective organisation of the various authorities involved on both the central and local level, in order to create injury controllers with a mandate to act in a coordinated manner.

An important task for the medical authorities is to create and maintain injury surveillance systems that enable setting priorities, following the trends and identifying factors contributing to accidents and injuries.

On both central and local levels, injury prevention action plans should be developed based on the existing knowledge on best practices and evidence-based strategies in collaboration between relevant authorities having responsibility on the various accident and injury types.

Injury prevention is a never-ending process. The new generation needs to be trained to master the dangers, new products will be introduced, and environments will change. There is a need to have institutions that can follow this field in order to ensure that we always will work towards building a safer world.

References

1. Murray CJL, Lopez AD (1997) Alternative projections of mortality and disability by cause 1990–2020: global burden of disease study. Lancet 349:1498–504
2. WHO (2009) World health statistics 2009. World Health Organisation, Geneva
3. Peden M, McGee K, Krug EG (eds) (2002) Injury: a leading cause of the global burden of disease. World Health Organization, Geneva
4. Last JM (ed) (2001) A dictionary of epidemiology, 4th edn. Oxford University Press, Oxford
5. Lund J. (2004) Epidemiology, registration and prevention of accidental injuries. Dissertation, University of Oslo, Oslo, Department of General Practice and Community Medicine
6. Gibson JJ (1961) The contribution of experimental psychology to the formulation of the problem of safety: a brief for basic research. In: Approaches to accident research. Association for the Aid of Crippled Children, New York, pp 79–89
7. Nordic Medical Statistical Committee (NOMESCO) (1984, 1990, 1997) Classification of external causes of injuries, 1st edn., 2nd edn., 3rd edn. NOMESCO, Copenhagen
8. Baker SP, O'Neill B, Karpf RS (1984) The injury fact book, 1st edn. Lexington Books, Lexington
9. Bonnie RJ, Guyer B (2002) Injury as a field of public health: achievements and controversies. J Law Med Ethics 30:267–80
10. Lund J, Aaro LE (2004) Accident prevention. Presentation of a model placing emphasis on human, structural and cultural factors. Saf Sci 43:271–324
11. Peden M, Oyegbite K, Osanne-Smith J, Hyder AA, Branche C, Rahman AKMF, Rivara F, Bartolomeos K (eds) (2008) World report on child injury prevention. World Health Organization, Geneva
12. Pollock DA, McClain PW (1989) Trauma registries. Current status and future prospects. J Am Med Assoc 262:2280–2283
13. Holder Y, Peden M, Krug E, Lund J, Gururaj G, Kobusingye O (eds) (2001) Injury surveillance guidelines. World Health Organization, Geneva. www.who.int/violence_injury_prevention/media/en/136.pdf. Accessed 26 Jan 2015
14. Frerichs RR (1991) Epidemiologic surveillance in developing countries. Annu Rev Publ Health 12:257–280
15. Dupré D (2000) Accidents at work in the EU in 1996. Stat Focus 4:1–8

16. Elvik R, Mysen AB (1999) Incomplete accident reporting: a meta-analysis of studies made in thirteen countries. Transp Res Rec 1665:133–140
17. World Health Organization: International Classification of External Causes if Injury (ICECI). www.who.int/classifications/icd/adaptations/iceci/en/. Accessed 26 Jan 2015
18. Bloemhoff A, Hoyinck S, Dekker R, Mulder S (2001) Data dictionary for minimum data sets on injuries. Consumer Safety Institute, Amsterdam
19. Lund J, Bjerkedal T, Gravseth HM, Vilimas K, Wergeland E (2004) A two-step medically based injury surveillance system: experiences from the Oslo injury register. Accid Anal Prev 36:1003–1017
20. Sethi D, Mitis F, Racioppo F (2010) Preventing injuries in Europe: from international collaboration to local implementation. World Health Organization, Copenhagen
21. Eurosafe (2013) Injuries in the European Union. Summary of injury statistics for the years 2008–2010. http://ec.europa.eu/health/data_collection/docs/idb_report_2013_en.pdf. Accessed 26 Jan 2015
22. Haagsma J, Belt E, Polinder S, Lund J, Atkinson M, Macey S, Lyons RA, van Beeck EF (2010) Integris WP5 injury disability indicators: towards a standardized methodology for measuring the burden of disability due to injury. Inj Prev 16:A139
23. Veiligheid, Letsels – Kerncijfers 2011 (Injuries: Key Figs. 2011, in Dutch). Veiligheid NL, Amsterdam (Consumer Safety Institute), 2012, Factsheet No. 28. http://www.veiligheid.nl/csi/veiligheidnl.nsf/content/37FDA3DFB5357093C1257AD10046D84C/$file/Factsheet%20kerncijfers%202011%20incl%20cover%20voor%20site.pdf. Accessed 26 Jan 2015
24. Myklestad I, Alver K, Madsen C, Ohm E, Hesselberg O, Baevre K, Sjolingstad A, Groholt E-K (2014) Skadebildet i Norge. Hovedvekt på personskader i sentrale registre. (Injury pattern in Norway with focus on injuries in central registers - in Norwegian). National Institute of Public Health, Oslo, Report 2014:2
25. Münchener Rückversicherungs-Gesellschaft (Munich Re) (2004) Assessing disability: an international comparison of workers' compensation systems. Munich Re, Munich. www.munichre.com/publications/302-04093_en.pdf. Accessed 26 Jan 2015
26. European statistics on road accidents. DG mobility and transport, road safety observatory (2012), EU road fatalities. http://ec.europa.eu/transport/road_safety/specialist/statistics/index_en.htm. Accessed 26 Jan 2015
27. Elvik R, Vaa T (2004) The handbook of road safety measures. Elsevier, Amsterdam
28. Safe Work Australia (March 2012) The cost of work-related injury and illness for Australian employers, workers and the community: 2008–09. http://www.safeworkaustralia.gov.au/sites/SWA/about/Publications/Documents/660/Cost%20of%20Work-related%20injury%20and%20disease.pdf
29. Gyllensvärd H (2010) Cost-effectiveness of injury prevention -a systematic review of municipality based interventions. Cost Eff Resour Alloc 8:17
30. Polinder S, Meerding WJ, van Baar ME, Toet H, Mulder S, van Beeck EF (Dec 2005) EUROCOST reference group. Cost estimation of injury-related hospital admissions in 10 European countries. J Trauma 59(6):1283–1290; (discussion 1290–1)
31. Robertson LS (1997) Injury control: some effects, principles, and prospects. In: Detels R et al (eds) Oxford Textbook of Public Health, 3rd ed, Oxford University Press, Oxford, pp 1307–1319
32. Spinks A, Turner C, Nixon J, McClure RJ (2009) The 'WHO Safe Communities' model for the prevention of injury in whole populations (Review). Cochrane Library 2009(3)
33. Erke A, Elvik R (2007) Nyttekostnadsanalyse av skadeforebyggende tiltak. (Cost-benefit analyses of injury prevention measures—in Norwegian). Institute of Transport Economics, Oslo
34. Peden M, Scurfield R, Sleet D, Mohan D, Hyder AA, Jarawan E, Mathers C (eds) (2004) World report on traffic injury prevention. World Health Organization, Geneva
35. Dyreborg J, Nielsen K, Kines P, Dziekanska A, Frydendal KB, Bengtsen E, Rasmussen K (2013) Review af den eksisterende videnskabelige litteratur om effekten af forskjellige typer tiltag til forebyggelse av arbejdsulykker. (Review of safety interventions for the Prevention

of Accidents at Work—in Danish). National Research Center for the Working Environment, Copenhagen

36. Michel FI, Bochud Y (2012) Haus und Freizeit. Unfall-, Risiko- und Interventionsanalyse. (Home and leisure. Accident-, risk- and prevention analyses. A condensed version translated to French, Italian and English). bfu—Beratungsstelle für Unfallverhütung, Bern
37. Kisser R, Bauer R (2012) The burden of sports injuries in the European Union. Research report D2h of the project "Safety in Sports". Austrian Road Safety Board, Vienna (Kuratorium für Verkehrssicherheit)
38. Steffen K, Andersen TE, Krosshaug T, Mechelen WV, Myklebust G, Verhagen EA, Bahr, R (2010) ECSS position statement 2009: prevention of acute sports injuries. Eur J Sport Sci 10(4):223–226
39. MacKay M, Vincenten J, Brussoni M, Towner L (2006) Child safety good practice guide. European Child Safety Alliance, Eurosafe, Amsterdam
40. Lund J and members of working group 4 (2006) Priorities for elderly safety in Europe Agenda for action. Medical School, Athens University, Athen

Chapter 11
Migrant and Ethnic Minority Health

M.L. Essink-Bot, C.O Agyemang, K Stronks and A Krasnik

Ethnic Inequalities in Health: A Conceptual Framework

Defining Migration, Ethnicity and Associated Terminology

Using country of birth, we use the terms "migrants" to refer to residents of a European country who were born elsewhere. "Non-Western migrants" were born in low- and middle-income countries outside of Europe, whereas "Western migrants" were born in another European country or in a highly developed country outside Europe (such as the USA, Japan, or Australia). The complementary term "local born" refers to residents born in the host country. In this chapter, we focus on non-Western migrants.

The different reasons for migration can be categorized as forced and unforced. Refugees and asylum seekers were forced to migrate from their home countries because of violence or political circumstances. Reasons for unforced migration include former colonization (e.g. Algerians migrating to France, or Surinamese to the Netherlands), economic reasons (labour migration, such as Turkish men to

M.L. Essink-Bot (✉) · C.O. Agyemang · K. Stronks
Department of Public Health, Academic Medical Center—University of Amsterdam,
PO Box 22660, Amsterdam 1100, The Netherlands
e-mail: m.l.essink-bot@amc.uva.nl

C.O. Agyemang
e-mail: c.o.agyemang@amc.uva.nl

K. Stronks
e-mail: k.stronks@amc.uva.nl

A. Krasnik
Faculty of Health Sciences Department of Public Health CSS, Danish Research Centre for Migration Ethnicity and Health (MESU) University of Copenhagen, Øster Farimagsgade 5, 1014 Copenhagen, Denmark
e-mail: alk@sund.ku.dk

S. Boccia et al. (eds.), *A Systematic Review of Key Issues in Public Health*,
DOI 10.1007/978-3-319-13620-2_11

Germany), family reunification (Turkish women and children following their husbands and fathers to Germany), work or study (e.g. Japanese students in Sweden). Migrants can live legally in a country or illegally as so-called undocumented migrants. Undocumented migrants constitute an especially disadvantaged group.

There is no commonly accepted definition of ethnicity, but current definitions all use ethnicity as a social construct. An ethnic group is defined as a group that shares a number of characteristics, including history, ancestry, identity, a geographical affiliation, culture and traditions, language and religious tradition [46].

European countries differ in the choice of indicators to translate this definition into measurable elements. In the UK, self-identified ethnicity is the indicator of choice. In mainland Europe, definitions based on country of origin are most commonly used. If nothing else is available, nationality may serve.

Ethnic minorities are ethnic groups who may have lived in a country for generations but differ from the majority population in one or more shared characteristics, such as language and cultural traditions. For specific attention to ethnic minority groups such as the Roma population in Central and Eastern Europe, we refer to the literature [14], but many causal mechanisms underlying worse health of migrants also apply to ethnic minorities within countries.

A Conceptual Model Linking Migration, Ethnicity and Health Outcomes

Disease patterns often differ between migrants and local-born people. Diverging epidemiology of diseases can be expected not only for communicable but also for non-communicable diseases. While some chronic conditions, such as diabetes mellitus (DM), occur more frequently among many migrant groups, lower risks have been reported for most types of cancer. Studies on specific diseases such as stroke have reported diverse epidemiology between migrant groups, with higher risk for migrants coming from Sub-Saharan Africa, the Caribbean and South Asia, and lower risks for those born elsewhere such as Morocco [40]. Migrants generally tend to be healthier in the first period after migration (healthy migrant effect), but after longer periods, migrant health is generally worse than that of the host population. Such inequalities in health apply not only to first-generation migrants but also to their offspring. The dynamic nature of health inequalities between migrants and the host population requires a life course approach for analysis, taking the migration process as well as life phases and generational developments into account.

The following model (modified from [49]) can be used to specify how ethnicity is linked to health (Fig. 11.1).

The model assumes that an individual's ethnic background influences health in two stages. First, ethnicity is associated with an uneven distribution of specific risk factors, also called proximal risk factors, as they are considered to be proximate to the onset of pathogenic processes. These include behavioural (e.g. smoking, diet), psychosocial (e.g. stress) and biological (e.g. hypertension) exposures that trigger

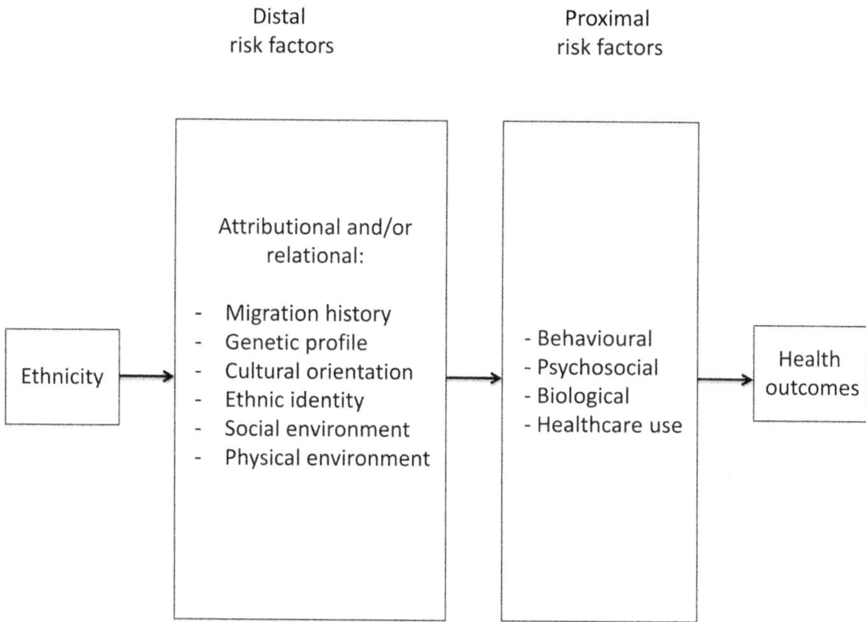

Fig. 11.1 Conceptual model [49]

pathogenic processes, and can therefore be perceived as a direct "cause" of a disease. If the outcome measure is health outcome rather than disease incidence, the proximal risk factors also include health care. The relevance of the proximal risk factors depends on the specific outcome measure under study. For example, ethnic inequalities in the incidence of type 2 diabetes might be due to an uneven distribution of behavioural risk factors such as dietary habits or lack of exercise, whereas ethnic inequalities in depression might arise from an uneven distribution of psychosocial stressors across ethnic groups.

Second, it is important to examine the causal pathways that link ethnicity to the proximal risk factors. It is not a coincidence that proximal risk factors are unevenly distributed across ethnic groups. This distribution is rooted in the characteristics of the individual people in an ethnic group, such as migration history, genetic profile, cultural orientation (that also partly determines the tendency to master the majority language), and the social and physical environmental conditions they are exposed to as a result of migration.

We explicitly consider the migration process, operationalized as "migration history", as one of the distal risk factors in the causal pathway between ethnicity and health. Migration histories are of course generally different for forced and unforced migration. Migration history includes premigration factors (e.g. hunger, war), the 'travel' (e.g. uncertainty, accidents) and postmigration factors (e.g. asylum-seeking procedures, formal migrant status and access to health care). Length of stay in the host country is also a postmigration factor, and includes generational differences (being a first-generation migrant or a descendant of migrants). As illustrated by the examples, the impact of premigration factors and the exposures during the journey (in that case, the flight) may generally be larger in forced migration. Also, the post-migration situation on arrival in the host country is quite different.

Ethnic identity points at the individual's feelings or emotional attachment towards a specific ethnic group. It is a psychological label that is related to the process of acculturation. As such, it is dynamic over time and may vary across various life domains.

The social environment points at the lower socioeconomic position of migrants and ethnic minority groups, but also to perceived and/or actual discrimination. The physical environment includes working conditions, but also exposure to the Western European diet.

Both distal and proximal determinants of health outcomes by ethnicity can be either attributional (i.e. the unique characteristics of a specific ethnic group, such as genetic profile or cultural orientation) or relational (i.e. the characteristics resulting from the interaction of an ethnic group with the majority society, including discrimination, a low socioeconomic position and an unhealthy diet). Some distal and proximal determinants can even be both attributional and relational. For example, ethnic identity is a characteristic of a specific group, but at the same time, it is formed by the interactions this group has with other groups in the host country.

The distal risk factors of ethnic groups thus explain why a certain proximal risk factor is unevenly distributed across ethnic groups. If, for example, a certain ethnic minority group has an increased prevalence of smoking, this may be due to the fact that the group is exposed to discrimination in the host country (relational), or to specific sociocultural values characteristic for that group (attributional). By placing the distribution of proximal factors in these causal pathways, scientific research will yield statements on the explanation of ethnic inequalities in health that are generalizable to other ethnic groups (including the majority population) with similar characteristics.

This conceptual model replaces one-dimensional explanations of ethnic inequalities in health. These include attribution to genetic causes only, to differences in culture or to lower socioeconomic status than the majority group. In fact, all these factors contribute to ethnic inequalities in health, and a singular cause is unlikely [27]. In European research and policy making, there may be a tendency to reduce "social determinants" of health to "socioeconomic determinants" and to ignore the role of ethnicity, migration and other factors in the creation of ethnic inequalities in health. However, an integrated approach, simultaneously taking account of socioeconomic status, migration and ethnicity as well as other determinants of ethnic inequalities in health, is essential. An integrated, intersectional, multivariate and multilevel approach will improve our understanding of ethnic health inequalities [27]. As of 2013, there is not very much empirical evidence available to quantify the relative contributions of the various factors to ethnic inequalities in health, and additionally, the relative contributions are likely to differ between the ethnic inequalities in various diseases. Large-scale multiethnic cohort studies such as the HELIUS study [49] are required to fill the gaps in empirical data and analyses.

Ethnic Inequalities in Cardiovascular Health and Diabetes as an Illustration

Ethnic inequalities in cardiovascular health have been widely documented and may also serve to illustrate the conceptual model above. A Danish study showed generally lower cardiovascular disease mortality among migrants compared with native Danes [37]. Incidence and mortality levels due to cardiovascular disease appear to vary between migrants from different countries of origin. For example, in the Netherlands, mortality from all cardiovascular diseases combined was found to be 13% higher among male migrants from Suriname, but 50% lower among male Moroccan migrants [13].

A more consistent view emerges when a distinction is made between the two main types of cardiovascular diseases: stroke and coronary heart disease (CHD). Below, we will discuss each disease type separately.

Stroke

For stroke, consistently higher mortality and incidence rates have been observed for migrants from Western African origin. In England, in 1999–2003, stroke mortality was almost 200% higher among male migrants from western Africa, and almost 100% higher among those from the Caribbean [26]. Similar findings come from the Netherlands, showing high stroke mortality of Surinamese and Antillean-born residents in the Netherlands [1, 48]. This common pattern has been attributed to high rates of hypertension among people from Western African origin. It is uncertain whether the high prevalence of hypertension in West Africans is mostly due to genetic factors or to environmental factors. A significant role of environment is suggested by studies that found a higher prevalence of hypertension of Western African migrants as compared to their counterparts who did not migrate from their countries of origin [2].

Although high stroke rates are not a universal pattern among migrant groups, they seem to be the rule rather than an exception. Hypertension contributes to the higher risks for many groups, although the available evidence indicates that hypertension prevalence is decreased in some migrant groups. This implies that increased stroke mortality levels may be partly linked to other factors, such as problems in the care for patients with hypertension or stroke. Although the evidence on this issue is yet inconclusive, there are indications for ethnic differences in control and treatment of high blood pressure [2].

Coronary Heart Disease

With regard to CHD, migrants from non-Western countries do not show consistently higher or lower mortality rates as compared to the local-born populations of

European countries. For example, in Sweden, the incidence of myocardial infarction was increased by 50 % among men born in Turkey or South Asia, but decreased by 20–30 % among men born in Northern Africa and Southeast Asia [40]. Similar patterns are observed in other European countries.

Several English studies have addressed the high rates of CHD mortality among residents born on the Indian subcontinent [11]. While the rates of CHD mortality of these migrants groups have declined in recent decades, as among local-born English population, the gap in CHD risk persisted or even widened [26]. The causes of the higher CHD risk are yet uncertain, and may in part be related to genetic factors. In addition, South Asian migrants have rates of overweight, together with a greater CHD risk, at similar levels of body mass index. Further, South Asians are less likely than local-born English to present themselves with the classic symptoms of CHD, which might hinder timely diagnosis and treatment [6].

By contrast, English studies have found a lower rate of CHD in West African descent migrants than the local-born population [25, 52]. Recent English data seem to indicate that the CHD advantage is diminishing rapidly. Harding et al.'s study (2008) spanning from 1979 to 2003 showed very disturbing trends. For the first time, Jamaican-born women had a higher directly age-standardized CHD death rate than those born in England and Wales. In 1979–1983, the age-standardized rate of CHD was lower in Jamaican-born women than in those born in England and Wales (RR = 0.63, 95 % CI: 0.52, 0.77). In 1999–2003, however, Jamaican-born women were more likely than those born in England and Wales to have CHD (RR = 1.23, 95 % CI: 1.06, 1.42). The gap between Jamaican-born men and those born in England and Wales is also closing rapidly. The age-standardized rate ratio of CHD in Jamaican-born men in 1979–1983 was 0.45 (95 % CI: 0.40, 0.50). In 1999–2003, the rate had increased to 0.81 (95 % CI: 0.73, 0.90). The convergence of CHD rates among Jamaican-born people bears resemblance to African Americans in the USA who now have a higher rate than the White Americans, reversing the previous pattern [5].

Diabetes Mellitus

High rates of CHD occurrence may be related to a high prevalence of DM. In almost all migrant groups, DM incidence, prevalence and mortality rates are much higher than among local-born residents [35]. The evidence for a higher occurrence of DM comes from both mortality studies and health interview surveys. For example, in the Netherlands, the occurrence of DM has been found to be higher among each of the main immigrant groups (i.e. those born in Turkey, Morocco, Suriname or the Antilles). For these groups combined, DM prevalence rates were two times higher than among the local born [51]. Even larger differences were observed in terms of DM mortality (i.e. deaths with DM as the "underlying" cause of death), with a threefold increase among men, and a fourfold increase among women in migrant groups as compared to the local-born population. Migrants of Surinamese origin had the highest prevalence as well as mortality rates [48].

Inequalities in the incidence of DM are likely to be reflected in similarly sized inequalities in both DM mortality and DM prevalence. If there are also ethnic differences in case fatality, the inequalities in DM mortality may exceed the incidence of inequalities. Unfortunately, due to lack of data sources, direct evidence on the DM incidence or case-fatality among migrants to European countries is scarce. One of the few examples is an English follow-up study that found that South Asian diabetic patients had excess diabetes mortality as compared to European diabetic patients, especially at younger ages [34].

A European overview study analysed ethnic inequalities in DM mortality [51]. Data were included from seven European countries on 30 different migrant groups in total. For the majority of the migrant groups, DM mortality was much higher than the rates for local-born residents. On average, DM mortality was increased by 90% for men and by 120% for women. This overview further illustrated that, of all non-communicable diseases for which ample data are available, DM is the only disease whose occurrence is strongly increased in virtually all immigrant groups.

The causes of the increased DM risk of migrants are manifold. At the level of proximal risk factors, lifestyle factors suggested to be involved include both physical inactivity and unhealthy diet ("behavioural factors" in the conceptual model). Their joint effect is to raise the prevalence of moderate overweight and obesity in many migrant populations as compared to local-born residents [35]. Obesity may be especially important as a factor contributing to increased insulin concentrations and decreased insulin sensitivity (biological factors). Moreover, metabolic control is poor among migrant groups with diabetes, and HbA1c in migrants is generally higher than in the local-born population [3, 32]. These findings suggest shortfalls in diabetes health care among migrant populations.

At the level of the distal risk factors, a genetic predisposition to diabetes is likely. A certain susceptibility to insulin resistance and abdominal adiposity, the intrauterine environment and biological imprinting all act synergistically to increase the risk of DM in migrant populations [39]. Probably, genetic predisposition interacts with migration, suggesting that migrants' excess DM prevalence is related to a change from a poor to an affluent environment [35]. According to this hypothesis, DM risk is raised because most migrants in non-Western countries have been raised in situations of poverty, and their bodies have been "programmed" to cope with starvation. As a result, later in life, they are especially susceptible to gaining weight in the obesogene (nutrient-rich and activity-poor) environments of the European host countries.

Diversity: Responsive Care as a Tool to Combat Ethnic Inequalities in Health

Ethnic inequalities in access and/or quality of care are likely to contribute to ethnic inequalities in health. Because most causes of ethnic inequalities in health are beyond the span of control of the health-care sector, it is unreasonable to expect that such inequalities could be erased by interventions from the health-care system only. However, it is a relatively "easy" way to intervene and to combat unnecessary health losses.

Health-Care Equity

Equity of care has been defined as: "equal access and quality across ethnic population subgroups; meaning equal access to available care for equal need, equal utilization for equal need, equal quality for all" [54]. Health care is deemed accessible if there are no financial, geographical, times or cultural barriers to health-care consumption. High quality of care means safe, effective, efficient, timely and patient-centred (or responsive) care [28].

Health care inequity can be horizontal or vertical. Horizontal inequity means that people with the same health care needs do not have access to the same level of services. Vertical inequity exists when people with greater needs are not provided with more health care services [47]. Hence, equal health care consumption across ethnic groups may in fact signify vertical inequity, if need differs by ethnic group [19, 47]. Empirical analysis of ethnic inequalities in health care outcomes potentially enables the identification of ethnic inequities in the process of care [19].

Internationally, ethnic inequalities in quality and accessibility of health care have been well established [29]. A review of European studies on utilization of health care suggested a diverging picture regarding utilization of somatic health care services by migrants compared to nonmigrants in Europe [36]. Overall, migrants tended to have lower attendance and referral rates to mammography and cervical cancer screening, more contacts per patient to general practitioner but less use of consultation by telephone, and a similar or higher level of use of specialist care as compared to nonmigrants. Emergency room utilization showed higher, equal, and lower levels of utilization for migrants compared to nonmigrants, whereas hospitalization rates were higher than or equal to those for nonmigrants.

For European health care contexts, empirical research on inequalities in health-care outcomes is scarce. For some diseases or care contexts, ethnic inequalities in outcomes, attributable to deficient care, have been shown. For example, Fransen et al. found that Turkish and Surinamese origin women in the Netherlands less often than Dutch women made an informed decision whether or not to participate in prenatal screening, due to underuse of interpretation services and translated information materials by their obstetric care providers [4, 23]. Alderliesten [4] found that the prevalence of substandard prenatal care varied among ethnic groups and that the prevalence of substandard care was highest among Surinamese mothers. Poeran et al. [38] showed that adverse perinatal outcomes among a Dutch urban population could be attributed to social deprivation in Western women, but that differential effectiveness of preventive services was the most likely cause in non-Western women. An exploratory study in the Netherlands showed ethnic differences in excess lengths of stay in hospital and unplanned readmission rates [15]. Excess length of stay (LOS) and readmission can possibly be interpreted as distal indicators of quality of care, but other interpretations, including a difference in nursing care needs, are possible.

Diversity-Responsive Care Provision

Diversity-responsive care is considered a strategy to decrease inequities in healthcare outcomes for migrants and ethnic minority patients. We prefer the term "diversity-responsive care" over the better known term "culturally competent care", because the latter may suggest that "cultural differences" are all that matter. The term "cultural competence" is derived from the USA and has started to appear in the literature during the 1990s. Originally, cultural competence training programmes stemmed from an urge to overcome cultural and linguistic barriers experienced between migrant patients and their care providers. These programmes focused on teaching about beliefs and characteristics of specific cultural and ethnic groups [8, 42].

It has been recognized that adequate diversity-responsiveness of a health care system requires at least adaptations at two levels, i.e. the patient–provider interaction and the level of health care organizations.

Diversity-responsiveness at the level of individual care providers is generally defined as the knowledge, attitudes and skills necessary to provide good quality of care for ethnic minority patients [44]. At the level of patient–provider interaction, many difficulties between care providers and ethnic minority patients were documented. Communication problems are the most prominent. Common causes of communication problems with ethnic minority patients are language barriers, sociocultural differences in explanatory models (EMs) of illness and low health literacy (HL) [7, 43]. Research also showed that prejudice, stereotyping and nonconscious biases impact on how medical professionals diagnose and treat ethnic minority patients [50]. Language barriers, low HL and discrimination are associated with worse health care outcomes such as therapy nonadherence, higher risk for adverse invents and lower levels of shared decision making.

Knowledge

- Knowledge of epidemiology and manifestation of diseases in various ethnic groups
- Knowledge of differential effects of treatment in various ethnic groups
- Attitudes
- Awareness of how culture shapes individual behaviour and thinking
- Awareness of the social contexts in which specific ethnic groups live
- Awareness of one's own prejudices and tendency to stereotype
- Skills

- Ability to transfer information in a way the patient can understand and to know when to seek external help with communication
- Ability to adapt to new situations flexibly and creatively
- Practical and concrete translation of cultural competence at the provider level (from Ref. [44]).

In fact, the required knowledge, attitudes and skills boil down to effective handling of the characteristics of ethnic groups that are considered as distal determinants of ethnic inequalities in health, see the conceptual model in Fig. 11.1.

Below, we illustrate some of the important attitudes and skills.

Language Barriers

The "ability to transfer information in a way the patient can understand and to know when to seek external help with communication" is often related to overcoming language barriers. All care providers will face migrants and ethnic minority patients who are not fluent in the language of their doctor. Use of professional interpretation services is recommended to bridge this language gap. Studies in the USA indeed found that professional interpreters improve clinical care for patients with limited English language proficiency [30, 33]. The use of family or friends as interpreters instead of professional interpreters carries the risk of errors in medical interpretation, with potentially serious clinical consequences [20–22]. Despite the demonstrated benefits of professional interpreters, care providers under-use professional interpretation and rather 'get by' with ad hoc interpreters [18].

Low Health Literacy

HL is defined as the degree to which individuals have the capacity to obtain, process and understand basic health information and services needed to make appropriate health decisions [41]. Subjects with low HL tend to be less likely to successfully manage chronic diseases [16, 17]. Conceptually, low HL is considered an important mediator of health disadvantages in lower socioeconomic groups. HL is related to educational level. Most migrant and ethnic minority groups tend to belong to lower socioeconomic groups in the host country. Language barriers and low HL add up to difficulties to navigate the health-care system effectively, and to make optimal use of the interaction with the health system, including preventive services. In the consultation room, diversity-responsive care providers should also have the skills to communicate effectively with low health literate persons. Care providers need to develop the skills to adapt their communications with low health literate patients effectively.

Explanatory Models

According to the theoretical model of the medical anthropologist Kleinman [31], health care providers and patients have different "EMs" of disease and treatment, including explanations for the aetiology of the condition, the timing and onset of symptoms, the pathophysiological processes involved, the natural course and severity and appropriate treatments. Awareness of the phenomenon of EMs is an example of "how culture shapes individual behaviour and thinking". Lay EMs vary according to personality and sociocultural factors, whereas those of health care providers rely more on scientific logic and evidence. Studies among ethnic minority populations suggest that cultural factors have an impact on the manner in which patients from these groups explain diseases such as hypertension [9, 10, 12, 53]. It has become increasingly recognized that doctors must improve their understanding of the EMs of their patients in order to increase patient adherence to treatment and to improve their self-management of disease.

Organizational Level

At the level of health care organizations, current conceptualizations suggest that organizational responsiveness to diversity in health care means ensuring equal access and providing appropriate care. Seeleman et al. [45] developed an analytic framework that defined several preconditions, such as demonstrating organizational commitment, developing a competent and diverse workforce, and fostering patient and community participation. One of the policy elements includes the explicit intention to monitor the organization's own equity performance, meaning that indicators for access and quality of care need to be analyzed by patients' ethnic origin. This, in turn, requires a standardized and safeguarded opportunity to link patients' ethnicity data to health care registries.

The organizational level even includes the existence of formal barriers related to migrant status. Being an undocumented migrant most often implies very limited access—i.e. restricted to acute care only or a few care facilities from voluntary organizations only. Asylum seekers in many countries are also provided with limited care facilities during the sometimes-lengthy asylum-seeking processes before final decision on permission to stay.

Recommendations for Policy Makers

We structured some recommendations to policy makers in three categories, for general health policies, for policy at the level of health care organizations and for research policy.

General Health Policy

- Migrant and ethnic minority health should be considered in general policy documents and guidelines at the national, regional, local and institutional level. This recommendation follows directly from the evidence shown above, implying that ethnicity is a relevant determinant of health and that health care equity requires care differentiation by ethnicity.
- Shift from focus on merely social determinants of health to also include ethnicity and migrant status.
- Ensure formal rights to health care to all groups of migrants and ethnic minorities, including refugees and asylum seekers.
- Facilitate cross-sectional and multidisciplinary collaboration between health care and social care.

Policies at the Level of Health Care Organizations

- Structurally implement strategies for diversity-responsive health care organizations, such as the culturally and linguistically appropriate services (CLAS) standards (developed in the USA) or the environmental quality standards (EQS; European).This implies, for example, the implementation of professional interpretation and professional education in diversity-responsive care provision.
- Consider inclusive instead of ethnicity-specific programs.

Research Policy

- Develop common international categories and indicators for studies of migrant and ethnic minority health
- Include migrant status and ethnic characteristics in population-based research
- Use an evidence-based theoretical model to analyze ethnic inequalities in health and health care to unravel the causal mechanisms at the level of the proximal determinants
- Comprehensively analyse factors with favourable as well as unfavourable effects on ethnic minority health.

References

1. Agyemang C, Addo J, Bhopal R, Aikins Ade G, Stronks K (2009) Cardiovascular disease, diabetes and established risk factors among populations of Sub-Saharan African descent in Europe: a literature review. Global Health 5:7

2. Agyemang C, Kunst A, Bhopal R et al (2010) A cross-national comparative study of blood pressure and hypertension between English and Dutch South-Asian- and African-origin populations: the role of national context. Am J Hypertens 23(6):639–648
3. Agyemang C, Kunst AE, Bhopal R et al (2011) Diabetes prevalence in populations of South Asian Indian and African origins: a comparison of England and the Netherlands. Epidemiology 22(4):563–567
4. Alderliesten ME, Stronks K, van Lith JM et al (2008) Ethnic differences in perinatal mortality. A perinatal audit on the role of substandard care. Eur J Obstet Gynecol Reprod Biol 138(2):164–170
5. American Heart Association (2001) 2002 Heart and stroke statistical update Dallas. American Heart Association, Texas
6. Barakat K, Wells Z, Ramdhany S, Mills PG, Timmis AD (2003) Bangladeshi patients present with non-classic features of acute myocardial infarction and are treated less aggressively in east London, UK. Heart 89(3):276–279
7. Betancourt JR (2006) Cultural competency: providing quality care to diverse populations. Consult Pharm 21(12):988–995
8. Betancourt JR, Green AR (2010) Commentary: linking cultural competence training to improved health outcomes: perspectives from the field. Acad Med 85(4):583–585
9. Beune EJ, Haafkens JA, Schuster JS, Bindels PJ (2006) 'Under pressure': how Ghanaian, African-Surinamese and Dutch patients explain hypertension. J Hum Hypertens 20(12):946–955
10. Beune EJ, Haafkens JA, Agyemang C, Schuster JS, Willems DL (2008) How Ghanaian, African-Surinamese and Dutch patients perceive and manage antihypertensive drug treatment: a qualitative study. J Hypertens 26(4):648–656
11. Bhopal R (2000) What is the risk of coronary heart disease in South Asians? A review of UK research. J Public Health Med 22(3):375–385
12. Brown CM, Segal R (1996) The effects of health and treatment perceptions on the use of prescribed medication and home remedies among African American and white American hypertensives. Soc Sci Med 43:903–917
13. Bos V, Kunst AE, Keij-Deerenberg IM, Garssen J, Mackenbach JP (2004) Ethnic inequalities in age- and cause-specific mortality in The Netherlands. Int J Epidemiol 33(5):1112–1119
14. Cook B, Wayne GF, Valentine A, Lessios A, Yeh E (2013) Revisiting the evidence on health and health care disparities among the Roma: a systematic review 2003–2012. Int J Public Health 47(3):268–272
15. de Bruijne MC, van Rosse F, Uiters E, et al (2013) Ethnic variations in unplanned readmissions and excess length of hospital stay: a nationwide record-linked cohort study. Eur J Public Health 23(6):964–971
16. DeWalt DA, Berkman ND, Sheridan S, Lohr K, Pignone MP (2004) Literacy and health outcomes: a systematic review of the literature. J Gen Intern Med 19:1228–1239
17. DeWalt DA, Hink A (2009) Health literacy and child health outcomes: a systematic review of the literature. Pediatrics 124(Suppl 3):S265–S274
18. Diamond LC, Schenker Y, Curry L, Bradley EH, Fernandez A (2008) Getting by: underuse of interpreters by resident physicians. J Gen Intern Med 24(2):256–262
19. Essink-Bot ML, Lamkaddem M, Jellema P, Nielsen SS, Stronks K (2013) Interpreting ethnic inequalities in healthcare consumption: a conceptual framework for research. Eur J Public Health 23(6):922–926
20. Flores G, Barton Laws B, Mayo SJ et al (2003) Errors in medical interpretation and their potential clinical consequences in pediatric encounters. Pediatrics 111(1):6–14
21. Flores G (2005) The impact of medical interpreter services on the quality of health care: a systematic review. Med Care Res Rev 62(3):255–299
22. Flores G, Abreu M, Barone CP, Bachur R, Lin H (2012) Errors of medical interpretation and their potential clinical consequences: a comparison of professional versus ad hoc versus no interpreters. Ann Emerg Med 60(5):545–553

23. Fransen MP, Essink-Bot ML, Vogel I, Mackenbach JP, Steegers EA, Wildschut HI (2010) Ethnic differences in informed decision-making about prenatal screening for Down's syndrome. J Epidemiol Community Health 64(3):262–268
24. Fransen MP, Wildschut HIJ, Mackenbach JP, Steegers EAP, Essink-Bot ML (2012) Midwiven unable to overcome language barriers in prenatal health. Italian J Public Health 9(3):1–9
25. Gill PS, Kai J, Bhopal RS, Wild S (2007) Black and minority ethnic groups. In: Stevens A, Raftery J, Mant J (eds) Health care needs assessment: the epidemiologically based needs assessment reviews. Radcliffe Medical Press Ltd, Abington, pp 227–239
26. Harding S, Rosato M, Teyhan A (2008) Trends for coronary heart disease and stroke mortality among migrants in England and Wales, 1979–2003: slow declines notable for some groups. Heart 94(4):463–470
27. Ingleby D (2012) Ethnicity, migration and the 'social determinants of health' agenda. Psychosoc Interv 21(3):331–341
28. Institute of Medicine (2001) Crossing the quality chasm: a new health system for the 21st century. National Academies Press, Washington
29. Institute of Medicine (2003) Unequal treatment. National Academies Press, Washington
30. Karliner LS, Jacobs EA, Chen AH, Mutha S (2007) Do professional interpreters improve clinical care for patients with limited English proficiency? A systematic review of the literature. Health Serv Res 42(2):727–754
31. Kleinman A, Eisenberg L, Good B (1978) Culture, illness, and care: clinical lessons from anthropologic and cross-cultural research. Ann Intern Med 88:251–258
32. Lanting LC, Joung IM, Mackenbach JP, Lamberts SW, Bootsma AH (2005) Ethnic differences in mortality, end-stage complications, and quality of care among diabetic patients: a review. Diabetes Care 28(9):2280–2288
33. Lindholm M, Hargraves JL, Ferguson WJ, Reed G (2012) Professional language interpretation and inpatient length of stay and readmission rates. J Gen Intern Med 27:1294–1299
34. Mather HM, Chaturvedi N, Fuller JH (1998) Mortality and morbidity from diabetes in South Asians and Europeans: 11-year follow-up of the Southall Diabetes Survey, London, UK. Diabet Med 15(1):53–59
35. Misra A, Ganda OP (2007) Migration and its impact on adiposity and type 2 diabetes. Nutrition 23(9):696–708
36. Norredam M, Nielsen SS, Krasnik A (2010) Migrants' utilization of somatic healthcare services in Europe–a systematic review. Eur J Pub Health 20(5):555–563
37. Norredam M, Olsbjerg M, Petersen JH, Juel K, Krasnik A (2012) Inequalities in mortality among refugees and immigrants compared to native Danes–a historical prospective cohort study. BMC Public Health 12:757
38. Poeran J, Maas AF, Birnie E, Denktas S, Steegers EA, Bonsel GJ (2013) Social deprivation and adverse perinatal outcomes among Western and non-Western pregnant women in a Dutch urban population. Soc Sci Med 83:42–49
39. Ramachandran A, Ma RC, Snehalatha C (2010) Diabetes in Asia. Lancet 375(9712):408–418. doi:10.1016/S0140-6736(09)60937-5
40. Rafnsson SB, Bhopal RS, Agyemang C et al (2013) Sizable variations in circulatory disease mortality by region and country of birth in six European countries. Eur J Public Health 23(4):594–605
41. Ratzan SC, Parker RM (2000) Introduction. In: Selden CR, Zorn M, Ratzan S, Parker R (eds) National library of medicine current bibliographies in medicine: health literacy. National Institutes of Health, U.S. Department of Health and Human Services, Bethesda, Pub. No. CBM 2000–1
42. Saha S, Beach MC, Cooper LA (2008) Patient centeredness, cultural competence and healthcare quality. J Natl Med Assoc 100(11):1275–1285
43. Schouten BC, Meeuwesen L (2009) Cultural differences in medical communication: a review of the literature. Patient Educ Couns 64(1–3):21–34
44. Seeleman C, Suurmond J, Stronks K (2009) Cultural competence: a conceptual framework for teaching and learning. Med Educ 43(3):229–237

45. Seeleman MC, Essink-Bot ML, Stronks K, Ingleby D (2015) How should health service organizations respond to diversity? A content analysis of six approaches (submitted)
46. Simon P (2012) Collecting ethnic statistics in Europe: a review. Ethn Racial Stud 13:1366–1391
47. Starfield B (2011) The hidden inequity in health care. Int J Equity Health 10:15
48. Stirbu I, Kunst AE, Bos V, Mackenbach JP (2006) Differences in avoidable mortality between migrants and the native Dutch in The Netherlands. BMC Public Health 6:78
49. Stronks K, Snijder MB, Peters RJ, Prins M, Schene AH, Zwinderman AH (2013) Unravelling the impact of ethnicity on health in Europe: the HELIUS study. BMC Public Health 13:402
50. Suurmond J, Uiters E, de Bruijne MC, Stronks K, Essink-Bot ML (2010) Explaining ethnic disparities in patient safety: a qualitative analysis. Am J Public Health 100(Suppl 1):S113–S117
51. Vandenheede H, Deboosere P, Stirbu I et al (2012) Migrant mortality from diabetes mellitus across Europe: the importance of socio-economic change. Eur J Epidemiol 27(2):109–117
52. Wild SH, Fischbacher C, Brock A, Griffiths C, Bhopal R (2007) Mortality from all causes and circulatory disease by country of birth in England and Wales 2001–2003. J Public Health 29:191–198
53. Wilson RP, Freeman A, Kazda MJ et al (2002) Lay beliefs about high blood pressure in a low- to middle-income urban African-American community: an opportunity for improving hypertension control. Am J Med 112:26–30
54. Whitehead M, Dahlgren G (2000) Concepts and principles for tackling social inequities in health: levelling up. Part 1. World Health Organization, Regional Office for Europe, Copenhagen

Chapter 12
Public Mental Health

Chiara Cadeddu, Carolina Ianuale and Jutta Lindert

Definition

Mental health is "a state of well-being in which the individual realizes his or her own abilities, can cope with the normal stresses of life, can work productively and fruitfully, and is able to make a contribution to his or her community" [1].

Mental health disorders refer to conditions characterized by deregulation of mood, thought, and/or behavior, as recognized by the *Diagnostic and Statistical Manual*, fourth edition (DSM-IV) of the American Psychiatric Association (APA) [2]. Two systems are currently applied to classify mental disorders: the "ICD-10 Chapter Mental and behavioral disorders" [3] and the "DSM-IV of Mental Disorders" of the APA. The global burden of disease attributable to neuropsychiatric conditions is 13.8 %. Depression alone accounts for 7 % of the disease burden and is among the leading causes of disability. The World Health Organization (WHO) has predicted that by 2030, neuropsychiatric conditions will cause the greatest overall increase in disability-adjusted life years (DALYs) [4]. Furthermore, having a mental

C. Cadeddu (✉) · C. Ianuale
Institute of Public Health, Section of Hygiene, Università Cattolica del Sacro Cuore, L.go F. Vito 1, 00168 Rome, Italy
e-mail: chiaracadeddu@yahoo.it

C. Ianuale
e-mail: carolina.ianuale@rm.unicatt.it

J. Lindert
Protestant University of Ludwigsburg, Paulusweg 6, 71638 Ludwigsburg, Germany

J. Lindert
University of Leipzig, Leipzig, Germany

J. Lindert
Harvard School of Public Health, Boston, USA

J. Lindert
e-mail: mail@jlindert.de

S. Boccia et al. (eds.), *A Systematic Review of Key Issues in Public Health*,
DOI 10.1007/978-3-319-13620-2_12

illness may increase the risk of developing other illnesses: evidences showed that mental disorders are associated with an excess of all-cause mortality, cardiovascular diseases, diabetes, and maternal and child diseases. Conversely, having a physical illness may increase the development of mental diseases [5].

In this chapter, we describe the most prevalent mental health disorders:

- Mood disorders, in particular *depressive disorder:* A state of sad mood and diminished interest in activities that can affect a person's thoughts, behavior, feelings, and physical well-being [6];
- *Anxiety disorders:* Excessive and unrealistic worry about everyday tasks or events, or about certain objects or rituals [7];
- *Schizophrenia:* A mental disorder characterized by a breakdown of thought processes and by poor emotional responsiveness [8];
- *Alzheimer's disease and other dementias:* A group of disorders typically characterized by decline in memory and other cognitive abilities [9].

Depressive Disorders

Depression is a term describing both a transient mood state that all individuals virtually experienced during their life and a medical disorder. It is a heterogeneous diagnosis, characterized by depressed mood and/or loss of pleasure in most activities. The DSM of mental disorders defined a major depressive episode as a depressive mood and loss of interest in pleasure and activities during a period of at least 2 weeks. Bipolar disorder is characterized by the occurrence of at least one manic or mixed-manic episode during the patient's lifetime. Finally, dystimia is a mood disorder less severe than major depressive disorder that lasts for at least 2 years [10]. Depressive disorders are pervasive with effects on affects and mood, neurovegetative functions, cognition, and psychomotor activities, causing great disability [11].

Depression is the most common mental health disorder in communities, and is among the leading causes of disability across the world: It is estimated to affect 350 million people worldwide [12]; in 1990, it was the fourth most common cause of loss of DALYs worldwide [13], and by 2020, it is estimated to become the second common cause [14].

The estimated prevalence rate for major depression among 16- to 65-year-olds in the UK is 21/1000 (males 17, females 25). Risk factors for depressive disorder are individual (e.g., age, gender, migration history), family factors, social factors (e.g., socioeconomic status), medical comorbidities, and life events. Moreover, the current period of economic crisis, accompanied by an increase of unemployment and poverty and cuts in welfare services, can influence people's mental health [15].

Depression is associated with economic consequences: the costs impact on many different parts of society, especially on individuals with depressive disorders and their families. In a recent European estimate, the overall annual cost of depression in Europe was estimated at € 118 billion in 2004, with a cost of € 253 per inhabitant. Direct costs (outpatient care, drug costs, and hospitalization) were estimated at

42 billion, whereas indirect costs due to morbidity and mortality were estimated at € 76 billion [16]. Depressed people lose 5.6 h of productive work every week when they are depressed [17], and 50 % of the loss of work productivity is due to absenteeism and short-term disability [18].

According to WHO, effective treatments for depression consist of psychosocial treatments for mild depression that can be associated with antidepressants and psychotherapy in moderate and severe depression. However, fewer than 25 % of those affected have access to effective treatments; the level of under diagnosis and inadequate care is higher in migrants due to linguistic differences that can constitute barriers to recognition of depression. Rates of incident depression can be reduced through the use of preventive interventions, including individual, family, and social factors, such as physical activity [19], improving of sleep quality and healthy dietary practices [20], family cognitive behavioral therapy (CBT) in children with parents affected by depression [21], health policies such as reducing economic disability and inequality, reducing work stress, supporting refugees and migrants, improving public education on mental health [22].

Anxiety Disorders

Anxiety is a universal human experience in all age groups and its evocation does not necessarily imply the presence of a clinically significant mental disorder, but anxiety disorders are common and costly [23]. Anxiety in the recent understanding refers to the brain's response to danger, with expressions falling from mild to severe. It becomes maladaptive and a mental disorder when it interferes with functioning, physical and psychological health, and behaviors. The differentiation between normal and pathological anxiety, however, can be difficult. Only in the past few decades, scientists and clinicians have been able to develop screening and diagnostic schemas to assess the prevalence of anxiety [24]. In these schemas, common elements of anxiety disorders include among others chest discomfort, palpitations and shortness of breath, uneasiness of mind over an anticipated illness, abnormal apprehension of fear, and self-doubt. According to these schemas, anxiety disorders are among the most prevalent disorders worldwide.

Anxiety disorders are described and classified in diagnostic systems such as the DSM of mental disorders [25] or the International Classification of Diseases (ICD, currently version 10, WHO). For anxiety disorders, a steady increase in the number of categories across editions of the DSM and the ICD can be noted. The new DSM-V has a number of changes to anxiety and anxiety disorders (Table 12.1).

Anxiety disorders are among the most widespread psychiatric disorders worldwide with a considerable variation in frequency depending on the type of disorder. Specific phobias are the most prevalent anxiety disorders, panic disorder the least prevalent. In an early literature review, prevalence rates were determined 3 % for panic, 6 % for agoraphobia, 3 % for generalized anxiety, 2.5 % for simple phobia, and 1.5 % for social phobia. Anxiety disorders develop early in life during childhood

Table 12.1 Overview of key features and changes to the definition of types of anxiety disorders introduced in the DSM-IV and in the DSM-V

Type of anxiety disorder	Number in the DSM-IV	Key features	Changes in the DSM IV	Changes in the DSM V
Anxiety disorder	300.00	–	–	–
Panic disorder	300.01	Recurrent unexpected panic attacks; persistent worry/concern about additional attacks or their consequences	Eliminations of panic severity specifiers; introduction of a panic typology	No significant changes, description of different kinds of panic disorders are removed and lumped together into two categories (expected/unexpected)
Panic disorder without history of agoraphobia	300.22	–	–	Panic disorders and agoraphobia are no longer linked together
Panic disorder with agoraphobia	300.21	Meets criteria for panic disorder; agoraphobia: fear/avoidance of situations in which panic attacks might occur	See panic disorder	Panic disorders and agoraphobia are no longer linked together
Social phobia (Renamed: social anxiety disorder)	300.23	Marked fear/avoidance of social situations because of possibility of embarrassment or humiliation	Diagnosis permitted in presence of unexpected panic attacks	Specifiers change: from more "most social situations" to "performance only"
Specific phobia	300.29	Fear avoidance of circumscribed objects or situations	Introduction of phobia types	Adults no longer must recognize that their anxiety or fear is excessive or unreasonable, duration criterion was introduced
Generalized anxiety disorder	300.02	Chronic excessive, uncontrollable worry about a number of events	Criterion of uncontrollable worry	Unchanged
Obsessive-compulsive disorder	300.3	Recurrent, thoughts, images, or impulses	Recognition of mental compulsions	Now included under the chapter on obsessive-compulsive and related disorders

Table 12.1 (continued)

Type of anxiety disorder	Number in the DSM-IV	Key features	Changes in the DSM IV	Changes in the DSM V
Separation anxiety disorder	309.21		Unchanged; age before 18 years is no longer necessary; duration criterion was introduced	Wording has been slightly changed
Selective mutism	–		Classified in the section "Disorders usually first diagnosed in infancy, childhood or adolescence"	Newly introduced as anxiety disorder
Acute stress disorder	308.3			Now in the chapter on trauma and stressor-related disorders
Posttraumatic stress disorder	309.81	Three clusters (reexperiencing, negative cognitions and mood, avoidance of stimuli associated with prior exposure)	Traumatic event criterion	Now in a new chapter on trauma- and stressor-related disorders, more behavioral symptoms included, four clusters (reexperiencing, negative cognitions and mood, avoidance of stimuli associated with prior exposure, arousal)

DSM Diagnostic and Statistical Manual of Mental Disorders

or in adolescence and often have a chronic recurrent course [26, 27], but may remit spontaneously. The chronic course differs by type of anxiety disorder with variation, in the age of onset, in periodicity of symptoms, and in severity of behaviours [26]. Symptoms and expressions of anxiety disorders change over the life course: Approximately one in three women and one in six men report a lifetime history of any mood and/or anxiety disorders. The risk factors for anxiety disorders may vary across the lifespan and research on potential similarities and differences between age groups is needed.

The development of anxiety after the onset of a physical disease is a common reaction (e.g., to myocardial infarction) [28]. Physical diseases may cause symptoms such as fatigue which, as a result, may compromise the individual's ability to manage even normal, everyday stressors. Certain medical conditions have demonstrated an association with anxiety disorders, such as gastrointestinal problems, respiratory conditions, and vestibular problems.

Many anxiety disorders develop between childhood and adulthood [29]. Indeed, 90 % of individuals who developed a primary anxiety disorder did so before the age of 41 and 75 % before the age of 21. In older age, symptoms of anxiety disorders may differ and assessment may be more difficult in older age groups than in younger age groups. There are some differences as well as limitations to the assessment of symptoms among older adults as anxiety disorders are highly comorbid with depression in older adults; and anxiety disorders are highly comorbid with a number of medical illnesses. It might be necessary to investigate further anxiety and depression among older individuals as associations between cognitive decline and anxiety have been observed. [29]

Clearly, anxiety disorders are prevalent among children and adolescents, adults, and older persons. Findings suggest that, overall, anxiety disorders are more prevalent among younger adults than older adults. Another significant problem with regard to incidence of anxiety disorders in late life is the overlap with and influence of significant medical illnesses or other life changes. [29]

Studies indicate that anxiety disorders are common. Much more research is needed for adequately understanding anxiety disorders and its impact on health and quality of life. Cross-sectional and longitudinal research suggests that anxiety is associated with cognitive decline and dementias. Some suggestions may be made as pathways for future research: [25-29] They include additional investigation on dimensional measures of anxiety to better elucidate the latent structure and interrelationships between anxiety disorders and anxiety disorders and further mental disorders and concurrent use of different measures to better understand validity of concepts and measures. In addition, there is a high need of longitudinal studies on nonclinical samples to better identify risk factors and develop tailored public health programs.

Schizophrenia

Schizophrenia is a devastating mental illness that impairs mental and social functioning and often leads to the development of comorbid diseases [30]. It is characterized by a breakdown of thought processes and by a deficit of typical emotional responses. Positive symptoms typically include auditory hallucinations, paranoid or bizarre delusions, or disorganized speech and thinking. Negative symptoms—i.e., flat or blunted affect and emotion, poverty of speech (alogia), inability to experience pleasure (anhedonia), lack of desire to form relationships (asociality), and lack of motivation (avolition)—prevent the patient from functioning in society and limit his/her ability to hold a job, attend school, take care of children, or form friendship [31].

Schizophrenia affects about 24 million people worldwide (7/1000 of the adult population) mostly in the age group 15–35 years. Though the incidence is low (about 0.2/1000 per year), the prevalence is high (about 5/1000) due to chronicity [32]. About 1 % of the population may suffer from an episode of schizophrenia lasting at least 6 months. Two thirds of those will have further episodes [31].

The most common risk factors for schizophrenia include: individual factors (age, with the risk declining with age; gender, men develop schizophrenia earlier and with more severe symptoms), family factors, social factors (schizophrenia occurs twice as often in unmarried and divorced people as in married or widowed individuals and eight times more often in the lowest socioeconomic groups), life events (discrimination), famine, and malnutrition (e.g., folate deficiency).

Schizophrenia ranks among the top ten causes of disability in developed countries worldwide. The majority of people with schizophrenia do not attain "normal" milestones in social functioning, productivity, residence, and self-care. Further, people with schizophrenia typically underperform compared to expectations based on the achievements of family members and their own functioning prior to diagnosis [33]. These impairments are present early in the illness [34] and are clearly detectable at the time the diagnosis of schizophrenia is confirmed [35]. These impairments also are stable and are not produced in most cases by psychosis, per se, in that disability can be present even during periods when symptoms of psychosis are controlled [36].

Schizophrenic subjects have a 50 times higher risk of attempting suicide than the general population and suicide is the first cause of their premature death, with an estimated 10–13 % of killing themselves and approximately 40 % attempting suicide at least once. Moreover, more than 50 % of patients are not receiving appropriate care [31, 32]. This is clearly demonstrated, especially in Europe [37].

About interventions for people with schizophrenia, they differ between and within countries. Between countries, in a 1-year prospective cohort set up in six countries (France, Ireland, Italy, the Netherlands, Portugal, and Spain), comparisons highlighted cultural differences concerning the interventions that were proposed [37]. Centres in Italy, Spain, and Portugal proposed many interventions even though they were relatively deprived in terms of resources, and the tendency seems to be the reverse for the Northern European countries. On average, one in four patients suffered from needs (on average six per patient) that were not adequately met by the mental health service in their region, which varied from psychotic symptoms to managing their own affairs. The number of interventions was not correlated to the need status. The availability of community-based treatment, rehabilitation, and residential care seems to predict smaller proportions of patients with unmet needs. Thus, there appeared to be a systematic relationship between the availability of community-based mental health care and the need status of schizophrenic patients: The fewer the outpatient and rehabilitation services available, the more unmet their needs were.

Schizophrenia has very significant economic consequences; the costs impact on many different parts of society, especially on individuals with schizophrenia and their families. In an English estimate, overall schizophrenia cost to English society was £ 11.8 billion per year and that to the public sector was £ 7.2 billion [38]. This amounts to an average annual cost to society of £ 60,000 and to the public sector of £ 36,000 per person with schizophrenia.

Affected people consume about 2.5 % of the total annual health-care expenditures and about 10 % of the totally or permanently disabled population [31, 32]. They are often unemployed, homeless, and substance misusers; have a disrupted education and physical health problems; and are overrepresented in the criminal justice system [39].

According to National Institute for Health and Care Excellence (NICE) guidelines about schizophrenia [40], zotepine is potentially the most cost-effective pharmacological treatment of those examined for relapse prevention in people with schizophrenia that is in remission. However, results were characterized by high uncertainty, and probabilistic analysis showed that no antipsychotic medication can be considered to be clearly cost-effective.

While some of the costs estimated in previous studies are unavoidable, given the nature of schizophrenia, there is nevertheless strong evidence that several interventions that are not currently in widespread use could reduce the overall cost of schizophrenia and improve health and quality-of-life outcomes for people with the illness and for their families [39].

Considering early interventions, it has been demonstrated that their introduction could produce savings for health service, public sector, and society as well [39].

Other interventions to be implemented as effective and cost-effective for schizophrenia patients are: individual placement (a type of supported employment aimed at helping those with severe mental health problems to gain paid competitive employment) and support schemes (Fig. 12.1), family therapy, criminal justice system diversion, interventions on physical health (reduction of weight, exercise therapy, smoking cessation), interventions for substance misuse, homelessness-targeted interventions/supporting housing, crisis teams, peer support workers, advanced treatment directives, and CBT (in Table 12.2 rehospitalization rates with CBT are shown with their estimated risk) [39].

Dementias

Dementia is a syndrome that can be caused by a number of progressive disorders such as Alzheimer's disease, Parkinson's disease, and vascular dementia that affect memory, thinking, behaviour, and the ability to perform everyday activities [42]. It must include decline in memory and in at least one of the following cognitive abilities [43]:

1. Ability to generate coherent speech or understand spoken or written language
2. Ability to recognize or identify objects, assuming intact sensory function
3. Ability to execute motor activities, assuming intact motor abilities, sensory function, and comprehension of the required task
4. Ability to think abstractly, make sound judgments, and plan and carry out complex tasks

The decline in cognitive abilities must be severe enough to interfere with daily life.

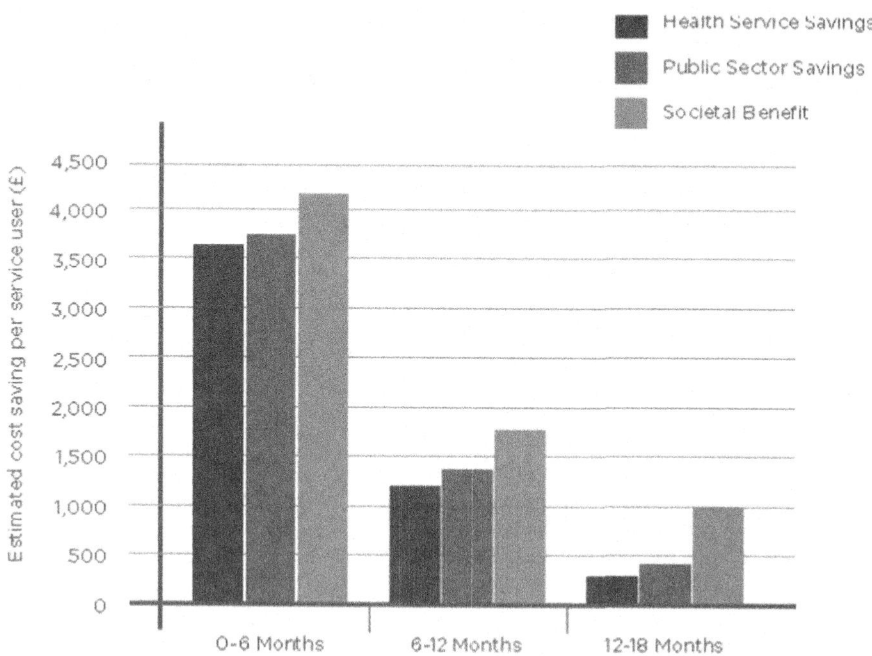

Fig. 12.1 Estimated cost savings per service user following the introduction of an Individual Placement and Support (IPS) service (Reproduced from London School of Economics [39])

Table 12.2 Rehospitalization rates with cognitive behavior therapy (CBT; Reproduced from Jonas et al. [41])

Rehospitalization	Pooled sample size	Estimated risk ratio	95 % confidence interval
Short term	136	0.36	0.11–113
Medium term	132	0.59	0.27–1.30
Long term	294	0.86	0.61–1.20

Different types of dementia have been associated with distinct symptom patterns and distinguishing microscopic brain abnormalities [44–48]. Alzheimer's disease is the most common type of dementia [49]. Other types include vascular dementia, Parkinson's disease, and frontotemporal dementia (Table 12.3) [43, 50].

Dementia mainly affects older people, although there is a growing awareness of cases that start before the age of 65. After age 65, the likelihood of developing dementia roughly doubles every 5 years [43].

Prevalence and incidence projections indicate that the number of people with dementia will continue to grow, particularly among the oldest old, and countries in demographic transition will experience the greatest growth. The total number of people with dementia worldwide in 2010 is estimated at 35.6 million and is

Table 12.3 Common types of dementia, typical characteristics, and epidemiological data about Europe [43, 49, 51–55]

Type of dementia	Characteristics	Prevalence rates (%)	Risk factors
Alzheimer's disease	Difficulty remembering names and recent events is often an early clinical symptom; apathy and depression are also often early symptoms. Later symptoms include impaired judgment; disorientation; confusion; behavior changes; and trouble speaking, swallowing, and walking	4.7	Advancing age, genetic (apolipoprotein E-e4)
Vascular dementia	Symptoms often overlap with those of Alzheimer's, although memory may not be as seriously affected	1.5	Advancing age, arterial stiffness, hypertension, diabetes mellitus, peripheral arterial disease, smoking
Parkinson's disease	Tremor, slowed movements, rigid muscles, impaired posture and balance, loss of automatic movements, speech and writing changes	0.3	Age, heredity, sex, exposure to toxins
Frontotemporal dementia	Typical symptoms include changes in personality and behavior and difficulty with language	1.2–3.6 (age range 40–59)	Family history of frontotemporal dementia

projected to nearly double every 20 years, to 65.7 million in 2030 and 115.4 million in 2050 (Fig. 12.2). The total number of new cases of dementia each year worldwide is nearly 7.7 million, implying one new case every 4 s [56].

Among 291 causes of DALY's per 100,000 persons, Alzheimer's disease and other dementias in 2010 ranked 49th globally. When viewed regionally, disability from Alzheimer's and other dementia ranked 19th in the high-income western Pacific region, 11th in Western Europe, 13th in Australasia, 12th in the high-income North American Region, 24th in Central Europe, and 26th in southern Latin America, all within the overall population of all ages [57]. Specific to Alzheimer's disease and other dementias, the GBD found that deaths from dementia in 2010 rose threefold over 1990. Looking at age-standardized rates of mortality, Alzheimer's had a 95.4 % increase in rates of death per 100,000 population over that same period of time [57].

Dementias challenge the health and social systems. The huge cost of the disease will challenge health systems to deal with the predicted future increase of prevalence. The total estimated worldwide costs of dementia were US $ 604 billion in 2010. In high-income countries, informal care (45 %) and formal social care (40 %) account for the majority of costs, while the proportionate contribution of direct medical costs (15 %) is much lower. In low-income and lower-middle-income countries, direct social care costs are small, and informal care costs (i.e., unpaid care provided by the family) predominate [56]. A broad public health approach is needed to improve the care and quality of life of people with dementia and family caregivers. The priority areas of action that need to be addressed within the policy

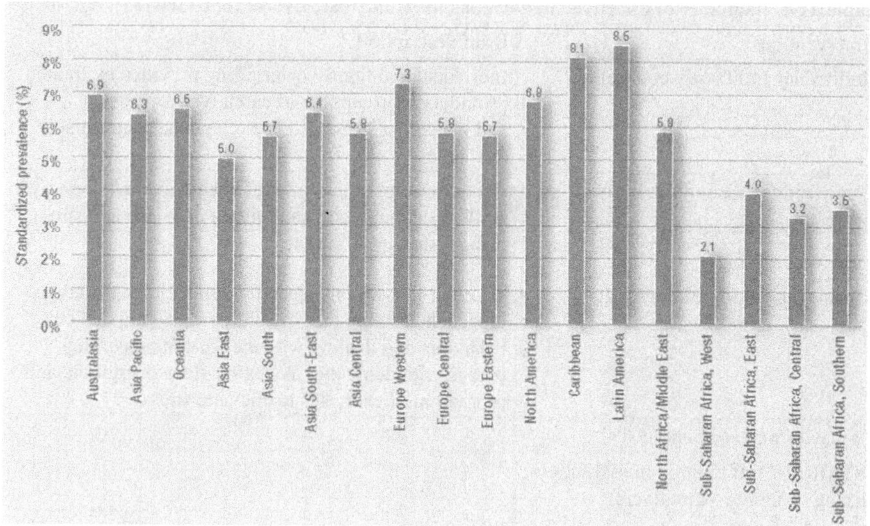

Fig. 12.2 Estimated prevalence of dementia for persons aged 60 and above, standardized to Western Europe population, by global burden of disease region. (Reproduced from WHO [56])

and plan include raising awareness, timely diagnosis, commitment to good-quality continuing care and services, caregiver support, workforce training, prevention, and research. The aims and objectives of this approach should either be articulated in a stand-alone dementia policy or plan or be integrated into existing health, mental health, or old-age policies and plans. Some high-income countries have launched policies, plans, strategies, or frameworks to respond to the impact of dementia [56]. In the WHO dementia survey, respondents from 12 countries stated that their country provided at least one program targeting dementia. The most frequently identified program areas were research (11 countries; 37 % of the total) and awareness raising (ten countries; 33 %). Risk-reduction programs (eight countries; 27 %), community care services (eight countries; 27 %), residential care (seven countries; 23 %), and education and training for the workforce (seven countries; 23 %) were also identified as important areas of action. Respondents from four (13 %) countries reported other programs such as improving management of people with dementia in emergency departments and training in management of behavioral and psychological symptoms of dementia [56].

Many studies, mainly conducted in high-income countries, attest to the wide-ranging benefits of caregiver interventions benefits to whom. The wideranging benefits of caregiver interventions to people affected by dementia are demonstrated by many studies, mainly systematic reviews and meta-analyses, conducted in high-income countries [58–63]. A recent review evaluated the evidence on the efficacy and effectiveness of psychological and psychosocial interventions [63]. These studies cover a wide range of intervention programs such as caregiver information and education, psychoeducational training (e.g., for self-management of moods), training in coping skills (e.g., implementing assistive technologies), support groups,

Table 12.4 Examples of effective interventions for family caregivers [56, 63, 64–83]

Interventions	Brief description
Individual and family counselling	Individual and family counselling provided by trained providers for treatment of careg iver depression and managing stress. Ad hoc telephone access also available
Psychoeducational programmes1, eg.:	Caregivers are taught a set of behavioral and cognitive skills for coping with care giving demands and stress, using a structural format
Coping with caregiving	
Sawy caregiving	
Specialized skill trainings, eg:	Training focuses on a specific issue related to caregiving, such as home modifications, managing difficult behaviors and dealing with the frustrations of the person with dementia, managing sleep disruption, and promotion of exercises to alleviate stress
Behavior management	
STAR-C (Staff training in assisted-living residences-caregivers)	
In-home modifications	
Multi component programmes (i. e. REACH II (Resources tor Enhancing Alzheimer's Caregiver Health II))2	A multicomponent programme that consists of home visits to create individualized plans tor caregivers to manage their stress, behavioral interventions, telephone support group calls, and access to various local resources
Psychotherapy/ cognitive behavioral therapy	Use of cognitive behavioral therapy to treat caregivets who are clinioally depressed or who have other significant mental health problems

[a]Psychoeducational and/or behavior management training programs have been used in Australia, India, Spain, UK, and some other parts of Europe. Work is ongoing in other regions of the world (e.g., China, Hong Kong Special Administrative Region)
[b]Adaptations of REACH II are currently in dissemination trials in many parts of the USA

counseling for primary caregivers and family (face-to-face, telephone, or video-link), psychotherapy (e.g., CBT), respite, and multicomponent studies. The review concluded that non-pharmacological treatments "emerge as a useful, versatile, and potentially cost-effective approach to improve outcomes and quality of life for both the person with dementia and caregiver" (Table 12.4).

Among best practices, experiences from Austria and the Netherlands will be described. The 2-week respite program for caregivers and persons with dementia in Austria [84, 85] provides care for both the caregiver and the person with dementia. Between 10 and 15 "pairs" (caregiver and person with dementia) join each program. While people with dementia receive individual stage-specific stimulation (e.g., cognitive and memory training, occupational therapy, physical training), caregivers take part in an intensive training course in which they learn about the disease and are trained in special communication techniques. They receive group and individual counseling. Caregivers also have the freedom to use the time as they please, to relax and take time off. The effectiveness of this program with regard to perceived burden and depressive symptoms of caregivers was evaluated in a single group, with pre–post-design assessing 104 caregivers. The results indicated that depressive symptoms and the burden related to symptoms of the disease were reduced during the treatment. The program was well received and accepted by caregivers and patients. More than 30 such courses have been held so far since 2000.

In the Netherlands, the government funded a program to stimulate integrated care by building dementia care networks [56]. This program met several barriers, including lack of professional participation at the social level (for instance general practitioners). Despite the barriers, the participants observed major improvements in integrated care in dementia and moderate changes in working conditions. With the client-centered approach, 86 % of the professionals reported improved familiarity with various informal caregivers' problems such as guilt and embarrassment about having coping difficulties. Of these professionals, 40 % found that the program helped them deal with these problems. Furthermore, 50 % of the professionals reported improvement in their knowledge of options for referring clients. The participants, especially the nurses, noted that their collaborative dementia care competencies improved. The WHO states about dementia that the time to act is now by [56]:

- Promoting a dementia-friendly society globally;
- Making dementia a national public health and social care priority worldwide;
- Improving public and professional attitudes to, and understanding of, dementia;
- Investing in health and social systems to improve care and services for people with dementia and their caregivers;
- Increasing the priority given to dementia in the public health research agenda.

References

1. WHO (2001) Strengthening mental health promotion. https://apps.who.int/inf-fs/en/fact220.html. Accessed 7 Aug 2013
2. Center for Disease Control and Prevention. Mental illness. http://www.cdc.gov/mentalhealth/basics/mental-illness.htm. Accessed 3 Aug 2013
3. ICD-10 Chapter Mental and behavioural disorders. http://www.who.int/classifications/icd/en/GRNBOOK.pdf. Accessed 6 Aug 2013
4. WHO (2004) Projections of mortality and global burden of disease 2004–2030. http://www.who.int/healthinfo/global_burden_disease/projections2004/en/index.html. Accessed 2 Aug 2013
5. Prince M, Patel V, Saxena S et al (2007) No health without mental health. Lancet 370(9590):859–877
6. Center of Disease Control (CDC). http://www.cdc.gov/mentalhealth/basics/mental-illness/depression.htm. Accessed 6 Aug 2013
7. Center of Disease Control (CDC). http://www.cdc.gov/mentalhealth/basics/mental-illness/anxiety.htm. Accessed 6 Aug 2013
8. Schizophrenia (2010) In E. A. Martin (Ed.), *Concise Medical Dictionary* (8th edition). Oxford University Press. Maastricht University Library. Retrieved 29 June 2010
9. CDC. http://www.cdc.gov/mentalhealth/basics/mental-illness/dementia.htm. Accessed 6 Aug 2013

10. American Psychiatric Association (2000) Diagnostic and statistical manual of mental disorders: DSM-IV-TR, 4th edn. American Psychiatric Association, Washington, D. C
11. Ormel J, Vonkorff M, Oldehinkel AJ, Simon G, Tiemens BG, Ustün TB (1999) Onset of disability in depressed and non-depressed primary care patients. Psychol Med 29(4):847–853
12. World Health Organization. Mental health—depression. http://www.who.int/mental_health/management/depression/en/. Accessed 1 Aug 2013
13. Murray CJ, Lopez AD (1996) Evidence-based health policy—lessons from the Global Burden of Disease Study. Science 274:740–743
14. Murray CJ, Lopez AD (1996) The global burden of disease: a comprehensive assessment of mortality and disability from diseases, injuries and risk factors in 1990 and projected to 2020. Harvard University Press, Cambridge
15. World Health Organization. Mental health—depression. http://www.who.int/mental_health/management/depression/en/. Accessed 1 Aug 2013
16. Sobocki P, Jönsson B, Angst J, Rehnberg C (2006) Cost of depression in Europe. J Ment Health Policy Econ 9(2):87–98
17. Stewart WF, Ricci JA, Chee E, Hahn SR, Morganstein D (2003) Cost of lost productive work time among US workers with depression. J Am Med Assoc 289(23):3135–3144
18. Kessler RC, DuPont RL, Berglund P, Wittchen HU (1999) Impairment in pure and comorbid generalized anxiety disorder and major depression at 12 months in two national surveys. Am J Psychiatry 156(12):1915–1923
19. Brown HE, Pearson N, Braithwaite RE, Brown WJ, Biddle SJ (2013) Physical activity interventions and depression in children and adolescents: a systematic review and meta-analysis. Sports Med 43(3):195–206
20. Reynolds CF 3rd, Cuijpers P, Patel V et al (2012) Early intervention to reduce the global health and economic burden of major depression in older adults. Annu Rev Public Health 33:123–135
21. Beardslee WR, Gladstone TR, Wright EJ, Cooper AB (2003) A family-based approach to the prevention of depressive symptoms in children at risk: evidence of parental and child change. Pediatrics 112(2):e119–e131
22. WHO. http://www.who.int/mental_health/evidence/en/prevention_of_mental_disorders_sr.pdf. Accessed 25 Aug 2013
23. Angst J (1995) History and epidemiology of panic. Eur Psychiatry 10(Suppl 2):57s–59s
24. Kessler RC, Calabrese JR, Farley PA et al (2013) Composite international diagnostic interview screening scales for DSM-IV anxiety and mood disorders. Psychol Med 43(8):1625–1637
25. Cairney J, Corna LM, Veldhuizen S, Kurdyak P, Streiner DL (2008) The social epidemiology of affective and anxiety disorders in later life in Canada. Can J Psychiatry 53(2):104–111
26. Hendriks SM, Spijker J, Licht CM, Beekman AT, Penninx BW (2013) Two-year course of anxiety disorders: different across disorders or dimensions? Acta Psychiatr Scand 128(3):212–221
27. Wardenaar KJ, Giltay EJ, van Veen T, Zitman FG, Penninx BW (2012) Dimensions of the inventory of depressive symptomatology as predictors of the course of depressive and anxiety disorders. J Psychiatr Res 46(12):1655–1661
28. Roest AM, Heideveld A, Martens EJ, de Jonge P, Denollet J (2013) Symptom dimensions of anxiety following myocardial infarction: associations with depressive symptoms and prognosis. Health Psychol doi:10.1037/a0034806
29. Beesdo-Baum K, Knappe S (2012) Developmental epidemiology of anxiety disorders. Child Adolesc Psychiatr Clin N Am 21(3):457–478
30. Schultz SH, North SW, Shields CG (2007) Schizophrenia: a review. Am Fam Physician 75(12):1821–1829
31. Mandal MK, Nizamie SH (2004) Current developments in schizophrenia. Allied Publishers, New Delhi
32. World Health Organization. Mental health—schizophrenia. http://www.who.int/mental_health/management/schizophrenia/en/. Accessed 23 Jul 2013

33. Wilk CM, Gold JM, McMahon RP, Humber K, Iannone VN, Buchanan RW (2005) No, it is not possible to be schizophrenic yet neuropsychologically normal. Neuropsychology 19(6):778–786
34. Reichenberg A, Harvey PD, Bowie CR et al (2009) Neuropsychological function and dysfunction in schizophrenia and psychotic affective disorders. Schizophr Bull 35(5):1022–1029
35. Caspi A, Reichenberg A, Weiser M et al (2003) Cognitive performance in schizophrenia patients assessed before and following the first psychotic episode. Schizophr Res 65(2–3):87–94
36. Keefe RS, Bilder RM, Harvey PD et al (2006) Baseline neurocognitive deficits in the CATIE schizophrenia trial. Neuropsychopharmacol 31(9):2033–2046
37. Kovess-Masféty V, Wiersma D, Xavier M et al (2006) Needs for care among patients with schizophrenia in six European countries: a one-year follow-up study. Clin Pract Epidemiol Ment Health 2:22
38. Mangalore R, Knapp M (2007) Cost of schizophrenia in England. J Ment Health Policy Econ 10(1):23–41
39. London School of Economics—PSSR (2012) Effective interventions in schizophrenia—the economic case. http://www.lse.ac.uk/LSEHealthAndSocialCare/pdf/LSE-economic-report-FINAL-12-Nov.pdf. Accessed 23 Jul 2013
40. National Institute for Health and Care Excellence (NICE) (2010) Schizophrenia—the NICE guideline on core interventions in the treatment and management of schizophrenia in adults in primary and secondary care, updated edition. http://www.nice.org.uk/nicemedia/live/11786/43607/43607.pdf. Accessed 23 Jul 2013
41. Jones C, Hacker D, Cormac I, Meaden A, Irving CB (2012) Cognitive behaviour therapy versus other psychosocial treatments for schizophrenia. Cochrane Database Syst Rev 4:CD008712
42. Alzheimer's Disease International (2010) World Alzheimer report 2010. The global economic impact of dementia. http://www.alz.co.uk/research/files/WorldAlzheimerReport2010.pdf. Accessed 24 Jul 2013
43. Alzheimer's association. 2009 Alzheimer's disease facts and figures. http://www.alz.org/national/documents/report_alzfactsfigures2009.pdf. Accessed 24 Jul 2013
44. Bassil N, Mollaei C (2012) Alzheimer's dementia: a brief review. J Med Liban 60(4):192–199
45. Tampellini D, Rahman N, Lin MT, Capetillo-Zarate E, Gouras GK (2011) Impaired β-amyloid secretion in Alzheimer's disease pathogenesis. J Neurosci 31(43):15384–15390
46. Gibb WR, Lees AJ (1988) The relevance of the Lewy body to the pathogenesis of idiopathic Parkinson's disease. J Neurol Neurosurg Psychiatry 51(6):745–752
47. Román G, Pascual B (2012) Contribution of neuroimaging to the diagnosis of Alzheimer's disease and vascular dementia. Arch Med Res 43(8):671–676
48. Korczyn AD, Vakhapova V, Grinberg LT (2012) Vascular dementia. J Neurol Sci 322(1–2):2–10
49. Román GC (2002) Vascular dementia may be the most common form of dementia in the elderly. J Neurol Sci 203–204:7–10
50. Alzheimer's Disease International (2010) World Alzheimer report 2010. The global economic impact of dementia. http://www.alz.co.uk/research/files/WorldAlzheimerReport2010.pdf. Accessed 24 Jul 2013
51. Alzheimer's Disease International (2009) World Alzheimer report 2009
52. Roman GC, The epidemiology of vascular dementia. In: Duyckaerts C, Litvan I (eds) *Dementias - Handbook of Clinical Neurology, vol 89 (3rd series).* Elsevier Edinburgh, 2008, pp 639-658.
53. Akinyemi RO, Mukaetova-Ladinska EB, Attems J, Ihara M, Kalaria RN (2013) Vascular risk factors and neurodegeneration in ageing related dementias: Alzheimer's disease and vascular dementia. Curr Alzheimer Res 10(6):642–653
54. de Lau LM, Breteler MM (2006) Epidemiology of Parkinson's disease. Lancet Neurol 5(6):525–535
55. Rosso SM, DonkerKaat L, Baks T et al (2003) Frontotemporal dementia in The Netherlands: patient characteristics and prevalence estimates from a population-based study. Brain 126(Pt 9):2016–2022

56. World Health Organization & Alzheimer's Disease International (2012) Dementia: a public health priority. http://apps.who.int/iris/bitstream/10665/75263/1/9789241564458_eng.pdf Accessed 24 Jul 2013
57. Alzheimer's Disease International (2012) Initial release of Global Burden of Disease 2010 Study in Lancet. http://www.alz.co.uk/media/121213 Accessed 24 Jul 2013
58. Pinquart M, Sorensen S (2006) Helping caregivers of persons with dementia. Which interventions works and how large are their effects? Int Psychogeriatr 8:577–595
59. Smits CH, de Lange J, Dröes RM, Meiland F, Vernooij-Dassen M, Pot AM (2007) Effects of combined intervention programmes for people with dementia living at home and their caregivers: a systematic review. Int J Geriatr Psychiatry 22(12):1181–1193
60. Brodaty H, Green A, Koschera A (2003) Meta-analysis of psychosocial interventions for caregivers of people with dementia. J Am Geriatr Soc 51:657–664
61. Lee H, Cameron M (2004) Respite care for people with dementia and their carers. Cochrane Database Syst Rev 2004:CD004396
62. Spijker A, Vernooij-Dassen M, Vasse E et al (2008) Effectiveness of nonpharmacological interventions in delaying the institutionalization of patients with dementia: a meta-analysis. J Am Geriatr Soc 56(6):1116–1128
63. Olazarán J, Reisberg B, Clare L et al (2010) Nonpharmacological therapies in Alzheimer's disease: a systematic review of efficacy. Dement Geriatr Cogn Disord 30(2):161–178
64. Mittelman MS, Ferris SH, Steinberg G et al (1993) An intervention that delays institutionalization of Alzheimer's disease patients: treatment of spouse-caregivers. Gerontologist 33(6):730–740
65. Mittelman MS, Ferris SH, Shulman E, Steinberg G, Levin B (1996) A family intervention to delay nursing home placement of patients with Alzheimer disease. A randomized controlled trial. JAMA 276(21):1725–1731
66. Mittelman MS, Haley WE, Clay OJ, Roth DL (2006) Improving caregiver well being delays nursing home placement of patients with Alzheimer disease. Neurology 67(9):1592–1599
67. Mittelman MS, Roth DL, Clay OJ, Haley WE (2007) Preserving health of Alzheimer caregivers: impact of a spouse caregiver intervention. Am J Geriatr Psychiatry 15(9):780–789
68. Mittelman MS, Brodaty H, Wallen AS, Burns A (2008) A three-country randomized controlled trial of a psychosocial intervention for caregivers combined with pharmacological treatment for patients with Alzheimer disease: effects on caregiver depression. Am J Geriatr Psychiatry 16(11):893–904
69. Sörensen S, Duberstein P, Gill D, Pinquart M (2006) Dementia care: mental health effects, intervention strategies, and clinical implications. Lancet Neurol 5(11):961–973
70. Gallagher-Thompson D, Coon D (2007) Evidence-based psychological treatments for distress in family caregivers of older adults. Psychol Aging 22:37–51
71. Hepburn K, Lewis M, Tornatore J, Sherman CW, Bremer KL (2007) The Savvy Caregiver program: the demonstrated effectiveness of a transportable dementia caregiver psychoeducation program. J Gerontol Nurs 33(3):30–36
72. Burgio LD, Collins IB, Schmid B, Wharton T, McCallum D, Decoster J (2009) Translating the REACH caregiver intervention for use by area agency on aging personnel: the REACH OUT program. Gerontologist 49(1):103–116
73. Teri L, Logsdon RG, Uomoto J, McCurry SM (1997) Behavioral treatment of depression in dementia patients: a controlled clinical trial. J Gerontol B Psychol Sci Soc Sci 52(4):P159–P166
74. Gitlin LN, Winter L, Corcoran M, Dennis MP, Schinfeld S, Hauck WW (2003) Effects of the home environmental skill-building program on the caregiver-care recipient dyad: 6-month outcomes from the Philadelphia REACH Initiative. Gerontologist 43(4):532–546
75. Farran C, Gilley D, McCann J, Bienias J, Lindeman D, Evans D (2004) Psychosocial interventions to reduce depressive symptoms of dementia caregivers: a randomized clinical trial comparing two approaches. J Mental Health Aging 10:337–350

76. Gitlin LN, Hauck WW, Dennis MP, Winter L (2005) Maintenance of effects of the home environmental skill-building program for family caregivers and individuals with Alzheimer's disease and related disorders. J Gerontol A Biol Sci Med Sci 60(3):368–374
77. Teri L, McCurry SM, Logsdon R, Gibbons LE (2005) Training community consultants to help family members improve dementia care: a randomized controlled trial. Gerontologist 45(6):802–811
78. Gonyea J, O'Connor M, Boyle P (2006) Project CARE: a randomized controlled trial of a behavioral intervention group for Alzheimer's disease caregivers. Gerontologist 46:827–832
79. Gitlin LN, Winter L, Burke J, Chernett N, Dennis MP, Hauck WW (2008) Tailored activities to manage neuropsychiatric behaviors in persons with dementia and reduce caregiver burden: a randomized pilot study. Am J Geriatr Psychiatry 16(3):229–239
80. Belle SH, Burgio L, Burns R et al (2006) Enhancing the quality of life of dementia caregivers from different ethnic or racial groups: a randomized, controlled trial. Ann Intern Med 145(10):727–738
81. Brodaty H, Gresham M, Luscombe G (1997) The Prince Henry Hospital dementia caregivers' training program. Int J Geriatr Psychiatry 12:183–192
82. Gallagher-Thompson D, Steffen A (1994) Comparative effects of cognitive/behavioral and brief psychodynamic psychotherapies for depressed in family caregivers. J Consult Clin Psychol 62(3):543–549
83. Charlesworth GM, Reichelt FK (2004) Keeping conceptualizations simple: examples with family carers of people with dementia. Behav Cogn Psychoth 32(4):401–409
84. Auer RS, Span E, Donabauer Y, Reisberg B (2009) A 10-day training program for persons with dementia and their carers: a practical nonpharmacological treatment program. Alzheimer's Dementia 5(4)(Suppl 1):406
85. Auer RS, Zehetner F, Donabauer Y, Span E (2007) Entlastung pflegender Angehöriger: Ein Programm der M.A.S Alzheimerhilfe. Zeitschrift für Gerontopsychologie Psychiatrie 20(2/3):169–174

Chapter 13
Urban Public Health

Umberto Moscato and Andrea Poscia

Definition

Urban health has been defined as "the study of the health of urban populations," including the description of the health of urban populations and understanding the determinants of population health in cities, with the objective of improving the health of urban dwellers [1]. In the past decade, it became of particular interest, as showed by the more than 1000 research papers that have been published since 1960, with over 60 % of them after 2000. Most of these articles analyze the relationship between urban environment and health outcomes, and several organizations (i.e., the World Health Organization, WHO) have focused their attention to addressing the challenges of urban health.

However, what is classified as "urban" varies considerably, without a universally accepted definition of what constitutes a city or an urban area. Small nations can consider "urban" all settlements with 1000 or more inhabitants, while for USA, it is an area densely populated by more than 50,000 people [2]; WHO uses in a recent report the word "city" to define urban areas with sizeable populations of more than 100,000 people [3], while the UN-HABITAT (the United Nations agency for human settlements delegated by the UN General Assembly to promote socially and environmentally sustainable towns and cities with the goal of providing adequate shelter for all) defines "megacities" as high-density metropolises of more than 10 million inhabitants and "metacity" or "hypercity," massive sprawling conurbations of more than 20 million people [4].

U. Moscato (✉) · A. Poscia
Institute of Public Health, Section of Hygiene, Università Cattolica del Sacro Cuore, L.go F. Vito 1, 00168 Rome, Italy
e-mail: umoscato@rm.unicatt.it

A. Poscia
e-mail: andrea.poscia@edu.rm.unicatt.it

S. Boccia et al. (eds.), *A Systematic Review of Key Issues in Public Health*,
DOI 10.1007/978-3-319-13620-2_13

However, according to Galea and Vlahov (2005), cities "can represent diverse conditions within which people live, and represent a range of human experiences," offering human beings the potential to share urban spaces, participate in public and private events, and exercise both duties and rights [5]. Cities can represent a positive determinant of health, but urban areas could be also unhealthy places to live, characterized by heavy traffic, pollution, noise, violence, and social isolation for elderly people and young families. In this sense, it will be important to promote the concept of "healthy city" as defined by WHO Europe since 1986: European cities and national networks that contribute to health and sustainable development and support politicians, public sectors, and other agencies in implementing strategies and action to address the growing health challenges in cities.

In this chapter, a comprehensive literature review is conducted using PubMed with the following keywords: "urban health, healthy city, healthy cities, urbanization." Only reviews published in peer-reviewed journals or international scientific society/agencies and written in English or Italian were included. No time restriction was set a priori. The initial research was done in July 2013 independently by two researchers: It highlighted 3.381 reviews (on 89.506 references). After applying the exclusion criteria and looking at the title or abstract, researchers selected and read the full text of 54 reviews and scanned all the references listed in the "Related article" section and in their bibliography. In parallel, an investigation of websites through Google and using the same keywords was done to also include important articles from gray literature and acknowledged international institutions (such as WHO, United Nations, etc). At the end of the process, authors reviewed and synthesized 76 references: 39 reviews, 32 documents from international agencies, and 5 books.

Burden

Urbanization, the demographic transition from rural to urban, is one of the major public health challenges of this century, as urban populations are quickly increasing: in 2010, more than half of all people, about 3.5 billion, lived in an urban area, and this proportion is projected to grow in the coming years (see Fig. 13.1) [6].

At the beginning of the last century, only two out of every ten people lived in an urban area, while, according to WHO projections, they will become six out of every ten people by 2030 and more than two thirds of the global population will be living in cities by 2050 (6.4 billion).

In the middle of the twentieth century, the urban growth reached a peak, with a population expansion of more than 3 % per year, while today the number of urban residents is growing by nearly 60 million every year, and it is expected to grow roughly 1.5 % per year between 2025 and 2030, mostly in developing countries. As a matter of fact, developing countries have known a great expansion between 1995 and 2005, around 165,000 people every day, and their annual urban population growth is projected to 1.55 % per year between 2025 and 2050, while in

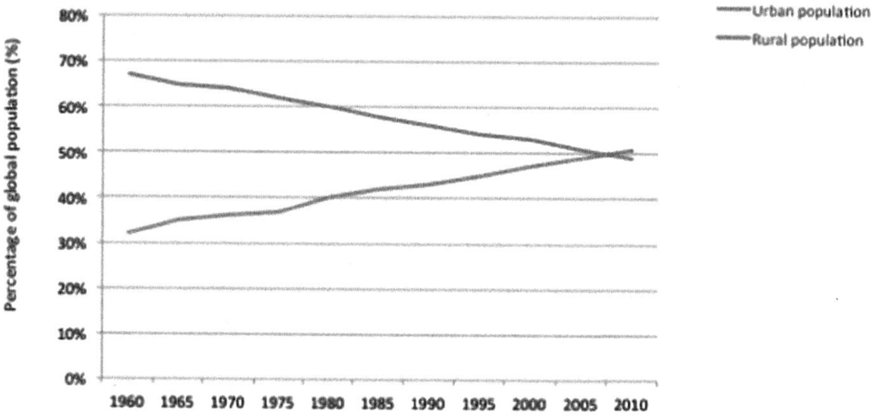

Fig. 13.1 Percentage of total population living in urban areas, 1960–2010. (Reproduced from [6])

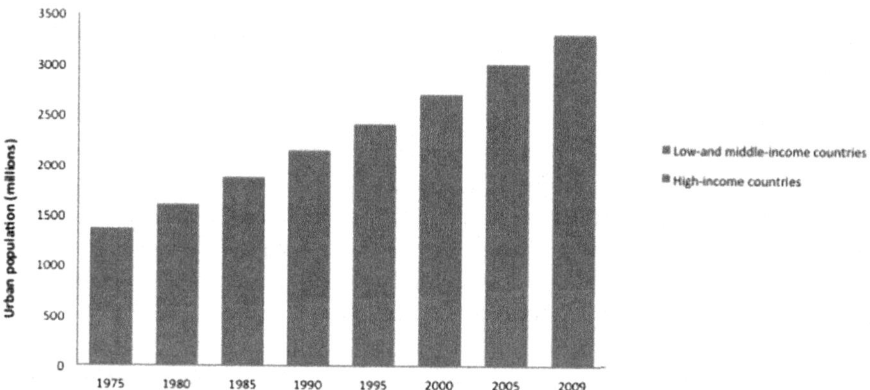

Fig. 13.2 Urban population in low-/middle- versus high-income countries, 1975–2009. (Reproduced from [7])

high-income countries, the increase for the next two decades is mainly linked to legal and illegal immigration (see Fig. 13.2) [7].

Accordingly, even Europe was historically the most urbanized region in the world for many centuries and London was the first city in the world to surpass one million residents in the mid-nineteenth century; nowadays, about 75 % of the population of the 27 member states of the European Union lives in urban areas, but many cities deal with measured growth or declining dwellers [7]. Besides, many of these cities are facing a conflicting phenomenon characterized by de-urbanization towards the newly developing suburbs versus re-urbanization due to the attractiveness of the city center, influenced in particular by immigration from poor to richer localities and from rural to urban areas.

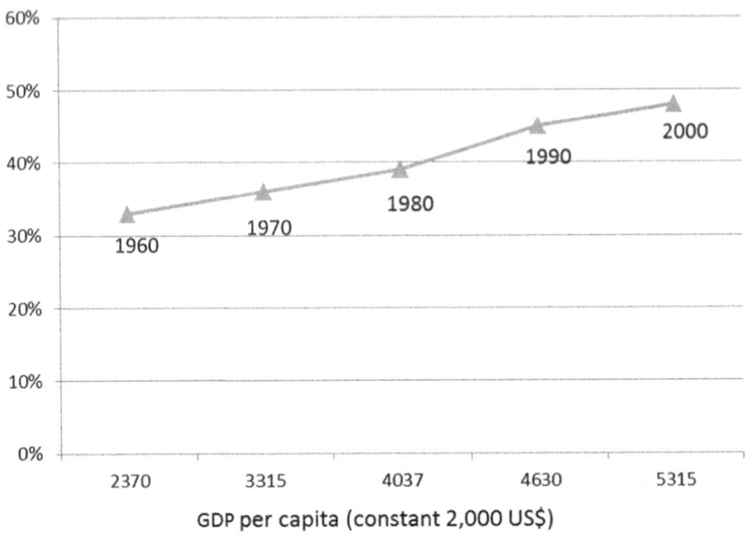

Fig. 13.3 Trends in urbanization and GDP per capita for all countries, 1960–2000. *GDP* gross domestic product. (Reproduced from UN-HABITAT, 2013 [7])

Besides urbanization, the population aging is another result of successful human development during last century and, together, also a major challenge for this century and for our cities. As a matter of fact, the proportion of the elderly residing in cities in developed countries matches that of younger age groups at about 80 % and it is speedily increasing, while in developing countries, they will increase 16 times, from about 56 million in 1998 to over 908 million in 2050 (one fourth of the total urban population) [8].

Another important characteristic of urbanization is that the highest growth will be in the smaller cities. Even if the number of megacities is likely to increase from 5 in 1975 to 23 by 2015, they have fewer than 10 % of urban dwellers, while around half of all urban dwellers are living in cities with between 100,000 and 500,000 people, and urbanization in these cities is more rapid than in the largest cities [3].

Urbanization has significant effects on population health: of course, it can and should be beneficial for health as urban areas can provide healthy living and working environment and concentrate opportunities, jobs, services, and technologies; part of the improvements over the past 50 years in mortality and morbidity in highly urbanized countries like Japan, Sweden, the Netherlands, and Singapore could be attributed to the potentially health-promoting features of these modern cities. Furthermore, several studies have shown the relationship between urbanization and richness (measured as gross domestic product—see Fig. 13.3) [7] with urban areas being economically more prosperous than rural areas.

Nevertheless, there are several economic, social, and environmental determinants, at both structural and intermediate level, which could have a great negative impact on health in urban areas. In all countries, there is an unequal social

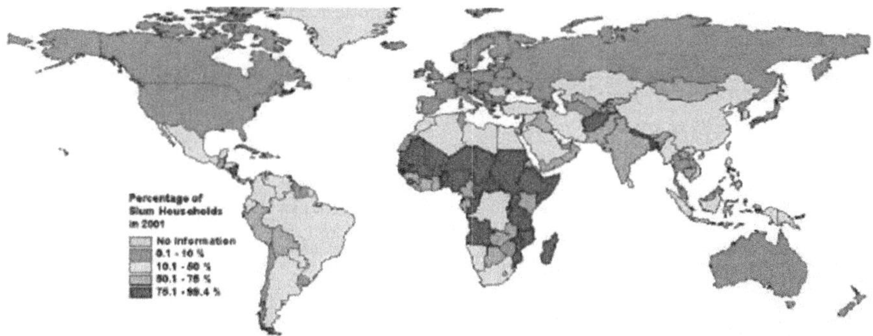

Fig. 13.4 Percentage of urban population living in slums in different countries. (Source: [3])

distribution of health, both within countries (the urban–rural divide) and within cities (the social gradient), and it can lead to a situation of urban disadvantage where health can be as bad as or worse than in rural poverty [9].

In fact, socioeconomic inequities in urban areas result in significant health inequalities, and the rapid growth of several cities, both for the fast migration from rural areas and for the overall population growth, could lead to basic infrastructure lack, putting further pressure on limited resources, especially in low-income countries [3].

The regions of the world with the fastest-growing urban populations are also the regions with the highest proportion of slum dwellers; this is in connection with the great role played by the governance, especially through policies that should address the key social determinants of health. According to WHO, the best local governance can help produce 75 years or more of life expectancy, while with bad urban governance, life expectancy goes down (even to 35 years) and informal settlements and slums grow up. As defined by the United Nations Human Settlements Programme (UN-HABITAT), a slum is a densely populated area with substandard housing and a low standard of living as depicted by the absence of one or more of the following: improved water supply, improved sanitation, sufficient living area, durability of construction, and security of tenure [9].

Nowadays, about one billion people, around one third of the world's urban population, are estimated living in slum conditions and they may double in coming decades without adequate policies for economic, social, and health equity. More than 90 % of slums are located in developing countries and they are no longer just marginalized neighborhoods but often the dominant type of human settlement (Fig. 13.4) [3].

Slum dwellers live in overcrowded, poorly constructed housing, often located in undesirable parts of the city (steep hillsides, riverbanks subject to flooding, industrial areas). The high population density, overcrowding, and lack of safe water and sanitation systems represent a flourishing environment for tuberculosis, hepatitis, dengue, pneumonia, cholera, and diarrheal disease [10].

Table 13.1 Infant and under-five mortality rates in Nairobi, Kenya, Sweden, and Japan. Reproduced from [12]

Location	Infant mortality rate (IMR)	Under-five moratlity rate (U5M)
Sweden	5	5
Japan	4	5
Kenya	74	112
Rural	76	113
Urban (excluding Nairobi)	57	84
Nairobi	39	62
High-income areas (estimate)	Likely < 10	Likely < 15
Informal settlements (average)	91	151
Kibera slum	106	187
Embakasi slum	164	254

In Sub-Saharan African cities, children living in informal settlements are more likely to die from entirely preventable respiratory and waterborne illnesses than children in rural areas [11]. Slums represent also an example of the growing disparities in health within cities as demonstrated by the strong gradient in infant and child mortality rates within Nairobi, Kenya, with rates in the slums more than three times higher than the city average and possibly ten or more times higher in the richer parts of the city (see Table 13.1) [12].

In urban areas of Africa, Americas, and Asia, children in the poorest 20 % population are twice as likely to die before their first birthday compared to children in the richest 20 % population, even if in these continents the infant mortality rate is decreasing comparing the 1990s with 2000–2007 (on average, from 99 to 70 per 1000 live births and from 81 to 51 per 1000 live births, respectively, in Africa and Asia) [13].

Furthermore, even if income inequalities in developed countries are low and little is known about inequalities in European urban areas specifically, several studies have shown differences in the life expectancy both in major American metropolitan areas, including Washington, DC, New York City, and Miami, and in the European cities (for example, in the Scottish Glasgow, male life expectancy in different wards of the same city differ from 54 to 82 years) [5, 14].

Surely, the widely described health, social, and economic inequalities within and between countries contribute a major part of the urban burden of disease that is characterized by several threats:

- Infectious diseases, exacerbated by poor living and working conditions
- Water availability and contaminations (physical, chemical, and biological)
- Chronic, noncommunicable diseases linked to lifestyles in cities, including mental health disorders
- Road accidents, violence, and crime
- Air pollution (indoor and outdoor air quality) and climate change

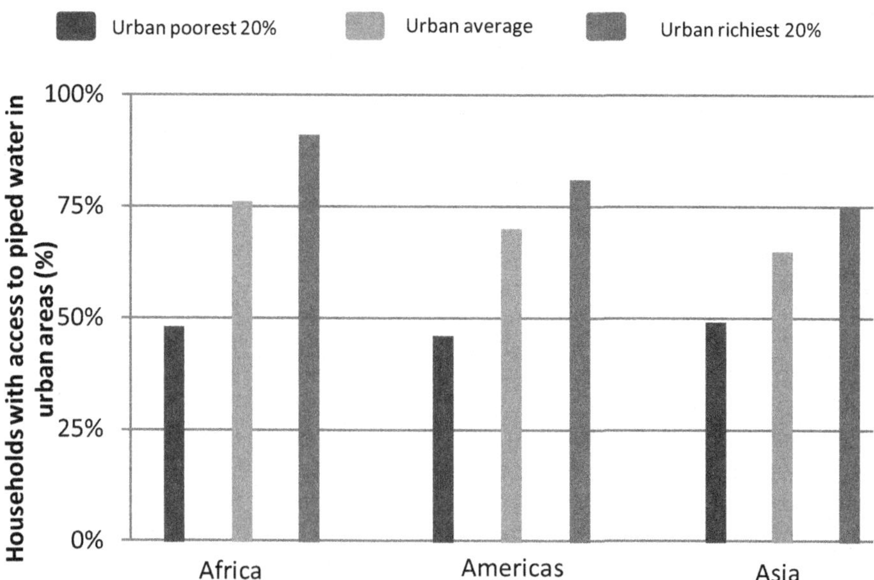

Fig. 13.5 Percentage of household with access to piped water in urban areas for 40 low- and middle-income countries. (Reproduced from WHO, 2000–2007 [19])

The communicable diseases remain an important urban health matter, especially among the urban poor, but more concern is due to the emerging diseases, especially respiratory diseases as severe acute respiratory syndrome (SARS) or avian flu, because they could endanger suddenly great part of the populations and spread quickly over the boundaries of cities and countries. Migration and increased mobility, crowding, insufficient drainage and improper disposal of solid waste, climate change and their impact on the ecology of urban environments, microbial adaptation to changes, and cessations in public health measures represent reasons to keep high the interest over long-standing and new communicable diseases [15–17]. In this sense, the main example is the reappearance of tuberculosis, documented in cities like Osaka (Bradford and Kawabata, 2006), often with multidrug-resistant strains, that impose important public health matters. HIV/AIDS, the plague of the latest 1980–1990s associated with several social determinants, is 1.7 times higher in urban than in rural settings, with higher prevalence in girls [18].

An important source of contamination is represented by *water:* access to piped and safe water dramatically reduces deaths from infections, while contaminated water and lack of water and sanitation facilitate the spread of diarrheal and worm infections. Also in this case, the developing countries are the most impaired (Fig. 13.5) and the poor, children, and women are the most vulnerable people [19].

This situation creates a great concern because it is far from a solution: access to piped water in Africa, Americas, and Asia is stable between the 1990s and 2000–2007 for the urban poorest 20 %, while it is showing a relevant decrease in the urban richest 20 %. WHO reports that almost half of city dwellers in Africa, Asia, and Latin America suffer from at least one disease caused by lack of safe water and sanitation, and that in Sub-Saharan Africa, poor people spend at least one third of

Table 13.2 The influence of urban planning and design on physical activities. Reproduced from [3]

Drivers	
Pro physical activity	Against physical activity
Residential density and land-use mix combined with street connectivity [31]; neighborhood safety from crime, traffic, injury, and a pleasing aesthetic; provision of and access to local public facilities and spaces for recreation and play, especially open green areas [25]	Pervasive advertising of motor vehicles and escalating reliance on cars or motorcycles [32]

their incomes for treatment of waterborne and water-related diseases. Several analyses in developed country have shown that the importance of water conservation is often under-recognized and lack of individual water-saving measures can amplify the waste of large volumes of water, especially in public buildings, due to faulty plumbing fixtures [20–22]. In this sense, another threat is related to the increasing risk of groundwater chemical contamination, especially in urban, industrialized, and intensive agriculture areas, that is strictly connected to the extensive exploitation of the water resource.

On the other hand, the population is aging, and this demographic transition is shifting the emphasis towards *chronic, noncommunicable diseases* in many urban settings, both in low-income countries as in developed one. The other chapters of this book are focused on chronic disease and aging, but there is some evidence about the link between these and lifestyles in cities. In low- and middle-income countries, the prevalence of hypertension is increasing with rates being higher in urban than in rural settings, and the prevalence of diabetes and obesity shows worrying social graduation among urban populations, increasing with decreasing social status, also in European and developed countries [23–26]. Several people are still afflicted by *undernourishment/malnutrition,* suffering from lack of food and for nutritional security: In Sub-Saharan Africa, the proportion of the urban population with energy deficiencies (underweight) was often above 40 % and even above (60 % in Ethiopia, Malawi, and Zambia), usually in slums [27]. The nutritional deprivation often ends towards the "urban nutrition transition" as defined by Dixon et al. or the "obesogenic" shifts in dietary composition, as defined by Mendez and Popkin, with low levels of fruits and vegetables and large increases in edible oils, animal source foods, and added sugar and caloric sweeteners [28, 29]. The nutrition transition typically begins in cities because urbanization encourages social and economic trends: access to nontraditional cheap foods; change in production and processing practices; rise of supermarkets and hypermarkets; processed foods; ready-to-eat meals; and snacks easy to buy from street vendors, restaurants, and fast-food outlets. Furthermore, evidence, usually from high-income countries, highlights the influence of urban planning, for example, open green space, and design on physical activities (Table 13.2) [3].

Among "new" chronic diseases, a growing evidence is about the urban predispositions for *mental health problems* linked to lack of control over resources, changing

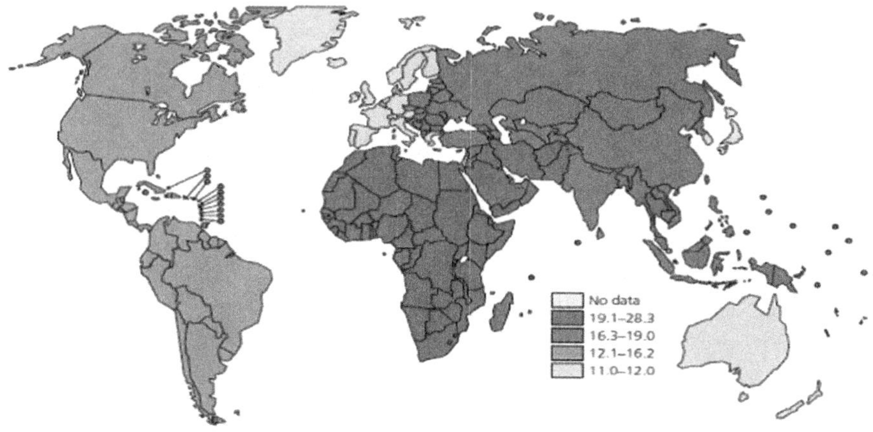

Fig. 13.6 Road traffic mortality rates (per 100,000 population) in WHO region, 2002. WHO World Health Organization. (Source: WHO, 2008 [33])

marriage patterns and divorce, cultural ideology, long-term chronic stress, exposure to stressful life events, and lack of social support [32]. In developing countries, the prevalence of some form of depression among urban adults ranges from 12 to 51 %, while in developed nations also loneliness has become a common concern, in addition to the increasing prevalence of major senility diseases, such as Alzheimer's disease [3]. Chronic stress and easy access to harmful products in the urban setting create also additional risks for substance abuse and dependency. Among these, excessive alcohol consumption represents at the meantime a symptom and a cause of poor mental health [3].

Another urban health concern is the increasing incidence of *road traffic injuries*. The Global status report on road safety 2013 indicates that worldwide the total number of road traffic deaths is about 1.24 million per year and between 20 and 50 million people sustain nonfatal injuries (Fig. 13.6) [33]. These numbers are forecast to increase significantly in the coming decades.

Vulnerable road users (pedestrians, cyclists, and riders of motorized two-wheelers and their passengers) account for half of all road traffic deaths globally and most of them are in low-income countries [33].

People living in urban areas are at greater risk of being involved in road crashes, but people living in rural areas are more likely to be killed or seriously injured if they are involved in crashes [34]. Deaths in traffic are sensitive to road infrastructure, traffic regulations, and enforcement, which are particularly lacking in low-income communities.

Urban violence and crime (*homicide, increasingly feminicide, robbery*) affect the poor and the rich in all countries, and they could have a devastating impact on people's health and livelihoods in many urban areas, contributing to generate feeling of fear and insecurity. They are more pronounced in urban areas, especially in

Data table
Member States
All ages
<5 years
Afghanistan 3 302 1 028
Albania 251 0
Algeria 1 941 35
Andorra 12 0
Angola 1 903 364
Antigua and Barbuda 2 0
Argentina 9 703 9
Armenia 1 931 3
Australia 1 479 0
Austria 1 235 0
Azerbaijan 1 390 12
Bahamas 10 0
Bahrain 49 0
Bangladesh 10 144 304
Barbados 1 0
Belarus 3 394 0
Belgium 1 557 0
Belize 13 0
Benin 916 123
Time animation
2004
2008
Map
Click on a country to display the distribution of deaths in the pie chart below. Hover your mouse on the pie slices to view the corresponding data.
Distribution of deaths by disease
Cardiopulmonary diseases
Lung cancers
Respiratory infections
Map legend
<100
101–500
501–1500
1501–5000
>5000
Not applicable

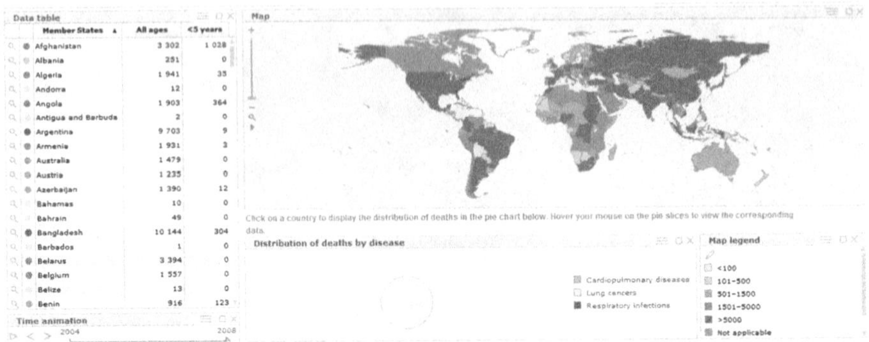

Fig. 13.7 Number of deaths from outdoor air pollution, 2008. (Source: [35])

slum areas: A recent study showed that 60 % of urban dwellers in developing and transitional countries had been victims of crime during a 5-year period. The WHO world report on violence and health indicates that for the 15–29-year age group, interpersonal injury ranks just below traffic fatalities, and in cities of Latin America, the whole population homicide rates in the late 1990s ranged between 6 and 248 per 100,000 depending on the degree of urban violence. In Washington, DC, the rate was 69.3 and in Stockholm 3.0. Associated with these conditions is a risk of substance abuse, including alcohol, and illicit drug use [3].

Next to the problem of the abovementioned traffic safety, there is concern about *quality of air and urban air pollution.* Outdoor air pollution is related to several sources: motor vehicles, industrial processes, power generation, and the household combustion of solid fuel. Each of them emits complex mixtures of air pollutants, many of which are harmful to health alone or in combination, and, recently, International Agency for Research on Cancer (IARC) has classified outdoor air pollution and one of its major components, particulate matter (PM), as carcinogenic to human beings (Group 1). Exposure to ambient fine particles (PM_{10} and $PM_{2.5}$) was recently estimated to have contributed to 3.2 million premature deaths worldwide in 2010, due largely to cardiovascular disease, and 223,000 deaths from lung cancer, most of them in China and other East Asian countries. Worldwide, urban air pollution is estimated to cause about 9 % of the lung cancer deaths, 5 % of cardiopulmonary deaths, and about 1 % of respiratory infection deaths (Fig. 13.7) [35].

The exposure level at city level for PM_{10} (PM with an aerodynamic diameter of 10 μm or less) ranges from 11 to over 100 μg/m^3 (average for the years 2003–2010), with many urban areas that have exceeded WHO's air quality guideline values and with important disparities in exposure between and within countries (Fig. 13.8) [36, 37].

In the modern urban environment, *air pollution from industry* is greatly limited by clean air legislation that have reduced industrial pollution with respect to the 1950s, but it remains still a problem in less developed countries, especially for the poor who live in unsafe locations, such as informal settlements or slum areas, built up too closely to industrial areas. Historical disasters have occurred because of co-location of industry and residential areas, for example, the Bhopal disaster (2000

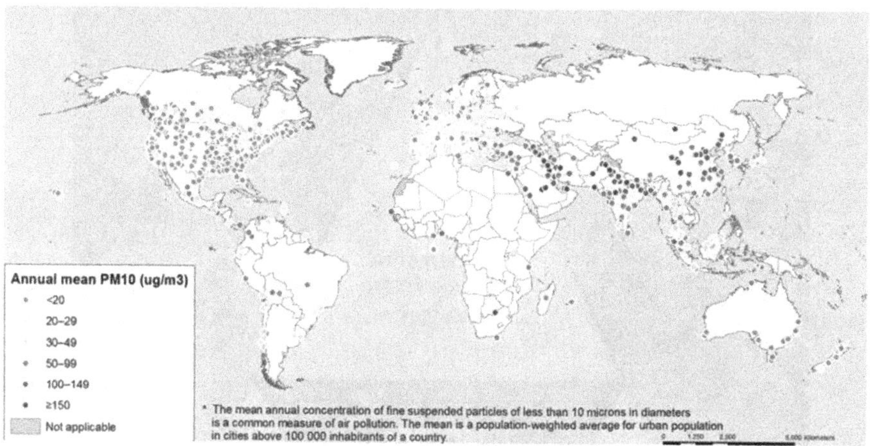

Fig. 13.8 Exposure to PM_{10} in 1100 urban areas in 2003–2010. (Source: WHO, 2013 [37])

people died and more than 200,000 were poisoned) or the Minamata disease caused by methyl mercury poisoning (with more than 2000 city residents in Minamata affected and 1784 deaths) [3].

Other well-known environmental concerns for cities are the acoustic quality, limited land resources with green areas, and open spaces under continuous threat due to more competitive land uses, and, more recently, the threat derived from the *global climate changes* [38].

Several authors point out that the observed and expected climate changes over the next century are likely to have a great impact on urban health, particularly in the poorest communities, which have contributed least to greenhouse gas emissions [39, 40]. Most of the health hazards, on which climate changes may play a role in amplification, regard the aspect described in the previous paragraph: vector-borne diseases, air pollution, increased severity of weather calamities (flooding risks, heat waves—exacerbated by the urban "heat island" effect), and water shortages. Even with the reasonable reservations due to the complexity of climate models and the uncertainties about biological and socioeconomic adaptation in the future, WHO estimates that climate change occurred since the mid-1970s may have caused over 166,000 deaths in 2000, and these numbers will increase, starting from the rural areas and the major cities, such as Mumbai, Rio de Janeiro, or Shanghai, settled near the coast (600 million people living in low-elevation coastal zones) or the rivers [3, 41].

Best Practices

The characteristics of our human-constructed physical environment (the built environment) have significant effects on population, especially in terms of urban health equity: All the aspects related to the urban physical form, its social infrastructure,

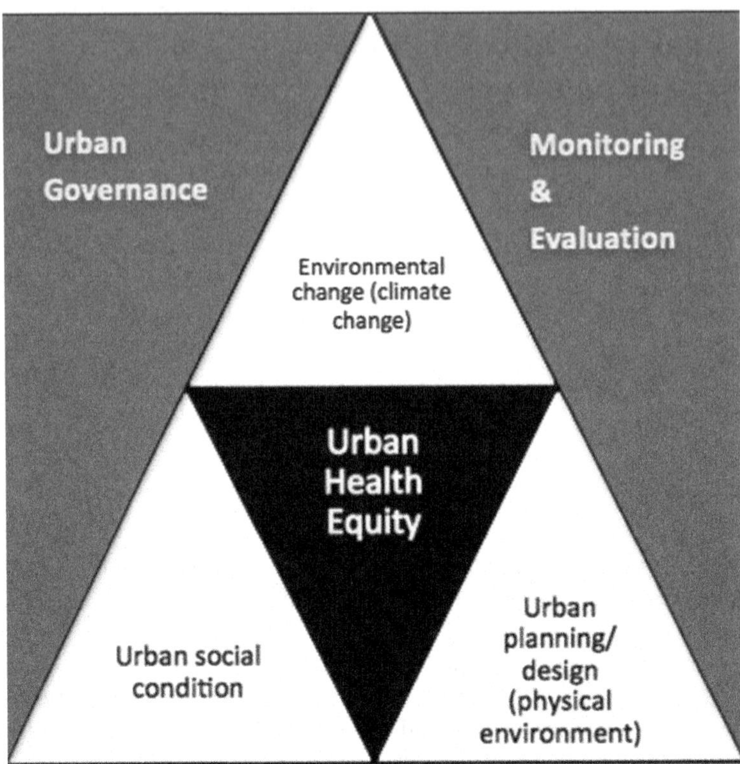

Fig. 13.9 Diagrammatic representation of Global Research Network on Urban Health Equity (GRNUHE) dimension of urban health equity. (Modified from Sharon et al., 2005 [9])

the added pressure of climate change, and the role of governance are essential to influence health benefits from urbanization (Fig. 13.9 and 13.10) [3, 9].

Modern research methods have allowed greater refinement on the question of how city living and urbanization may (or may not) affect health. However, it is difficult, and often misleading, to evaluate the relationship between urban life and health, as well as the effect that one has on the other. In fact, using comparable methodology, higher prevalence of mental illness, heart disease, or cancer in urban areas has been documented in some countries (for example, in the UK and USA), but not in others (i.e., in Canada) [42–48].

Arguing that all features of the urban context are modifiable, some of them may be more easily modifiable, with far greater and relatively short-term improvement in urban population health than others: this consideration strongly suggests to *focus interventions about problems that are commonly key determinants of health in cities* in this direction, as, for example, poor sanitation and inadequate clean water supply [49].

In the following discussion, we report strategies and some examples to be pursued to achieve best practices in urban health, with particular focus on cost-effectiveness. First of all, there is evidence that investments in *urban health can create*

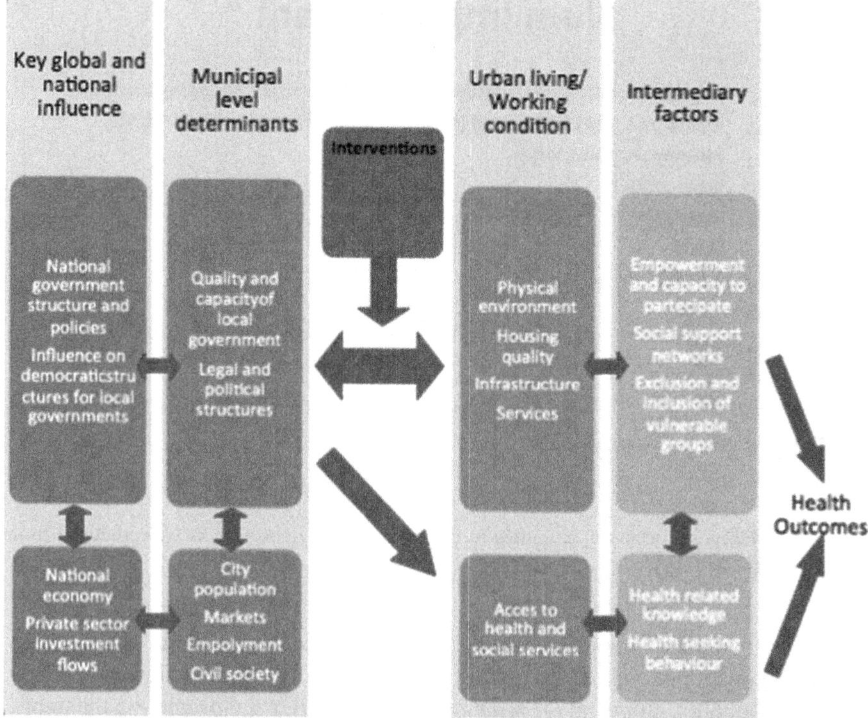

Fig. 13.10 A conceptual framework for urban health. (Reproduced from [3])

major returns for the economy, but the same is true for the opposite. Furthermore, experience shows that interventions concerning the physical environment become best practice only when they *integrate the social dimension.* So, pro-health policies need to be developed and implemented at supranational, national, and local levels, looking for a "healthy governance," empowering *all levels of society* and promoting *social cohesion* to ensure a control more shared and appropriated over resources for health [3]. In this sense, the demographic and epidemiological changes should require a life-course approach, rethinking cities as "global age-friendly," starting from the children to oldest olds [8]. UNICEF (2009) defines a "child-friendly city" as *a city or any local system of governance where policies, laws, programmes and budgets are committed to fulfilling children's rights, following the Convention on the Rights of the Child at the local level,* while WHO assumes that an "age-friendly city" *encourages active aging by optimizing opportunities for health, participation, and security in order to enhance quality of life as people age,* adapting its structures and services to be accessible to and inclusive of older people with varying needs and capacities [50, 8]. For both, children and olds, it is essential to: influence decisions about their city; support the affective and social relationship; protect them from exploitation, violence, and abuse; assure safe roads, sustaining in the meanwhile also unpolluted environment; and the development of green areas.

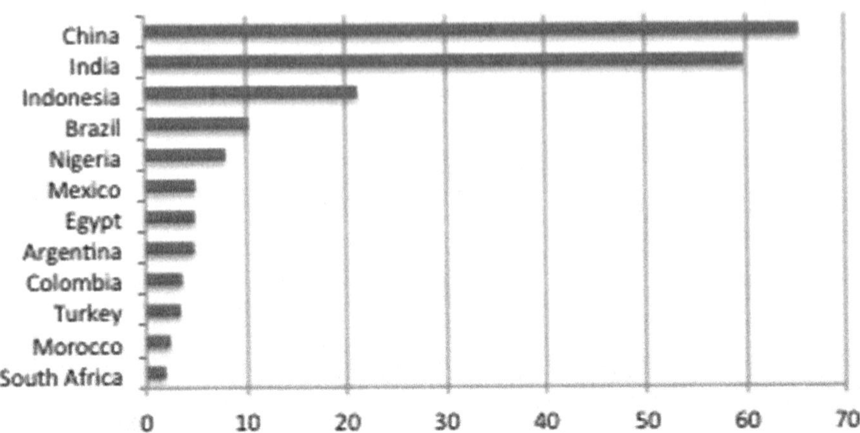

Fig. 13.11 The most successful countries in addressing slum improvement. (Reproduced from UN-HABITAT, 2009 [5])

Even if the best way to address public investment is often difficult to define, urban development policies and programs should explicitly acknowledge and address equity and equality, aiming at *the reduction of inequalities* and promoting the public good rather than private interests. According to a recent review of Laurence, while it is unrealistic to achieve income equality in market economies, it is realistic to promote the quality of life of citizens by ensuring access to education, leisure facilities, health care, community parks and gardens, and public transport [7]. Furthermore, cities are ideal context for interventions concerning the promotion and facilitation of good nutrition and physical activity, to reach the aim of "gaining health," according to the European Strategy for the Prevention and Control of Noncommunicable Diseases. In the same direction, it is essential to counteract urban violence, with increasing attention to gender- and age-related violence, and substance abuse (including smoking, alcohol, and illicit drugs). WHO indicates prevention as the most cost-effective strategy against violence and newer approaches such as conflict transformation, crime prevention through environmental design and community-based approaches to rebuilding trust and social capital, and tactics (early closing of nightclubs and bars, gun control, community awareness programs, and community policing) [3, 51, 52]. An analysis of more than 1700 initiatives from nearly 200 countries recorded from 1996 by UN-HABITAT shows the best practices that effectively address the top four critical problems in human settlement concerning the environment, housing, urban governance, and urban planning. In developing countries, important interventions address, i.e., slum upgrading (through the provision of basic infrastructure and services and tenure security, see Fig. 13.11) [5],solid waste management (in Durban, South Africa, a new approach to the construction of landfills allows for greenhouse gases to be captured to generate renewable energy instead of contributing to global warming.), etc.

An analysis of cost–benefit of different interventions to improve water access, quality, and sanitation indicated that in the developing regions of WHO, the benefit of a US$ 1 investment was in the range US$ 5–28.

The Fourth European Ministerial Conference on Environment and Health (Budapest, 2004) endorsed a high priority to housing and health. This conference asserts that layout, design, and maintenance of residential environments should meet the requirements of all groups of the population, including the increasing number of people with special needs, especially the most vulnerable in society, like homeless, elderly who need domiciliary care, people with disabilities, single-parent households (that may require access to particular child-care services), refugees, and migrants. In this sense, municipal housing programs have played an important input to provide these needs. So, at the moment, local authorities are planning guides and programs both for new construction and for those to be restored to promote better living conditions and health of vulnerable occupants [7]. An example from the Thai government's Community Organizations Development Institute has set a target of improving housing, living, and tenure security for 300,000 households in 2000 poor communities in 200 Thai urban centers.

Returning to the main issue, improving the lives of at least 100 million slum dwellers was a Millennium Development Goal target relevant to sustainable cities. More structurally sound, safe, and energy-efficient housing design, including good use of natural ventilation, can also help reduce domestic injuries and vulnerability to extreme weather/disasters. Besides, improving housing quality can reduce exposures to conditions of excessive heat, cold, dampness, and indoor air pollution, which are risk factors for a range of cardiopulmonary diseases (both infectious and noncommunicable). Progress in improving urban air quality can be easily measured and translated into quantifiable health ($PM_{10/2.5}$ is significantly associated with premature mortality from cardiopulmonary disease) and economic benefits; in fact, particulate air pollution, in many developing cities, causes about 1.3 million deaths annually [53]. One of the consequences of urban pollution is the increased incidence of asthma in children living in city. Therefore, a best practices in this direction is the urban health plan (UHP) that implemented a comprehensive asthma management program that has resulted in sustained improvements in patient outcomes, i.e., asthma, in the South Bronx [54].

Other best practices in air pollution management come from Linköping (Sweden), where they were able to reduce air pollution, greenhouse gas emissions, landfill waste, and vulnerability to oil price fluctuations, fueling public buses with biogas, and from Portland (USA), where, thanks to a collaboration between the national and local level, they decreased greenhouse gas emissions through improvements to public transport, creation of marketplaces for trading locally produced food, collection of recyclable and organic waste, and production of local renewable energy [55].

Investment in improved public transport can create great improvements in air pollution exposure, as well as traffic crash injury prevention and improved daily physical activity for public transport users. Besides, nonmotorization, using a wide range of technological and planning options that supply mobility needs, is compatible with high levels of prosperity, even if the opposite is true. For example, the proportion of people walking or cycling to work varies from about 30 % in Copenhagen and Santiago, to about 1 % in Tokyo and Brasilia [3].

Transport is one of the key points on which action must be taken to improve urban health. In fact, efficient transport is advantageous not only from the economic point of view but also from a healthy point of view, defining a healthy transport, because transport indicators thus reflect powerful aspects of a cities' overall "energy, health, and safety" scorecard. Therefore, cities served by transportation and dedicated walking/cycling networks are more energy efficient, safer, and healthy (reducing mortality risk for cardiovascular disease) for pedestrians and cyclists, as demonstrated by some studies that show that cities built around transit and active transport offer efficient and equitable access to jobs and health facilities [53].

In this regard, a study estimated the health risks and benefits of the transfer from car to cycling and public transport in Barcelona (Spain), demonstrating a significant increase in deaths averted (about 76 annually) for a shift of 40 % of the car trips to cycling and public transport. These interventions can, also, help to reduce greenhouse gas emissions and the energy utilization [56].

To reduce energy consumption, but also to help combat climate change, we can follow the example of The District Climate Change Plan that, thanks to three energy audits, led to the drawing up of a District Energy Plan, covering all the town's amenities of Valle de Elorz, which forecast the installation of eight renewable energy facilities and a change in energy consumption trends [55].

The reduction of energy consumption, and resources in general, cannot be separated from the reduction in water consumption; in this regard, the example of New York (USA) is reported, where the identification of planned land patterns and watershed management has resulted in ensuring a supply of clean water [57].

Most cities have significant vacant land within city limits; these areas should be exploited through infill development, that is, the process of developing unoccupied or underutilized land within vacant urban areas. These vacant areas could be used for the construction of public buildings or for the creation of green space. Indeed, many studies have associated, since 1845, the green areas to a better health condition and to more pleasant living environment. Other studies have shown that living in areas with walkable green spaces was linked with greater probability of promoting physical activity, higher functional status, lower cardiovascular disease risk, and longevity among the aged people [58]. Other examples of reutilization and conversion of urban space into green space come from Vauban eco-village (Germany) that today houses 5000 people, supplies 500 jobs, has ample green areas where food is grown nearby, and produces surplus energy [59]. Also the "StEP Klima," in Berlin (Germany) has previously shown the importance of existing urban green spaces and parks for city and people health [57].

The cities supply to geographic clustering of high-risk patients, creating a chance for deploying interventions where they can be most effective, like for both low-income elderly and adult disabled persons, as has been done, for example, in Durham (North Carolina). Besides, cities allow the concentration of technologies that could be used to implement the urban and people health, like in Boston (Massachusetts) where the Breathe Easy at Home program offers clinicians with a link in the patient's electronic medical record to initiate referrals to the Boston Inspectional Services Department [60].

A healthy city, besides, should provide to break down barriers to health care, starting from access to health facilities which should be equal for all the people, regardless of their social status [61]. Furthermore, it needs to implement violence prevention and health promotion, particularly in the most deprived areas because urban hospitals, in this neighborhoods, are often unprepared to handle emergency conditions (i.e., acute chemical or pesticide poisoning, drug intoxication, poisoning, gunshot wounds, maternal hemorrhage, or trauma) as well as against natural disasters (floods, earthquakes, etc.) [62].

Urban Health: "The Future...Today?"

The cities we live in, a synthesis of the cultural, ethnic, social, economic, technological, scientific, and cultural evolution, are essentially to be rethought in the light of the expectations and needs of the third millennium. Nevertheless, the old cultural paradigm (which sees the problems, or solutions, of the city, fragmented only in relations between traffic, pollution, and distribution of districts) still dominates the public imagination, not only of the population but also of the government's systems. Therefore, when we hypothesize the cities of the future, yet we use design models of the past, often valid in the past decades, but today no longer justifiable. More than anything else, this is because there is still no new consensus on the future of urban evolution: redesigning old street, reimagining or reinventing cultural, scientific, and green spaces or buildings according to the current and not future needs, thinking about how to reduce traffic without changing the context in which the traffic is generated, etc. Of course, this highlights the growing inertia that characterizes the urban planning choices compared to the speed with which technology or the scientific and health evidence evolve. In this lack of certainty, health should be at the center of the inspiring values for each sector and for each stakeholder in order to create a healthy and sustainable city: not only absence of disease, encompassing socioeconomic, physical, and mental well-being, but also appreciation of the nature and influence of the environmental, energy, social, biological, and political determinants of health, considering them as common and undifferentiated impact on the development of both the individual and of urban society level in which we live. As Z. Jakab has well defined, although the cities are the focus of job opportunities, cultural, scientific, and economic development, they are also: "...the nexus of negative economic, environmental and economic forces jeopardizing the lives and health of many inhabitants..." [63]. So that, according to A. Tsouros: "...living and working in urban areas affects health and health prospects both positively and negatively, through a complex array of exposures and mechanisms....," and therefore, although cities represent the center of the research development and entrepreneurship growth, they can also be a negative element of poverty aggregation, unemployment, and sources of risk for diseases related to lifestyle, occupational, and communicable diseases, often related to each other, as well as unrecognized or underestimated [64–66]. The importance that local governments represent in the city policy and management resides in and performance is measured by leadership functions that these governments are able to express, because many determinants of health operate at the local and community level. They can promote the health and well-being of their citizens through their influence in many contexts, including education, economy, security, social services and transport, environment, housing, tourism, culture, and, mainly, health [67].

The leadership of a city, conceived in the prevention and in the health view of its citizens, can be expressed through different types of interventions and policy, aimed at avoiding the risks and to promote good behavior. In particular, paying attention to the social categories that are more sensitive and susceptible (children, pregnant women, disabled and elderly people, immigrants, etc.), as well as avoid the social exclusion and racial, ethnic, cultural, religious, social, and economic inequity. So healthy and active living, in compliance with health policies aimed at increasing the empowerment of the community towards the determinants of health than towards those habits which constitute the risk factors for communicable and chronic degenerative diseases (policies to reduce or ban on alcohol consumption, especially among young people, of tobacco smoking, intake of foods and drinks, high in sugar and fat, etc.), are the priorities of a careful political leadership and governance of urban health, enhancing at the same time policies attentive to healthy and active living for safety, working conditions, reducing exposure to hazards in a "pollutionless environment." Thus, basics become both sharing processes and participatory involvement of citizens in the policy of urban health, and healthy urban planning and design, resulting in a new culture for the development of [64, 68]:

- A new global information and communication technology (through the use of new social tools like biosciences application of geographic information systems and global mapping).
- A new networking system that enables just-in-time manufacturing and connects our economies and ecological principles to urban habitat into a single interlinked and homogeneous network; through sharing experiences, networks with new information and communication technology support innovation while cities avoid risks and can achieve a capillary and preventive health care, through the use of *eHealth* approach and new technology tools.
- New concepts in energy use, amplifying the culture of reducing waste and consumption by aiming the use of renewable energy, preparing to deal with the profound consequences of climate change, which will have a major impact on the infinitesimal fabric of the same conception of the city for the future, and so…
- … New design programs, planning, and concepts for the built environment: breaking down the architectural and perceptive barriers, having as its first objective the needs of people with disabilities (considering that among these, we should put all the people who, in industrialized countries, will become increasingly older), giving them the opportunity to experience the city without any limitation; neighborhood planning, programming a new way of thinking about the

neighborhoods, in particular peripheral, aimed at reducing inequity and inequality and not only designed based on the availability of building land, building, or industrial needs, opening the suburb for a renaissance; developing the preferred way to achieve maximum accessibility and proximity of services, reducing traffic. Utmost importance and attention should be given to indoor environments, especially houses, schools, health facilities, and public utilities and services. Are needed a new culture of design and new methods of construction, with attention to eco-friendly and low toxicological impact materials and furnishings. This is because many of these environments are outdated, built with nonecological materials and favoring the emission of toxic or carcinogenic substances, resulting in an unjustified exposure since the adolescent age, that can be cause for the chronic degenerative and neoplastic diseases during adulthood age [69].

- A new mode to rethink the traditional problems of a modern city, which persist in the limitations arising from the overlap of the past inheritance and future needs: it is no longer possible to conceive a city where green spaces are inserted as "isolated patches on a tablecloth," but like a "total and integrated green city" to grow in terms of these "lungs for the urban habitat"; so, it is no longer possible to conceive a city where traffic is controlled only by closing the accessibility to the historical centers of most polluting cars. We need to rethink a new mode of transport, but also new systems of viability closely related to technological developments in transport and the future needs. The evolution of systems of road network and traffic control, in the last millennium, has not gone in tandem with the technological evolution of motor vehicles and renewable energy sources, that could be used as driving forces. Multiple economic interests and a high degree of inertia in decision making are still the primary cause of significant environmental pollution that is visible in all modern cities, with an exponential growth directly correlated to urbanization and the rise of the territorial extension.

It is intuitive, but it is always good to reiterate, that any evolution (new materials, new energy, although renewable, new ways of transportation, construction, manufacturing, etc.) should always be tested and demonstrated, with scientific evidence, to have a low impact on health at all or, at least, reduce the likely health effects due to what is to be replaced not to risk, as has often happened in the past, that many economic investment, a lot of resources and time are spent without there being real innovation to a urban health. "*…Or even to occur as the new to be worse than the old* (wrongly or, consumerist, considered obsolete)…"

Health 2020 puts a strong emphasis on new information and communication technology systems, promoting cities to consider socioeconomic networking as an important aspect of "smart governance":

> …Approaches need to be adaptive and mirror the complexity of causality, because complex and wicked problems have no simple linear causality or solution…. Interventions should be iterative and integrate continuous learning….[70]

Obviously, without us, forget or underestimate the role of active prevention breakthrough on the environment and in the community (which, to date, cannot be resolved by virtual digital or computer technology, etc.).

Of course, in a millennium in which next to the advancement of health technologies (*digital,* with the development of nanotechnology; *social and cultural,* with the emergence of new values that should be conjugated with the old; *scientific and medical,* through imaging and the study of genomics, proteomics, and metabolomics; etc.) there is a global crisis of the world economy, it is fundamental to strengthen and use the assets of *individual and community resilience* (most definitions of resilience refer to notions—derived from physics—of rebound, or bouncing back, from deformation or distress), also because action to improve community health requires the coordination and the cooperation of decision makers in many sectors responsible for shaping wider determinants, and also because the traditional management of policy may be ineffective to address the problems of the "future cities" and requires an institutional change, given the discrepancy that can exist between technological innovation, scientific evolution, and adaptive flexibility of governance systems. So, while the concept of *individual resilience* has evolved in psychology and the behavioral health sciences as a means to understand what adaptive capacities allow some individuals to continue functioning effectively and display positive outcomes in the face of adversity, instead *community resilience* is much more than the summation of individual resiliencies, and it has been defined as the sustained ability of a community to withstand and recover from adversity (e.g., economic stress, pandemic influenza, man-made or natural disasters, etc.) [71]. It represents a paradigm shift in public health emergency preparedness in emphasizing an assessment of community strengths not simply describing vulnerabilities [72, 73]. Therefore, probably, the measure of the ability of leadership and governance required *to ensure political support and adequate resources,* aimed *to plan and implement viable structures to facilitate the achievement of goals related to health cities,* is given by the resilience of the urban systems promoted by the integration of individuals and communities.

Conclusion and Key Messages for Decision Maker

In conclusion, what has been until now described can also be summarized through the WHO "Healthy City" approach that represents an example of a European comprehensive best practice for implementing in our cities the principles of the WHO strategy for "Health for All" and the "Ottawa Charter for Health Promotion" (1986) [74]. The WHO European Healthy Cities Network, established in 1986, is represented now by more than 90 members (cities and towns) from 30 countries and 30 national healthy cities networks across the WHO European Region, that have more than 1400 cities and towns as members, and embodies an ideal platform for the generation and spread of healthy urban policies [64, 75]. Urbanization is one of the major public health challenges of this century, considering that urban populations are quickly increasing and it is projected to reach more than two thirds of the global population, over 6.4 billion people by 2050. Moreover, population aging and the associated demographic transition are another great challenge that requires, suddenly, public health intervention for ensuring "global age-friendly cities," both for children and for oldest old. Urban areas have contributed to improve the mortality and morbidity rates in the highly industrialized and urbanized countries, providing healthy living and healthy working environment (although, of course, much is still to be done), concentrating opportunities, jobs, services, and technologies, and promoting prosperous economy. Besides, urbanization may pose a risk to health, deepening social and economic inequalities between and within countries and cities, as difference in life expectancy (especially infant mortality); growing slums and informal settings; communicable diseases, especially emerging and "re-emerging" infectious diseases; water availability and physical, chemical, and biological contaminations; chronic, noncommunicable diseases linked to lifestyles in cities; road traffic and accidents; violence and crime; indoor and outdoor air pollution; and climate changes. The right investments in urban health are directly related with returns for the economy and vice versa, and several interventions has been demonstrated, especially in developing countries; cost-effective (i.e., improve water access, quality, and sanitation) highlights the importance that urban development policies and programs address the reduction of inequalities. Healthy cities needs an integration of health considerations into urban planning, processes, strategic programs and policies to support health, recreation, and well-being, safety, social interaction, easy mobility, a sense of pride and cultural identity, by means of green and open spaces, for recreation and physical activity, encouraging walking and cycling; affordable transport and road systems; and anticipate implications of the climate changes, getting ready in case of public health emergencies. So, best practice in *urban health* can lead to "healthy cities," and *the key messages* are [76]:

- A clean safe high-quality environment, including affordable housing *and healthy schools or workplaces.*
- A stable and a *sustainable* ecosystem, *with increasing attention to the green energy with low impact on health, with attention to issues related to climate change, in which technology and environment are integrated, and outdoor–indoor living is healthy.*
- A strong, mutually supportive, and nonexploitative community, *where the overcoming of ethnic, religious, cultural, social, and economic inequity is a major goal.*
- Much public participation in and control over decisions affecting life, health, and well-being, *with a focus on leadership chosen and the governance system implemented.*
- The provision of basic needs (food, water, shelter, income, safety, and work) for all people *with shared access to resources, services, and community health.*
- Access to a wide range of experiences and resources with the possibility of multiple contacts, interaction, and communication, *through implementation of technologies at low cost.*
- A diverse, vital, and innovative economy, *supported by shared ethical principles.*
- Encouragement of connections with the past, with the varied cultural and biological heritage, and with other groups and individuals, *overcoming differences and inequalities.*

- A city form (design) that is compatible with and enhances the proceeding characteristics; *a design of age-friendly cities (accessible, affordable, flexible, adaptive) introducing holistic policies addressing the health needs of children, older people, but also migrants and vulnerable people, in particular by addressing disabilities and eliminating perceptive, psychical, social ,and architectural/physical barriers*
- An optimum level of appropriate public health and care services accessible to all, *developing and implementing programs aiming to strengthen the health literacy skills of the population, with attention to* "prevention and environmentally sustainable health systems."
- A high health status (both a high positive health status and low disease status), *supporting healthy lifestyles, especially in schools and workplaces, promoting the factors and conditions that support well-being and happiness, reduce stress, and enhance the resilience of communities.*
- *Governance and administration actions aimed to prevention, public and health care based on the criteria of transparency, accountability, sharing of knowledge, and new technologies.*
- *Policies and plans to deal with all aspects of violence and injuries in cities, including violence involving women, children and older people, vulnerable road users, and immigrants.*

Acknowledgment We would like to thank Dr. Daniele Ignazio La Milia for the support to the scientific literature review and research and Dr. Carolina Ianuale for the editing of the entire book.

References

1. Galea S, Vlahov D (2005) Urban health: populations, methods and practice. In: Galea S, Vlahov D (eds) Handbook on urban health: populations, methods and practice. Springer, New York
2. Frye V, Putnam S, O'Campo P (2008) Whither gender in urban health? Health Place 14(3):616–622
3. WHO (2008) Our cities, our health, our future: acting on social determinants for health equity in urban settings. World Health Organization, Geneva
4. United Nations Human Settlements Programme (UN-HABITAT) (2006). Urbanization: Mega & Meta Cities, New City States? http://www.unhabitat.org/documents/media_centre/sowcr2006/SOWCR%202.pdf. Accessed 2 Oct 2013
5. United Nations Human Settlements Programme (UN-HABITAT) (2010). State of the World's Cities 2010/2011: Bridging The Urban Divide. http://www.unhabitat.org/documents/SOWC10/L1.pdf. Accessed 2 Oct 2013
6. WHO (2013) http://www.who.int/gho/urban_health/situation_trends/urban_population_growth/en/index.html. Accessed 2 Oct 2013
7. Lawrence RJ (2007) Urban health challenges in europe. J Urban Health 90(S1):23–36
8. WHO (2007) Global age-friendly cities: a guide. World Health Organization, Geneva
9. Friel S, Akerman M, Hancock T, Kumaresan J, Marmot M, Melin T, Vlahov D, GRNUHE members (2011) Addressing the social and environmental determinants of urban health equity: evidence for action and a research agenda. J Urban Health 88(5):860–874. doi:10.1007/s11524-011-9606-1

10. WHO - UNHABITAT. PART ONE. THE DAWN OF AN URBAN WORLD. In: HIDDEN CITIES: UNMASKING AND OVERCOMING HEALTH INEQUITIES IN URBAN SETTINGS. World Health Organization, The WHO Centre for Health Development, Kobe, and United Nations Human Settlements Programme (UN-HABITAT), 2010
11. United Nations Human Settlements Programme (UN-HABITAT) (2006) State of the worlds' cities 2006/7. The millennium development goals and urban sustainability. Earthscan, London
12. African Population and Health Research Center (APHRC) (2002) Population and health dynamics in Nairobi's informal settlements. African Population and Health Research Center, Nairobi
13. Global Health Observatory (GHO). Infant mortality. Available at: http://www.who.int/gho/urban_health/outcomes/infant_mortality_text/en/index.html. Accessed 2 Oct 2013
14. WHO Commission on Social Determinants of Health (2008) Closing the gap in a generation: health equity through action on the social determinants of health. Final report of the Commission on Social Determinants of Health. World Health Organization, Geneva
15. Yassi A et al (2001) Basic environmental health. Oxford University Press, New York
16. Wilson ME (1995) Infectious diseases: an ecological perspective. Br Med J 311:1681–1684
17. Morse S (1995) Factors in the emergence of infectious diseases. Emerg Infect Disord 1(1):7–15
18. UNAIDS (2006) Report on the global AIDS epidemic. UNAIDS, Geneva
19. WHO - Global Health Observatory (GHO). Access to piped water. Available at: http://www.who.int/gho/urban_health/determinants/safe_water/en/index.html. Accessed 2 Oct 2013
20. Roccaro P, Falciglia PP, Vagliasindi FG (2011) Effectiveness of water saving devices and educational programs in urban buildings. Water Sci Technol 63(7):1357–1365
21. Willis RM, Stewart RA, Panuwatwanich K, Williams PR, Hollingsworth AL (2011) Quantifying the influence of environmental and water conservation attitudes on household end use water consumption. J Environ Manage 92(8):1996–2009
22. Azara A, Moscato U (2009) Rapporto Osservasalute Ambiente 2008. (Eds. Ricciardi G). Prex, Milano
23. Addo J, Smeeth L, Leon D (2007) Hypertension in sub-Saharan Africa: a systematic review. Hypertension 50(6):1012–1018
24. Evans GW, Jones-Rounds ML, Belojevic G, Vermeylen F (2012) Family income and childhood obesity in eight European cities: the mediating roles of neighborhood characteristics and physical activity. Soc Sci Med 75(3):477–481
25. Fleischer N, Diez Roux A, Alazraqui M, Spinelli H (2008) Social patterning of chronic disease risk factors in a Latin American city. J Urban Health 85(6):923–937
26. Friel S, Chopra M, Satcher D (2007) Unequal weight: equity oriented policy responses to the global obesity epidemic. Br Med J 335(7632):1241–1243
27. Ruel MT, Garrett JL (2004) Features of urban food and nutrition security and considerations for successful urban programming. Electron J Agric Develop Econ 1(2):242–271
28. Dixon J, Omwega AM, Friel S, Burns C, Donati K, Carlisleet R (2007) The health equity dimension of urban food systems. J Urban Health 84(S1):118–129
29. Mendez M, Popkin B (2004) Globalization, urbanization and nutritional change in the developing world. Electron J Agric Develop Econ 1(2):220–241
30. Frank L, Kavage S, Litman T (2006) Promoting public health through Smart Growth: building healthier communities through transportation and land-use policies and practices. Vancouver BC SmartGrowth BC, Beaconsfield
31. Kjellstrom T, Hinde S (2007) Car culture, transport policy and public health. In: Kawachi I, Wamala S (eds) Globalization and public health. Oxford University Press, New York
32. Harpham T (1994) Urbanization and mental health in developing countries: a research role for social scientists, public health professionals and social psychiatrists. Soc Sci Med 39(2):233–245
33. WHO (2013) Global status report on road safety. World Health Organization, Geneva
34. Nantulya VM et al (2003) Introduction: the global challenge of road traffic injuries: can we achieve equity in safety? Inj Control Saf Promot 10:3–7

35. WHO—Global Health Observatory (GHO) (2013) http://gamapserver.who.int/gho/interactive_charts/phe/oap_mbd/atlas.html—Accessed 4 Nov 2013
36. WHO—Global Health Observatory (GHO) (2013) http://www.who.int/gho/phe/outdoor_air_pollution/exposure/en/. Accessed 4 Nov 2013
37. Pascal M, Corso M, Chanel O et al (2013) Assessing the public health impacts of urban air pollution in 25 European cities: results of the Aphekom project. Sci Total Environ 1(449):390–400
38. Donatiello G (2001) Environmental sustainability indicators in urban areas: an Italian experience. Joint ECE/Eurostat Work Session on Methodological Issues of Environment Statistics Working Paper 16. Ottawa
39. Campbell-Lendrum D, Corvalan C (2007) Climate change and developing country cities: implications for environmental health and equity. J Urban Health 84(3)i109–i117
40. Oxfam (2007) Adapting to climate change. What's needed in poor countries and who should pay? Oxfam briefing paper 104, Oxford
41. McMichael A et al (2004) Climate Change. In: Ezzati M, Lopez A, Rodgers A, Murray C (eds) Comparative quantification of health risks: global and regional burden of disease due to selected major risk factors. World Health Organization, Geneva
42. Paykel ES, Abbott R, Jenkins R et al (2002) Noise exposure and public health. Environ Health Perspect 108(S1):123–131
43. Parikh SV, Wasylenki D, Goering P et al (1996) Mood disorders: rural/urban differences in prevalence, health care utilization, and disability in Ontario. J Affect Disord 38:57–65
44. Blazer D, George LK, Landerman R, et al (1985) Psychiatric disorders: a rural/urban comparison. Arch Gen Psychiatry 42:651–656
45. Blazer DG, Kessler RC, McGonagle KA, Swartz MS (1994) The prevalence and distribution of major depression in a national community sample: the National Comorbidity Survey. Am J Psychol 151:979–986
46. Kessler RC, McGonagle KA, Zhao S et al (1994) Lifetime and 12-month prevalence of DSM-III-R psychiatric disorders in the United States. Arch Gen Psychiatry 51:8–19
47. Hwu H-G, Yeh E-K, Chang L-Y (1989) Prevalence of psychiatric disorders in Taiwan defined by the Chinese diagnostic interview schedule. Acta Psychiatr Scand 79:136–147
48. Yamamoto S, Watanabe S (2001) Geographic characteristics and mortality profiles in the JPHC study. Japan public health center-based prospective study on cancer and cardiovascular diseases. J Epidemiol 11(S6):S8–23
49. Vlahov D, Gibble E, Freudenberg N, Galea S (2004) Cities and Health: history, approaches, and key questions. Acad Med 79:1133–1138
50. UNICEF National Committees and Country Offices (2009) Child friendly cities promoted. Fact sheet, Geneva
51. Fowler PJ, Braciszewski JM (2009) Community violence prevention and intervention strategies for children and adolescents: the need for multilevel approaches. J Prev Interv Community 37(4):255–259
52. WHO (2007) Preventing injuries and violence. World Health Organisation, Geneva
53. WHO (2012) Health indicators of sustainable cities. In the context of the Rio+20 UN conference on sustainable development. Initial findings from a WHO expert consultation. World Health Organisation, Geneva
54. Lester D, Mohammad A, Leach EE, Hernandez PI, Walker EA (2012) An investigation of asthma care best practices in a community health center. J Health Care Poor Underserved 23(S3):255–264
55. United Nations Human Settlements Programme (UN-HABITAT) (2012) Urban patterns for a green economy. Optimizing infrastructure. http://www.unhabitat.org/pmss/listItemDetails.aspx?publicationID!!/span>=3343. Accessed 04 Nov 2013
56. Rojas-Rueda D, de Nazelle A, Teixidó O, Nieuwenhuijsen MJ (2012) Replacing car trips by increasing bike and public transport in the greater Barcelona metropolitanarea: a health impact assessment study. Environ Int 15(49):100–109

57. United Nations Human Settlements Programme (UN-HABITAT) (2012) Urban patterns for a green economy. Working with nature. http://www.unhabitat.org/pmss/listItemDetails.aspx?publicationID!!/span>=3341. Accessed 04 Nov 2013
58. Galea S, Vlahov D (2005) Urban health: evidence, challenges and directions. Annu Rev Public Health 26:341–365
59. United Nations Human Settlements Programme (UN-HABITAT) (2012). Urban patterns for a green economy. Leveraging Density. http://www.unhabitat.org/pmss/listItemDetails.aspx?publicationID!!/span>=3342. Accessed 04 Nov 2013
60. Stine N, Chokshi D, Gourevitch M (2013) Improving population health in US cities. J Am Med Assoc 309(5):449–450. doi:10.1001/jama.2012.154302
61. Lee IM, Rexrode KM, Cook NR, Manson JE, Buring JE (2001) Physical activity and coronary heart disease in women: Is "no pain, no gain" passè? J Am Med Assoc 285:1447–1454
62. Campbell T, Campbell A (2007) Emerging disease burdens and the poor in cities of the developing world. J Urban Health 84(S1):54–64. doi:10.1007/s11524-007-9181-7
63. Jakab Z (2012) Contextualizing health: accounting for the urban environment. Harvard Int Rev 34(1): 46–51
64. Tsouros A (2013) City leadership for health and well-being: back to the future. J Urban Health 90(S1):4–13. doi:10.1007/s11524-013-9825-8
65. United Nations, Department of Economic and Social Affairs, Population Division (2010) World urbanization prospects, the 2009 revision: highlights. United Nations, New York
66. World Health Organization/UN HABITAT (2010) Hidden cities: unmasking and overcoming health inequities in urban settings. WHO, Kobe
67. Whitfield M, Machaczek K, Green G (2013) Developing a model to estimate the potential impact of municipal investment on city health. J Urban Health 90(S1):62–73. doi:10.1007/s11524-012-9763-x
68. Mau B (2011) Urbanity, revised: to imagine the future we must rethink the meaning of a city, Megalopolis. World Policy J 27(4):17–22
69. Ministry for the Environment, L and and Sea-Italy and Regional Environmental Center (2013) School environment and respiratory health of children. Summary of SEARCH II results and conclusions. http://search.rec.org/publications/airing-ideas/196. Accessed 2 Oct 2013
70. World Health Organization Regional Office for Europe (2012) Health 2020: policy framework and strategy. EUR/RC62/8. WHO, Copenaghen
71. Castleden M, McKee M, Murray V, Leonardi G (2011) Resilience thinking in health protection. J Public Health (Oxf) 33(3):369–377
72. Nuwayhid I, Zurayk H, Yamout R, Cortas CS (2011) Summer 2006 war on Lebanon: a lesson in community resilience. Glob Public Health 21:1–15
73. Plough A Fielding JE, Chandra A et al (2013) Building community disaster resilience: perspectives from a large urban county department of public health. Am J Public Health 103(7):1190–1197. doi:10.2105/AJPH.2013.301268
74. WHO (1986) The Ottawa charter for health promotion—first international conference on health promotion. WHO, Geneva
75. WHO Regional Office for Europe (2013). Healthy cities. http://www.euro.who.int/en/health-topics/environment-and-health/urban-health/activities/healthy-cities. Accessed 2 Oct 2013
76. Hancock T, Duhl T (1988) Promoting health in an urban context. WHO Healthy Cities Papers No. 1, WHO Regional Office for Europe, Copenhagen

Chapter 14
Genomics and Public Health

Stefania Boccia and Ron Zimmern

Introduction

Genomics and molecular biology have developed at an ever-increasing pace over the last decade. Building on the achievements of the Human Genome Project, and aided by advances in sequencing and information technology, groundbreaking discoveries in genomics and molecular biology are reported almost daily in the scientific and popular literature, suggesting multiple opportunities for improving the health of populations. Divergent claims about the utility of genomics for improving population health, however, have been released. On the one hand, genomics is viewed as the harbinger of a brave new world in which novel treatments rectify known causes of disease. A major promise of the 'omics' research is that of delivering new information that can transform health care through earlier diagnosis, more effective prevention programmes, and a higher precision in the treatment of disease. Targeting treatments and interventions will, arguably, enable the intelligent use of ever more pressed resources to allow the better identification of those susceptible to ill health, and provide opportunities for personalized treatments (with the concomitant reduction in drug and health professional-induced adverse events). On the other hand, the predominant social and environmental causes of disease should not be forgotten, particularly in low- and middle-income countries; and any focus on individual genetic variation should always have regard to the combined effects of genetic and environmental factors in the pathogenesis of disease.

Amid these competing visions of what advances in genomic science might entail, there is also a lack of consensus about the scope of public health. Traditionally

S. Boccia (✉)
Institute of Public Health, Section of Hygiene, Università Cattolica del Sacro Cuore, L.go F. Vito 1, 00168 Rome, Italy
e-mail: sboccia@rm.unicatt.it

R. Zimmern
PHG Foundation, 2 Worts' Causeway, Cambridge CB1 8RN, UK
e-mail: ron.zimmern@phgfoundation.org

S. Boccia et al. (eds.), *A Systematic Review of Key Issues in Public Health*,
DOI 10.1007/978-3-319-13620-2_14

in the developed world, public health has been concerned with interventions made at population level to promote better health, such as improving sanitation, or reducing exposure to infectious agents which might cause disease. Yet genomic medicine seems to promote a vision for health care which encourages individualism at the expense of the population. But this tension is not new. Geoffrey Rose wrote of the distinction between high risk and population prevention; but he also pointed out that 'causes of incidence' were to be distinguished from 'causes of cases', by which he meant that the factors that determine the cause of disease in individuals within a population needed to be distinguished from the causes of disease between populations. Thus, genomic and personalized medicine have the potential to challenge the rationale which underpins existing public health, as well as the methods with which it is conventionally delivered.

Against this background, a multidisciplinary expert meeting was held in Bellagio, Italy, in 2005 to assess the potential implications of these developments for population health. Public health genomics (PHG) has been defined as 'the responsible and effective translation of genome-based knowledge and technologies into public policy and health services for the benefit of population health' (Bellagio Statement). More recently, a larger international PHG meeting was held at Ickworth House, Suffolk, UK [8]. Nevertheless, although exactly how public health professionals should engage with this scientific agenda is at present not entirely clear, there was a consensus among those attending those meetings that public health professionals had to engage with the genomics agenda and to recognize its potential for disease prevention and health improvement. In this chapter, we summarize the potential for a personalized health care approach, and the challenges to address to facilitate its implementation in an effective and efficient manner.

In doing so, we assume that readers have an understanding of the basic principles of genetics.

The Potential for Genomics in Improving Population Health

With rapid advances in molecular and cellular biology and in genomics and related sciences, it has become increasingly evident that susceptibility to disease is not uniform in all individuals and/or populations. Susceptibility is based on complex interactions of social, biological (including genetic), and environmental determinants within a broader political and economic context. Furthermore, if disease does occur, its severity, outcome, and response to treatment are also influenced by various social, biological, and environmental factors.

From a philosophical point of view, the incorporation of the genomic discoveries into public health practice deals with an apparent paradox. While the mission of public health is to improve health from a population perspective, with its unit of intervention being the population, the approach of personalized medicine that focuses on individuals appears odd [36]). The example of newborn screening for the inherited metabolic disease phenylketonuria (PKU), however, illustrates how genomics came together with public health during the 1960s. Although this genetic disease was rare, screening was recognized as a public health responsibility because early diagnosis and treatment of affected infants could prevent serious mental and physical disability in the population. Thus, a dual rhetoric has emerged both about the transformative power of 'personalized' medicine to improve health at the level of the individual and the proper role of public health in that quest, as the role of public health includes the stratification of populations into groups rather than the provision of individualistic outcomes.

The scope and context of genomic applications have evolved since the completion of the Human Genome Project a decade ago, and the use of genetic and genomic tests for improving population health is currently broad. Between October 2009 and March 2014, more than 500 new genomic tests were identified from horizon scanning by the US Centers for Disease Control and Prevention [18]. A sober analysis of the current landscape, however, tempers the enthusiasm for any quick embrace of personalized medicine as broadly transformative in the realm of patient care and public health. An ultimate objective for those wishing to apply genomics in public health would be the ability to use genotypic information to identify groups of individuals who are at increased risk of disease and who could be offered opportunities to reduce their risk by means of interventions aimed at modifiable environmental factors such as diet. However, although not a simple goal to attain, evidence is building to suggest that modern public health practice should in certain cases take into account genetic variation in individuals as a tool for more efficient and effective action.

The first problem in using genotypic information for prevention is the low penetrance of most of the alleles implicated in susceptibility to common disease [26]. Individually, such alleles are typically associated with relative risks of around 1.1–2.0, though rarer alleles may confer higher risks [25]. For this reason, the positive and negative predictive values of tests for single alleles are likely to be low.

It has been suggested that the predictive power of genotypic information would be increased if more alleles were considered together. This approach is called genomic profiling [35]. Although individuals who carry multiple risk alleles will have a very high risk of disease, these individuals constitute a very small percentage of the population. For the bulk of the population, genomic profiling will be extremely complex, depending on the number of risk genotypes tested for, the spectrum of risk alleles an individual carries, and the odds ratios associated with each of them [24]. Pleiotropic effects of susceptibility genes must also be taken into account. For example, the apolipoprotein E4 (*APOE4*) variant increases risk for both Alzheimer's dementia and coronary heart disease but reduces risk for macular degeneration. Interventions aimed at preventing the negative effects of a gene variant might increase risk for another disease.

Another relevant issue is behavioural responses to genomic risk information. Is risk information based on genetic factors is likely to be effective in motivating the sustained behavioural change that would be needed to achieve health benefits? Current evidence on this issue is limited and more research is needed. The availability of an effective intervention is also important, as is the individual's assessment of his or her ability to achieve behavioural change; this assessment, in turn, is strongly dependent on the person's familial and social environment. There is some evidence that reactions to genetic risk information may differ from those to other types of risk information. For example, a recent study of individuals recently diagnosed with familial hypercholesterolemia through DNA testing found that perceived risk and perceived efficacy of medication were higher than the 'no genetic predisposition' control sample [11]. This points to the need to present genetic risk information in such a way that it does not undermine the individual's belief in the efficacy of behavioural change.

Concerning secondary prevention, there may be scope to refine existing screening programmes by the incorporation of genomic information, though so far success in the search for effective strategies using polygenic inheritance data has been limited [10]. Evans and colleagues have recently proposed, however, some ways in which the potential of PHG might be realized [17]. Rapid and inexpensive sequencing of genes can currently identify individuals carrying individually rare mutations that confer dramatic predisposition to preventable diseases. This concerns, for example, the use of *BRCA* 1 and 2 gene testing for the hereditary breast cancer: The combined prevalence of these mutations is around 0.2–0.3 % of the general population, but they may in some families confer a >70 % lifetime risk for breast and ovarian cancer. Also, the four Lynch-associated genes are present in 0.2 % of subjects and confer >80 % risk for colon cancer. Even though the public health benefit of screening for rare diseases might seem a paradox, early detection of carriers can lead to a large benefit in term of mortality reduction from cancer diseases that so far are identified by waiting until these individuals, or some of their family members, develop such diseases. For breast cancer, there are algorithms, based on family history, to assess whether a woman should receive genetic counselling, and if indicated, genetic testing; these tools, however, are not applied systematically in the primary care setting.

The Translation Agenda

A major challenge is to bridge the gap that currently exists between genome-based discovery and the realization of clinical and public health benefit. A measure of the optimal translation agenda might be the ease with which novel genome-based discoveries may be implemented by health services and made available to the public. This is influenced by a host of different factors, such as the availability of research funding, research capacity and expertise, the prevailing regulatory climate, and competing resources.

The translation of genomic research into interventions has been categorized into four phases (T1–T4), as represented in Fig. 14.1. In higher-income countries, a well-developed infrastructure exists to support the translation of novel drug targets from animal to human subjects. This phase of translation (T1) is managed through the clinical trial system, and is relatively generously funded because drug

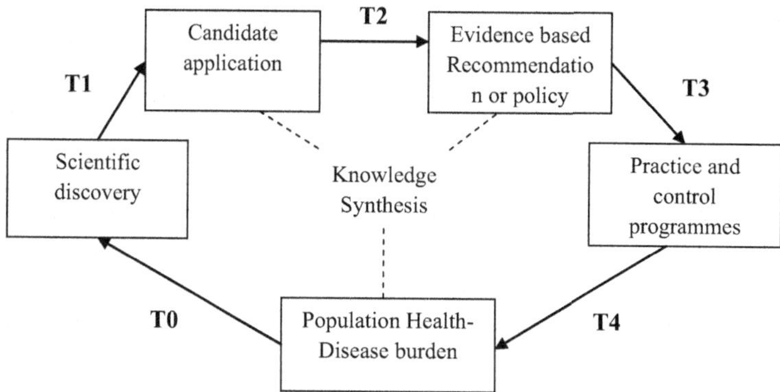

Fig. 14.1 Knowledge synthesis—the engine of translational research

development has a well-defined route, and for the minority of blockbuster drugs that make it to market, the patent system guarantees a financial reward.

With novel genomic discoveries however, the process is less well defined. Although the T1 phase is relatively well funded, subsequent phases of translation (T2–T4) lack the necessary infrastructure and funding for effective implementation. This is particularly the case for translational research that does not result in a marketable product, such as new models of service delivery that emphasise cost savings. There is also a lack of political will for translation at these levels. Finally, the application of new knowledge to reduce the population health disease burden can also result in new understanding that can feed back into basic scientific understanding (T0). There was very strong support for developing outcomes-driven research that focuses upon the evaluation of public health programmes (T3) and that builds capacity, growth, and development through population-based research.

Evaluation of Genetic and Genomic Tests

Public health programmes have an important role in ensuring that any diagnostic, predictive, or pharmacogenetic test used in health practice is properly evaluated in order to protect the public's health and assure validated health services. A genetic test (or any other clinical test) is a complex process that is part of an overall regime of disease prevention or management for a specific individual in an intended clinical scenario [30]. The first attempt to devise an evaluation framework for genetic tests was the ACCE evidentiary framework [20], using criteria originally proposed by the 1997 Task Force on Genetic Testing [22]. ACCE is an acronym standing for **A**nalytical validity, **C**linical validity, **C**linical utility, and **E**thical, legal, and social implications. It has been acknowledged that ethical, legal, and social implications such as potential discrimination, stigmatization, and psychosocial consequences form part of the assessment of the overall utility of a test [8, 19], and there has been a trend away from regarding them as a separable set of issues. The *analytical* *validity* is the means by which an assay is evaluated. It is defined as the assay's ability to measure accurately (in the case of a genetic test) the genotype of interest. It is important to define the genotype precisely. *Clinical validity* is the ability of a test to diagnose or predict a specific phenotype (usually, a specific disease); here, the reference standard is a clinical one. Parameters such as sensitivity, specificity, positive and negative predictive values, likelihood ratios, and the receiver operating characteristic (ROC) curve can be measured as diagnostic test performance. *Clinical utility* refers to the likelihood that a test will lead to an improved health outcome, by way of reduced mortality or morbidity or improved health care. Factors that may be considered include the clinical risks and benefits of testing, such as the availability of an effective intervention and the risks associated with any interventions [4, 6, 7], and health economic assessment. Clinical utility has proved very difficult to assess in practice, with Burke and Zimmern using criteria based on Donabedian's work on the quality of medical care to orientate the clinical utility evaluation [13, 14].

The full evaluation of a genetic test is a complex process that requires significant resources. Because it is not possible to apply the full process to all tests, different levels of evaluation may be applied, depending on the nature of the test, its purpose, and the population in which it is to be carried out. For example, most tests for rare disorders require a less stringent programme of evaluation than tests for common disorders or population screening. This is because, when penetrance is high, the association between a positive test and ultimate outcome is more predictable, and the rarity of the condition means that the number of tests will be small.

In the USA, an ongoing model initiative of the CDC, the Evaluation of Genomic Applications in Practice and Prevention [16], is spearheading the integration of various models of genetic test evaluations, including in-depth assessments and fast-track evaluation.

Evidence-Based Classification of Recommendations on Use of Genomic Tests in Practice

As the number of genetic tests increases, the task to evaluate the available evidence has become ever more challenging and data- and labour-intensive, suggesting a need for a system to classify genomics applications with a view to their readiness for public health action. Those who produce evidence (e.g. genomics test providers, scientists) and those who evaluate evidence (e.g. public health practitioners, regulatory scientists, social scientists) need to maintain an analytical distance for credibility and impartiality of decisions to transition (or not) candidate genomics applications to practice. The range of evidence taken into consideration may include prospective randomized controlled trials (RCTs) but often extend beyond so as to include observational and user-driven qualitative evidence, particularly on clinical utility of genomics tests. In addition, the existing binary (up or down) evidence-based recommendation for use of genomics tests often returns 'insufficient evidence' of clinical validity and utility for their use in clinical practice. The problem of insufficient evidence is not unique to genomics tests but is exacerbated by the lack of comparative effectiveness research [27, 28]. Binary or insufficient evidence recommendations do not permit refined decision-making, especially for clinicians who need to provide advice in the face of insufficient evidence. Khoury et al. [29] have recently suggested a three-tier evidence-based classification of recommendations for use of genomic tests:

- Tier 1: 'Use in practice'
- Tier 2: 'Promote informed decision-making'
- Tier 3: 'Discourage use'

The intermediate category of promoting informed decision-making is particularly notable because it provides interim guidance for clinical and public health practice. The framework for assigning genomics applications to one of the above three tiers requires consideration, in the context of intended use, of the analytic validity, clinical validity, and clinical utility of the test, and the existence of an evidence-based recommendation.

Tier 1 applications demonstrate analytic validity, clinical validity, clinical utility, and there are evidenced-based guidelines encouraging their use.

Tier 2 applications demonstrate analytic and clinical validity, display potential for clinical utility (e.g. well-designed trials with appropriately selected endpoints are known to be in progress), but there are no evidence-based guidelines recommending clinical use.

Tier 3 applications have not yet demonstrated adequate analytic validity, clinical validity, or clinical utility, or have demonstrated evidence of harms. The use of such applications is discouraged.

An updated list of the tier 1 genomics applications is available on the US CDC [33] website.

Delivering Genomics Within Health-Care Systems and Services

As public health evolves from a twentieth-century model into one that takes account of twenty-first-century advances in scientific understanding, we will need to update and strengthen the methodological framework for public health interventions as well as develop a more rigorous approach to ranking competing health care interventions. Public health comprises a range of interventions which act variously upon individuals and upon populations. An integrated approach which takes into account interventions at all these levels seems to be necessary to optimize health gains for the population. Though environmental and social factors continue to be of the greatest importance in the determination of health and disease in populations, public health practice in the twenty-first century can no longer ignore the knowledge derived from genomics, cell and molecular biology; and biological and social models of disease must be regarded as complementary paradigms by public health practitioners in their efforts to improve population health. Ethical considerations demanded that where effective interventions existed, patients should not be deprived of these just by virtue of the fact that they had a rare form of disease. However, it is necessary to be mindful of the costs and benefits of competing interventions in order to prioritise services; comparative effectiveness research has recently emerged as a helpful tool.

Within health-care systems, genomic tools are already used in the prevention, diagnosis, and treatment of disease. To ensure effective and efficient development will however require modification to the organisation of health-care services. In some clinical areas, this may build on the considerable expertise in specialist genetics services, which will be well placed to show substantial leadership. The role of new genomic technologies in clinical specialties such as cancer, haematology, and infectious diseases must be explored, including, in all cases, consideration of how the necessary massive expansion of bioinformatics support can be developed and sustained. Any strategy should explicitly address how clinical and laboratory personnel can be trained and employed, so to retain expertise and competence while enabling increases in capacity. This may involve reconfiguration of laboratories, clinical services, and their supporting systems. This is already starting within the UK's National Health Service, where the 100,000 genomes project is being used as a driver for genomic and personalized medicine, and for a reconfiguration of laboratories so as to be able to use whole genome sequencing and other genome-based technologies more efficiently for patient benefit. The potential for genomics to improve public health systems was thought to be relatively modest in the short term. However, the possibility that in the medium and longer term, genomics might play a more substantive role in public health systems suggests that a strategic review needs to be taken now to assess what infrastructure might be needed to prepare for future developments. This could run in parallel with the work on health systems, with experience being shared in the two areas. For both, effective change management will also require engagement with health-care professionals and the public.

Public Health Genomics, Infectious Diseases, and Vaccinomics

Infectious Disease

The complete genomes of many important human pathogens have been sequenced, including those of the organisms implicated in tuberculosis, malaria, plague, leprosy, diphtheria, cholera, and typhoid. Genomic information is being used to develop new diagnostics, vaccines, and drug treatments [34]. Pathogen genomics is already on CDC's top five list for 2013, and it is noteworthy on the PHG list. While the prospects for using human genome-based testing in clinical care and prevention are exciting, the emergence of powerful sequencing and bioinformatics tools has completely changed the landscape in the public health fight against infectious diseases. There are numerous applications for pathogen genomics, including diagnosing infection, investigating outbreaks, describing transmission patterns, monitoring antimicrobial resistance, and developing interventions such as vaccines. The new field of metagenomics promises to uncover entire communities of microorganisms, often including species never before cultured in the laboratory, that may be detected and characterized, opening the door to understanding the role of environmental, animal, and human microbiomes in health and disease.

The process of infection involves not just the pathogen genome but also that of the host organism. The genomes of human populations have co-evolved with those of the pathogens that infect them, and resistance or susceptibility to infection has been a strong selective pressure in human evolution. A wide range of human genes, including the highly polymorphic genes of the immune system, is involved in human responses to pathogens. In some cases, a single genetic variant appears to be significantly associated with susceptibility or resistance to a disease. For example, a specific polymorphism in the gene encoding the cell-surface receptor molecule CCR5 is associated with resistance to infection by human immunodeficiency virus (HIV). Analysis of genomic variants in resistant individuals may suggest new mechanisms and targets for drug development, or strategies for enhancing protective immunity in exposed populations.

In 2013, CDC launched the Advanced Molecular Detection initiative, which aims to build critical molecular sequencing and bioinformatics capacities at national and state levels to support public health efforts to control infectious diseases.

Examples of public health benefits resulting from these enhanced capacities include more rapid and accurate disease diagnoses and enhanced recognition of antimicrobial resistance, enabling better targeting of prevention and treatment measures (e.g. quickly identifying infections and their susceptibility or resistance to antibiotics); improved surveillance information on the transmissibility of infections and the extent and spread of outbreaks, leading to faster and more effective control efforts.

Vaccinomics

Vaccines are the most powerful measures to prevent the burden of infectious diseases, and represent the greatest successes in the history of public health, especially for microbial pathogens that are unable to evade the host immune detection and/or do not exhibit extensive variability. Vaccinomics is a rapidly emerging frontier in genomics medicine and twenty-first-century public health. Although immune response to vaccines can be influenced by several parameters, host immune genetic variations and host–pathogen interactions are thought to strongly influence the variability in vaccine responsiveness. Immune responses to vaccines are known to be influenced by several parameters, but host genetic variations are recognized as main culprits for variable vaccine responsiveness among vaccine recipients. Even with standard immunization schedules, for example, 5–10 % and 2–10 % of healthy individuals fail to respond to hepatitis B or measles vaccine, respectively. Although the genetic control of both humoral and cellular immune responses to vaccines remains largely unknown, immunogenetics studies revealed that single-nucleotide polymorphisms (SNPs) in human leucocyte antigen (HLA) class I and class II, cytokine, cytokine receptor, and innate immune response (e.g. toll-like receptor) genes may in part account for the inter-individual variability with respect to the markers of vaccine-induced protective immunity, including neutralizing antibodies.

In a recent analysis of the new field of vaccinomics, Bernstein et al. (2011) [2] noted 'despite the historic successes of vaccines, or perhaps because of these successes, vaccinology has evolved to rely almost entirely on an empirical, trial-and-error process, in which the pathways to protective immunity remain largely unknown'. Enabled with systems-oriented omics health technologies, vaccinomics offers unprecedented promise to transform vaccine R&D and health promotion in twenty-first century, with novel vaccines for common infectious pathogens (e.g. tuberculosis, HIV, malaria) as well as therapeutic vaccines for non-communicable diseases (NCDs;). By virtue of broad applications in both preventive and therapeutic contexts, vaccinomics brings about a broadening in the scope and ethos of vaccine-based health interventions. The US NIH Clinical Trials registry identifies over 20 clinical trials at phase III stage for therapeutic cancer vaccines [31]. The first therapeutic cancer vaccine (Sipuleucel-T) for castration-resistant prostate cancer was approved by the US Food and Drug Administration (FDA). The US National Comprehensive Cancer Network recognized this agent as a category 1 (highest recommendation) in 2010 [31].

A recent systematic reviews and meta-analyses synthesized the knowledge on the association of allelic variants or SNPs within immune response gene regions with vaccine responses in humans. While results showed that individuals with a particular HLA allelic composition are more likely to respond efficiently to vaccines, authors suggested that in future larger and collaborative studies should be encouraged to further elucidate the link between genetic variation and variability of the human immune response to vaccines.

Challenges

The potential of genomics to improve human health has been overstated in the past, and this hype has contributed to a lack of clarity and transparency about what PHG is capable of delivering in the future. Realistic expectations for what genomics will achieve in the next decade or so are likely to include the identification of specific genetic tests that are useful in clinical care (of which at present the most promising are in inherited disorders, cancer care, infectious diseases, and pharmacogenetics). The most effective agenda for public health in an age of personalized medicine involves multiple strategies.

First, a sustained drive to collect relevant evidence about the scientific and clinical validity and utility of genomics approaches, so that effective comparisons can be made with other public health interventions, and to make this available to citizen, patient, and physician alike. The requirement for a sound evidence base also applies to other clinical and public health interventions, for which evidence may also be weak or non-existent [8].

Second, to focus pragmatically upon areas which can make a real difference to population health. In the short term, this is likely to involve targeting single-gene disorders, and inherited subsets of common complex disorders. Early benefits are also likely in infectious diseases and pathogen sequencing. The sequencing of cancer genomes and the identification of specific driver mutations that can lead to targeted therapies will lead to improvements in cancer survival. It was recognized that even where evidence of utility is lacking, that there may still be independent indirect benefits of investing in these technologies (such as increased knowledge of disease pathology and building technical expertise).

Third, in both the developed and the developing world, public health professionals must be prepared for the impact genomics will have on their practice [1, 5, 23]. In addition, a working knowledge of basic genetics, they will need an understanding of human genome epidemiology and the criteria for evaluation of genetic tests, and an appreciation of the ethical, legal, psychosocial, and policy dimensions of applications of genomics and genomic technologies. A set of competencies in genomics for the US public health workforce has been developed [9]. Competencies are documented for the workforce as a whole and for specific groups, including leaders/administrators, clinicians, epidemiologists, health educationalists, laboratory staff, and environmental health workers. In addition, some individuals will require an in-depth knowledge of PHG, for example, those involved in screening and other preventive programmes, health service development and evaluation, public health education, and policy analysis and development. Educational programmes in PHG are already underway at some centres.

And fourth, to understand the tension between the long-term promise that must eventually come from our increased scientific knowledge of the genome and molecular mechanisms at a cellular level, and the hype of associated premature interventions presented to health-care funders and providers as well as individual citizens. Public health practice must engage with this new scientific agenda and give it some priority over the coming years.

Conclusions

Genomics is already having an impact on all areas on medicine, and will undoubtedly do it in an increasing fashion. New technologies that enable rapid and inexpensive sequencing of whole genomes promise to improve the ability to identify genetic mutations responsible for single-gene disorders, as well as genetic polymorphisms able to profile each individual subject. We should be alert to the unjustified hype, but also to developments that offer clear, evidence-based benefits. A key element of such evidence would be a better understanding of the relationship between genetic risk information and health-related behaviour.

In the course of these important changes brought upon by new genomics technologies and conceptual frameworks, PHG must take on the 'steering' role for the long haul as knowledge strands converge and coalesce from public health and data-intensive genomics sciences [12, 15, 21, 37]. However, there is a need now to establish integrated and inter-generational capacity for both discovery and infrastructure science for the decades ahead. Leadership, sharing of resource, and knowledge through international networks such as the PerMed [32], programmes of professional education and training, and engagement with public policy development for genomics will all contribute to timely progress. Health systems, especially those parts relating to pathology services, will also need to be re-engineered to take account of the new knowledge and technologies deriving from genomic science.

Public health practitioners have a responsibility to ensure that genome-based testing and interventions are evidence based and ethically applied to benefit the health of individuals and populations. In this senses, PHG should bring modern biology and science to public health to address population heterogeneity in disease and health intervention outcomes. Absent such knowledge, we risk a public health practice that delivers inadequate and suboptimal responses to the extant disease burden in the population, not to mention health interventions such as drugs and vaccines with poor safety and effectiveness. In a situation where there is a profound gap between our ability of interrogating the human genome, and the ability to use that information to improve health, public health practitioners should take a more active role and embrace the changes by welcoming the innovation and the personalization of health care to ensure that it works for the benefit of population health [3].

References

1. Austin MA, Peyser PA, Khoury MJ (2000) The interface of genetics and public health: research and educational challenges. Ann Rev Public Health 21:81–89
2. Bernstein A, Pulendran B, Rappuoli R (2011) Systems vaccinomics: the road ahead for vaccinology. OMICS 15(9):529–531
3. Boccia S (2014) Why is personalized medicine relevant to public health? Eur J Public Health 24(3):349–50
4. Burke W (2002) Genetic testing. N Engl J Med 347:1867–1875
5. Burton H (2003) Addressing genetics, delivering health. Public Health Genetics Unit, Cambridge
6. Burke W, Zimmern R (2007) Moving beyond ACCE: an expanded framework for genetic test evaluation. Paper prepared for the UK Genetic Testing Network.
7. Burke W, Atkins D, Gwinn M et al (2002) Genetic test evaluation: information needs of clinicians, policy makers, and the public. Am J Epidemiol 256:311–318
8. Burke W, Burton H, Hall AE et al (2010) Extending the reach of public health genomics: what should be the agenda for public health in an era of genome-based and "personalized" medicine? Genet Med 12(12):785–791
9. Centers for Disease Control and Prevention: website. http://www.cdc.gov/genomics/about/reports/2001.htm. Accessed 31 March 2014
10. Chowdhury S, Dent T, Pashayan N et al (2013) Incorporating genomics into breast and prostate cancer screening: assessing the implications. Genet Med 15(6):423–432

11. Claassen L, Henneman L, van der Weijden T, Marteau TM, Timmermans DR (2012) Being at risk for cardiovascular disease: perceptions and preventive behavior in people with and without a known genetic predisposition. Psychol Health Med 17:511–521
12. Davey SG, Ebrahim S, Lewis S, Hansell AL, Palmer LJ, Burton PR (2005) Genetic epidemiology and public health: hope, hype, and future prospects. Lancet 366:1484–1498
13. Donabedian A (1978) The quality of medical care. Science 200:856–864
14. Donabedian A (2005) Evaluating the quality of medical care. Milbank Q 83:691–729.
15. Dove ES, Faraj SA, Kolker E, Ozdemir V (2012) Designing a post-genomics knowledge ecosystem to translate pharmacogenomics into public health action. Genome Med 4(11):91
16. Evaluation of Genomic Applications in Practice and Prevention (EGAPP): Implementation and Evaluation of a Model Approach: website. http://www.egappreviews.org/default.htm. Accessed 31 March 2014
17. Evans JP, Berg JS, Olshan AF, Magnuson T, Rimer BK (2013) We screen newborns, don't we?: realizing the promise of public health genomics. Genet Med 15:332–334
18. GAPP Finder by CDC's Office of Public Health Genomics: website. http://64.29.163.162:8080/GAPPKB/topicStartPage.do. Accessed 31 March 2014
19. Grosse SD, Khoury MJ (2006) What is the clinical utility of genetic testing? Genet Med 8:448–450
20. Haddow J, Palomaki G (2004) ACCE: a model process for evaluating data on emerging genetic tests. In: Khoury M, Little J, Burke W (Eds) Human genome epidemiology. Oxford University Press, Oxford, p 217–233
21. Halliday JL, Collins VR, Aitken MA, Richards MP, Olsson CA (2004) Genetics and public health – evolution, or revolution? J Epidemiol Community Health 58:894–899
22. Holtzman NA and Watson MS (1997) Promoting safe and effective genetic testing in the United States. Final report of the Task Force on Genetic Testing, http://www.genome.gov/10001733. Accessed 31 March 2014
23. Hotez PJ (2011) New antipoverty drugs, vaccines, and diagnostics: a research agenda for the US President's Global Health Initiative (GHI). PLoS Negl Trop Dis 5:e1133
24. Janssens ACJW, Khoury MJ (2006) Predictive value of testing for multiple genetic variants in multifactorial diseases: implications for the discourse on ethical, legal and social issues. Ital J Public Health 4:35–41
25. Janssens ACJW, van Duijn CW (2008) Genome-based prediction of common diseases: advances and prospects. Hum Mol Genet 17(R2):R166–173
26. Janssens ACJW, Pardo MC, Steyerberg EW, van Duijn CM (2004) Revisiting the clinical validity of multiplex genetic testing in complex disease. Am J Hum Genet 74:585–588
27. Khoury MJ, Coates RJ, Evans JP (2010a) Evidence-based classification of recommendations on use of genomic tests in clinical practice: dealing with insufficient evidence. Genet Med 12:680–683
28. Khoury MJ, Feero WG, Valdez R (2010b) Family history and personal genomics as tools for improving health in an era of evidence-based medicine. Am J Prev Med 39(2):184–188
29. Khoury MJ, Bowen MS, Burke W et al (2011) Current priorities for public health practice in addressing the role of human genomics in improving population health. Am J Prev 40:486–493
30. Kroese M, Zimmern RL, Sanderson S (2004) Genetic tests and their evaluation: can we answer the key questions? Genet Med 6:475–480
31. O'Meara MM, Disis ML (2011) Therapeutic cancer vaccines and translating vaccinomics science to the global health clinic: emerging applications toward proof of concept. OMICS 15(9):579–588
32. Personalized Medicine 2020: website. http://www.permed2020.eu/index.php. Accessed 31 March 2014
33. US Centers for Disease Control and Prevention website: http://www.cdc.gov/genomics/gtesting/tier.htm. Accessed date 31st March 2014

34. Warnich L, Drögemöller BI, Pepper MS, Dandara C, Wright GE (2011) Pharmacogenomic research in South Africa: lessons learned and future opportunities in the rainbow nation. Curr Pharmacogenomics Person Med 9:191–207
35. Yang Q, Khoury MJ, Botto L, Friedman JM, Flanders WD (2003) Improving the prediction of complex diseases by testing for multiple disease susceptibility genes. Am J Hum Genet 72:636–649
36. Zimmern RL (2011) Genomics and individuals in public health practice: are we luddites or can we meet the challenge? J Public Health (Oxf) 33(4):477–482
37. Zimmern RL, Khoury MJ (2012) The impact of genomics on public health practice: the case for change. Public Health Genomics 15:118–124

Chapter 15
Health Impact Assessment: HIA

Roberto Falvo, Marcia Regina Cubas and Gabriel Gulis

HIA Definition

What is Health Impact Assessment?

Health impact assessment (HIA) could be defined as a combination of procedures, methods and tools by which a policy, a programme or a project may be judged as to its potential effects on the health of a population and the distribution of those effects within the population [1]. HIA identifies appropriate actions to manage those effects [2].

HIA can be considered as a multidisciplinary and comprehensive governance tool in a wider Health in All Policies vision, as reaffirmed during the Finnish presidency of the European Union [3, 4]:

- HIA involves working with a range of decision-makers and stakeholders to support the building of healthy public policy (*multidisciplinary*).
- It studies upstream health determinants in an integrated way, rather than concentrating on single risk factors, and is a resource for environment and health risk governance (*comprehensive*).

R. Falvo (✉)
Section of Hygiene, Institute of Public Health, Università Cattolica del Sacro Cuore,
Largo. go F. Vito 1, 00168 Rome, Italy
e-mail: falvoroberto@gmail.com

M. Regina Cubas
Pós-Graduação em Tecnologia em Saúde, Pontifícia Universidade Católica do Paraná,
Rua Imaculada Conceição, 1155, CEP 80215-901 Curitiba, PR, Brazil
e-mail: m.cubas@pucpr.br

G. Gulis
Unit for Health Promotion Research, University of Southern Denmark,
Niels Bohrs Vej 9-10, 6700 Esbjerg, Denmark
e-mail: ggulis@health.sdu.dk

S. Boccia et al. (eds.), *A Systematic Review of Key Issues in Public Health*,
DOI 10.1007/978-3-319-13620-2_15

- It aims to *identify what potential changes in health determinants might result from a new policy or project.*
- It contributes to *reduce health inequalities* by informing policy makers about the potential impacts of a proposed policy on different population groups.

According to the International Association of Impact Assessment (IAIA) and the World Health Organization (WHO), the principles and values that inspire the HIA are the following [2–5]:

- *Democracy:* allowing people to participate in the development and implementation of policies, programmes or projects that may impact on their lives. The HIA method should then involve and engage the public and inform and influence decision-makers.
- *Equity:* HIA assesses the distribution of impacts from a proposal on the whole population, with a particular reference to how the proposal will affect vulnerable people.
- *Sustainable development:* both short and long-term impacts are considered to meet the needs of the present generation without compromising the ability of future generations to meet their own needs.
- *Ethical use of evidence:* the best available quantitative and qualitative evidence must be identified and used in the assessment. A wide variety of evidence should be collected using transparent and rigorous methods and recommendations should be developed impartially.
- *Comprehensive approach to health:* emphasizing that physical, mental and social well-beings are determined by a broad range of factors from all sectors of society (known as the wider determinants of health).

Typologies of HIA

According to the moment in which the HIA is conducted, it is possible to identify three main typologies of HIA: *prospective* (before a policy is implemented), *concurrent* (during the implementation of a policy) and *retrospective* (after a policy has been implemented) [6]. Performing a prospective HIA may maximize beneficial effects and minimize any harmful effect on health, whereas through a concurrent HIA, it would be possible to act promptly to counter any negative effect associated with the implementation of the proposal and to monitor the accuracy of predictions about potential health impacts; a retrospective HIA would be useful for the development of future proposals and HIA analysis [7].

According to the HIA definition stated before, HIA relates to prediction, so concurrent and retrospective HIA should be considered more appropriately as monitoring and evaluation analysis [8]. According to the availability of time and resources, the appraisal of the potential health effects/impacts and the duration of the analysis, HIAs can be also classified as: *Mini* (rapid), *Standard* (intermediate) or *Maxi* (comprehensive) [9, 10] (see Table 15.1).

Table 15.1 Typologies of HIA according to duration and availability of resources. (The Authors 2013)

	Mini HIA	Standard HIA	Maxi HIA
	Rapid	Intermediate	Comprehensive
Duration	Days or weeks (1–6)	Months (>3)	>6 months–year
Resources	Limited	Sufficient	Available
Costs	Limited	Contained	High
Methodology	Restricted panel of experts, decision-makers and representatives of those potentially affected by the proposed policy sharing existing knowledge and experiences Usually there is no participation of people affected	Requires a broad range of multidisciplinary expertise and a combination of various methodologies Review of the available evidence, exploration of the opinions, experience and expectations of those who may be affected are included and, if needed, an analysis of new data is provided	It implies a more in-depth examination and the participation of the full range of stakeholders An extensive literature search, a secondary analysis of existing data and the collection of new data are provided

HIA health impact assessment

Table 15.2 HIA steps (WHO 2013 [11])

No	Phase	Explanation
1	*Screening*	Determining whether an HIA is valuable and feasible
2	*Scoping*	Identifying what to do and how to do it
3	*Appraisal*	Identifying health hazards and considering evidence of impact
4	*Reporting*	Synthesize and communicate findings; develop recommendations
5	*Monitoring*	Verify whether the HIA has influenced the decision-making process

The Steps of HIA

Generally, HIAs include five sequential phases that together define the HIA procedure [11] (Table 15.2):

Phase 1: Screening (HIA Yes or Not?)

Screening should be the *starting point* of an HIA but due to resource and organizational issues, it is used only when an organizational commitment to HIA is present (basically when a management allows time and resources to screen each project, policy or programme). Major economic outcome and epidemiological issues should be assessed and criteria to be followed in order to decide whether to proceed with an HIA or not [12] (see Fig. 15.1):

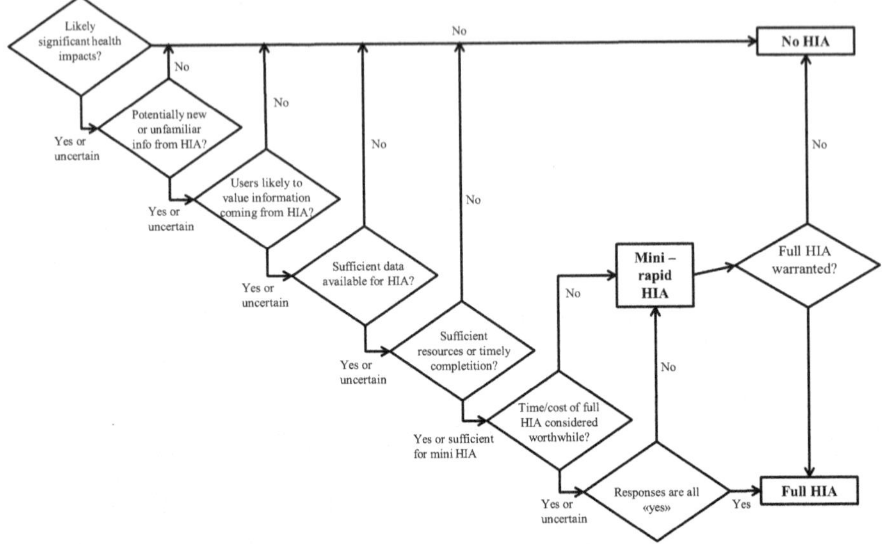

Fig. 15.1 Screening algorithm to guide decisions on whether to conduct an HIA [12]. *HIA* health impact assessment

- The significance of potential health impacts: likelihood and magnitude of health impacts
- Value of added information from an HIA: evidence to support the analysis
- Feasibility of conducting an HIA: availability of resources in terms of money, time, personnel, etc.

Ideally, steps for screening could be the following:

1. Define the policy, programme or project to be analyzed.
2. Identify screening tools to use (e.g. checklists). Review criteria for selection (including general HIA screening criteria and additional criteria relevant to a particular policy, locale or agency).
3. Team members evaluate the proposed HIA on each of the screening criteria and document their conclusions.
4. Make a preliminary assessment on whether to proceed with HIA.
5. Review decision and supporting documentation with stakeholders.

Phase 2: Scoping (What to do, How to do It)

This phase involves determining health issues for analysis, individuating the temporal and spatial boundaries for the appraisal of health impacts and defining research questions and methods. It establishes firm foundations for the subsequent appraisal phase and it is commonly brought forward by a steering group. Key tasks involved in scoping are also agreeing the way in which the appraisal will be managed; allocating responsibility for decision making and agreeing how to monitor and evaluate the HIA process and outcomes [13].

Phase 3: Appraisal (Assessment of Health Effects)

It refers to the use of data, expertise and qualitative and quantitative research methods in order to judge the magnitude and likelihood of potential health impacts, identifying appropriate mitigations and designing alternatives. Impact analysis should proceed using a logical, replicable sequence as shown in the example below [14]:

Task 1: Evaluate and weigh evidence of causal effects

- Utilize empirical literature and literature reviews to understand the nature of the relationship between the decision, health determinants and health effects
- Evaluate whether evidence demonstrates a cause and effect relationship and assess the generalizability of the evidence
- Conduct original research (e.g. surveys, interviews, focus groups, epidemiologic analysis) in affected communities, if needed

Task 2: Collect and synthesize data on baseline conditions

- Enumerate and characterize the affected population in the area affected by the decision
- Identify measurable indicators for health determinants and health outcomes, and access and synthesize existing data on these determinants and outcomes

Task 3: Forecast health effects quantitatively where feasible

- Identify suitable prediction models (e.g. exposure response functions, regression equations)
- Evaluate whether data are available to estimate effects quantitatively
- Compute estimated health effects for each decision alternative, based on the prediction model, baseline conditions and changes in risk or resilience factors

Task 4: Characterize expected health effects

- Characterize the likelihood, severity, magnitude and distribution of health effects for each decision alternative, using causal models, empirical evidence, the baseline conditions assessment and quantitative forecasting tools

Task 5: Evaluate the level of confidence or certainty in health effect characterizations

- Judge the confidence in the effect characterization, considering data limitations and assumptions with regard to population enumeration, exposure assessment, exposure assignment, evidence for cause and effect relationships, validity of dose response function and unmeasured mediating factors
- Evaluate how alternative assumptions may alter effect estimates and characterizations

Table 15.3 Modification of pending decisions according to health, equity, community aspects, inputs. (Adapted from Wismar et al. 2007 [16])

Yes	Direct effectiveness	General effectiveness
Health/equity/community adequately acknowledged	HIA-related changes in the decision Project is dropped due to the HIA Decision was postponed	Reasons provided for not following HIA recommendations Health consequences are negligible or positive HIA has raised awareness among policymakers
NO	Opportunistic effectiveness	No effectiveness
	The decision would have been taken anyway	HIA was ignored or dismissed

Phase 4: Reporting (Sum Up Results, Strategies and Recommendations)

It includes the synthesis of the assessment findings and the communication of results. Usually a report is prepared including the potential impacts and recommendations for enhancing the positive and minimizing the negative effects. The report, disseminated by written forms, media and digital means, is made public to give those who have legitimate interest an opportunity to become acquainted with the content of the report and express their opinion about it [15].

Phase 5: Monitoring (Has the HIA Influenced the Decision-Making Process?)

It is the last but not less important phase, conducted after a decision is taken. It aims to verify whether the HIA has influenced the decision-making process and to assess the accuracy of predictions made during appraisal. It is also very useful since it helps to modify future proposals so as to achieve health gain.

HIA: Effectiveness, Cost-Effectiveness and Sustainability

HIA: Effectiveness and Cost-Effectiveness

The effectiveness of HIA can be measured in terms of capacity to influence decision-making process and modify pending decisions according to health, equity, community aspects and inputs. There are four main types of HIA effectiveness [16] (see Table 15.3):

- *DIRECT effectiveness:* HIA has contributed to a modification in the pending decision.
- *GENERAL effectiveness:* The results of a HIA are taken adequately into consideration by decision-makers, but there is no modification in the pending decision.

- *OPPORTUNISTIC effectiveness:* When an HIA seems to have an effect on the decision, but in fact, it was only initialized because it was expected to support a preferred policy option.
- *NO effectiveness:* HIA was ignored or dismissed.

HIA Sustainability: How Much Does an HIA Cost?

HIAs can be initiated by public health practitioners, community groups and advocacy organizations, affected stakeholders, responsible public agencies or policy-makers who are concerned with the consideration of health in a decision-making process, or with environmental impact assessment (EIA) regulations. The following four are the main sources of sustainability of HIA:

- Government grants
- Public and private foundations
- Fee-for-service funding
- Use of funds by government agencies

The question "How much does an HIA cost?" is *difficult to answer* precisely as the nature of specific policies, programmes and projects is so varied (as is the extent of the HIAs proposed for them). Methods are available in the areas of environmental health and, to a lesser extent, traffic accidents, infectious diseases and behavioural factors. The methods are diverse and their reliability and validity are uncertain [17].

HIAs are highly tailored to work with individual budgets so quantification is comparatively rare in HIA; there is no standard cost for conducting one; anyway, costs can be estimated by HIA calculators. It can be estimated that rapid HIAs can cost as little as US$ 10,000 [18] while comprehensive HIAs can cost upwards of US$ 150,000 [19]. Similar costs have been estimated by the Merseyside Guidelines according to which the mean cost of the comprehensive health impact assessment approach of three projects was £ 12,650 (of which £ 10,497 (83 %) represented the actual costs of assessor/support staff time) [20].

The health consequences of a decision can be characterized according to their economic or monetary valuation. Although monetary effects clearly are not health effects themselves, many decision-makers and stakeholders may give substantial consideration to the economic value of effects, and economic valuation of health effects can facilitate comparison with the costs and benefits of competing alternatives [21]. It is important to maintain the distinction between HIA, which provides judgments of health effects, and cost–benefit analysis, which provides a more comprehensive analysis of all economic benefits and costs of a decision; unlike HIAs, cost–benefit analysis aims to provide a "bottom line" evaluation of the value of alternative choices using a common, monetary metric: This assumes that all important effects of a decision, positive and negative, can be valued and expressed adequately in monetary terms [22]. Economic valuation may undervalue some human health and welfare effects or may value the health of different populations differently (e.g. populations not in the labour force or immigrant workers) [23].

Regardless of the advantages, relying exclusively on quantitative estimation in HIA presents some drawbacks. First, quantification has high information requirements given the breadth of health effects potentially considered in HIA. Second, because quantification can be resource-intensive, it may require more time than allowed for the evaluation of a policy, plan, programme or project. Third, a quantitative approach has implications for communicating the process and results to a wider audience because the methods are typically highly technical and include assumptions that may be difficult to communicate outside the technical team [24].

Identification of the Best Practice

Depending on the sociopolitical environment of the place where it is conducted, characteristics of the particular policy questions to which it is applied, disciplinary backgrounds of practitioners and expectations of stakeholders who use its results, HIA has taken on a wide variety of forms. Canada was one of the first countries to develop an HIA within the public policy, particularly, HIA was integrated into existing procedures for EIA [25]. After that, several countries such as Sweden [26], Germany [27], Australia [28] and New Zealand [29] have been trying to introduce HIA into the public policy planning process. In UK, HIA tends to focus on projects rather than broad policies and has placed a strong emphasis on identifying impacts that affect health inequalities and facilitating participatory and inter-sectorial decision making [30]. In USA, although most HIA examples reflect applications in the transportation, housing or urban-planning sectors, there is growing awareness that HIA may play a substantive role in emphasizing the importance of the emerging issues to public health and to policymakers and stakeholders [31–33].

At the moment, HIA has been applied to a wide range of policies, programmes and projects around the world and has had a significant influence on policy making and planning; in fact, a wide array of decisions including some of those made in almost all government sectors on local, state, national and international scales may be appropriate candidates for HIA [34].

A series of completed HIAs can be found on institutional websites, see Table 15.4: Two examples of HIA are reported and summarized below in Boxes 1 and 2.

Table 15.4 HIAs on institutional websites (the Authors 2013)

Institution	Websites
WHO	http://www.who.int/hia/examples/en/
USA	http://www.hiaguide.org/hias http://www.healthimpactproject.org/resources#reports www.cdc.gov/healthyplaces/hia.htm
EU	http://www.euro.who.int/en/what-we-do/health-topics/environment-and-health/health-impact-assessment http://www.health-inequalities.eu/HEALTHEQUITY/EN/tools/health_impact_assessment/
UK	www.dh.gov.uk/hia http://www.apho.org.uk/default.aspx?RID=44538 www.publichealth.ie/eventsandresources/hiapublications
Australia	www.hiaconnect.edu.au/index.htm
Canada	http://www.ncchpp.ca/54/Health_Impact_Assessment.ccnpps
New Zealand	http://www.health.govt.nz/publications/health%20impact%20assessment

Box 1. A Health Impact Assessment of the Healthy Families Act of 2009

Human Impact Partners and San Francisco Department of Public Health, 2009 [35]

Screening:

In Spring 2009, the San Francisco Department of Public Health in collaboration with the Human Impact Partners determined that:

1. The 2009 Healthy Families Act had significant potential to affect the health of the entire population.
2. The legislation could address health disparities associated with income, class and occupational status.
3. An HIA could document the breadth, magnitude and certainty of potential health benefits associated with policies such as paid sick days.
4. An HIA could be completed in a timely manner.
5. The decision-making process would be receptive to an analysis of the health impacts of the proposed legislation.

Scoping:

Based on a preliminary review of health research on paid sick days and comments made in public testimony, the authors identified six hypothetical scenarios that illustrated the potential pathways between paid sick days and health outcomes.

Based upon the scenarios, the authors selected a set of research questions that focused on the evaluation of potential pathways, then developed research methods, workplan and timeline based on available resources.

Assessment:

The HIA was conducted using reviews of existing secondary data sources and empirical literature, analyses of 2007 National Health Interview Survey data and findings from California survey and California and Wisconsin focus groups.

The authors found that more than one third of flu cases are transmitted at schools and workplaces each year and that guaranteed paid sick days would reduce the spread of pandemic and seasonal flu by enabling workers to comply with public health advice if they or their family members show signs of illness.

The study found that 48 % of private-sector workers, 79 % of low-income workers (the majority of whom are women) and 85 % of restaurant workers do not have access to paid job-protected sick days. Researchers found that workers risked losing much-needed wages or possible termination if they stayed at home sick or to care for a sick child, yet risked infecting others if they came to work sick.

According to the Centers for Disease Control and Prevention, nearly 122,000 people fell ill from food-borne disease outbreaks and another 18,030 illnesses occurred in institutional and workplace setting involving an infected food handler between 2003 and 2007. According to the study, infected workers staying at home could reduce the spread of the pandemic flu virus by up to 34 %. However, without preventative strategies like paid sick days, a serious flu outbreak could kill more than two million people.

The HIA acknowledged that although paid sick days would require employers to cover the cost of absence due to illness, there were significant potential savings from reduced disease transmission to other workers and illness-related lost productivity.

Reporting:

Report authors developed a four-page summary of report findings and a full report detailing all stages of the HIA, including detailed descriptions of the methodology used. HIA findings received national attention after one of the report authors testified at a hearing of the US House Committee on Education and Labor on the proposed legislation.

Outcomes:

Before the HIA, the public health value of paid sick days was not broadly recognized.

The HIA resulted in greater attention to this value by the media and policy advocates.

The HIA also was used by policy advocates in advancing paid sick days legislation at the state and local level.

Decision:

The Healthy Families Act of 2009 proposed to guarantee that workers in the USA at firms that employ at least 15 employees accrue at least 1 h of paid sick time for every 30 h worked.

Box 2. Health impacts of transit-oriented development (TOD): Pittsburg Railroad Avenue Specific Plan Health Impact Assessment [36]

Screening

Pittsburg is a small suburb of the San Francisco Bay Area with a population of approximately 60,000. Due to high housing costs in the Bay Area, the more affordable Pittsburg has experienced a surge in population and the need to plan for a higher growth rate than the surrounding community. The City of Pittsburg supports Bay Area Rapid Transit (BART) plans to begin a four-stop extension, including a station at Railroad Avenue, with transit-oriented development (TOD) surrounding each station.

Pittsburg has a large Latino population with incomes slightly lower than surrounding suburbs. The Great Communities Collaborative (GCC), whose members advocate for TOD projects across the Bay Area, chose Pittsburg as a priority projects and one that a health lens could help in terms of improving the project's goals and mitigating any negative health outcomes.

The Plan Under Consideration

The Pittsburg Railroad Avenue Specific Plan includes a new BART station, extending from the current end of one of the lines. The new BART station would be located in the middle of State Highway 4, and would be surrounded by TOD: almost 1600 units of multiunit housing, 450,000 sq. ft of retail and commercial space and pedestrian and bike improvements. All new construction would be within a 1/2-mile of the proposed BART station.

HIA Scoping

The scope was decided in collaboration with the steering committee which included TransForm, a transportation and land use advocacy group, Contra Costa Interfaith Supporting Communities Organizing (CCISCO), and Human Impact Partners, with input from community meetings.

Scoped priority areas for research included housing, livelihood, transportation, retail and services, air quality and noise. Methods included air quality modelling, noise modelling, transportation predictive tools for vehicle trips and BART ridership, retail geographic information system (GIS) mapping with a predictive tool for where a grocery store should ideally go, Pedestrian Environmental Quality Index (PEQI) maps and data analysis and literature review.

Findings

Housing: Not enough affordable housing to accommodate demand; recommended increasing the amount.

Transportation: Increase in BART ridership from the current 8.4–16 % in the project area, an increase in risk of pedestrian injury in the BART station area, an increase in vehicle trips due to increased population but much less in comparison to a non-TOD project for a similar amount of people.

Air quality: An improvement in regional air quality but negative health effects for those living in the station area if no high-quality heating, ventilation, air conditioning (HVAC) system mitigations were included. Findings include a quantitative estimate of percentage increase in hospitalizations and illness.

Noise: Annoyance and sleep disturbance due to freeway and BART noise would affect residents of new housing if no mitigations were included in the design.

Retail: Community has high priority for a grocery store and a site equidistant for station area residents was mapped; retail and public services were quantified.

Jobs: Project area jobs from construction of this 15-year project would improve the health of local residents, particularly if provided for the large proportion of day labourers.

Outcomes and Decisions

The Pittsburg Specific Plan HIA was completed in June 2008. There were many positive outcomes.

The Specific Plan incorporated HIA recommendations for high-quality HVAC systems and noise mitigations. The city also increased the amount of affordable housing included in the project. Later, some Pittsburg residents did not want affordable housing to be built on the basis of air-quality impacts, but the city showed they had followed the HIA's recommendations for air-quality mitigations. Even later, one city councillor proposed to delete one of the affordable housing sites and add a park instead. Residents testified that affordable housing would be better for their health and that, as seniors, they would rather be close to public transportation. The affordable housing site was saved.

The HIA was a successful political tool, as it secured funding for housing and infrastructure improvements. The process improved city staff relationships and partnerships in the community.

Key Elements for Decision-Makers

- HIA is a multidisciplinary and comprehensive tool to support decision-makers in choosing between policies, programmes and projects according to their potential impacts on health of a population as well as on social and environmental issues.
- HIA promotes equity, sustainability and healthy public policy and should be considered as a fundamental tool to be used in the actual socioeconomic context of crisis and limited resources in order to act on determinants of health, such as education, air quality and housing.
- HIA encourages public participation in public policy issues and strategic planning
- HIA is effective and sustainable and may maximize beneficial effects and minimize any harmful effect on health

References

1. European Centre for Health Policy-WHO Regional Office for Europe (1999) Health Impact Assessment: main concepts and suggested approach. Gothenburg consensus paper
2. Quigley R, den Broeder L, Furu P et al (2006) Health Impact Assessment International Best Practice Principles. Special Publication Series Number 5, International Association for Impact Assessment: Fargo USA. http://iaia.org/publicdocuments/special-publications/SP5.pdf. Accessed 20 May 2013
3. Kemm J (2008) Health impact assessment: an aid to political decision-making. Scand J Public Health 36(8):785–788
4. Stahl T, Wismar M, Ollila E, Lahtinen E, Leppo K (2006) Health in all policies: prospects and potentials. Finnish Ministry of Social Affairs and Health, Helsinki
5. WHO (2010) Why use HIA? Values. http://www.who.int/hia/about/why/en/index.html. Accessed 21 May 2013
6. WHO (2010) Glossary of terms used. http://www.who.int/hia/about/glos/en/index.html. Accessed 21 May 2013
7. Taylor L, Gorman N, Quigley R (2003) Evaluating health impact assessment: learning from practice bulletin. Health Development Agency, London
8. Kemm J (ed) (2012). Health Impact Assessment: Past Achievement, Current Understanding, and Future Progress. Oxford: Oxford University Press
9. Furber SE, Gray E, Harris-Roxas BF et al (2007) Rapid versus intermediate health impact assessment of foreshore development plans. NSW Public Health Bull 18(10):174–176. doi:10.1071/NB07076
10. Chilaka MA (2010) Vital statistics relating to the practice of Health Impact Assessment (HIA) in the United Kingdom. Environ Impact Assess Rev 30(2):116–119
11. WHO (2010). Health Impact Assessment (HIA) tools and methods. http://www.who.int/hia/tools/en/. Accessed 21 May 2013
12. Cole BL, Shimkhada R, Fielding JE, Kominski G, Morgenstern H (2005) Methodologies for realizing the potential of health impact assessment. Am J Prev Med 28(4):382–389
13. Bhatia R (2010) A guide for health impact assessment. CDPH 10:17–20. http://www.cdph.ca.gov/pubsforms/Guidelines/Documents/HIA%20Guide%20FINAL%2010-19-10.pdf. Accessed 5 June 2013
14. Bhatia R (2011) Health impact assessment: a guide for practice. Human Impact Partners, Oakland. http://www.humanimpact.org/component/jdownloads/finish/11/139/0. Accessed 5 June 2013
15. SFPHES. http://www.sfphes.org/publications/HIA_Guide_for_Practice.pdf. Accessed 5 June 2013
16. European Observatory on Health Systems and Policies (2007) The effectiveness of health impact assessment: scope and limitations of supporting decision-making in Europe. The Cromwell Press, Trowbridge. http://www.euro.who.int/__data/assets/pdf_file/0003/98283/E90794.pdf. Accessed 6 June 2013
17. Veerman JL, Barendregt JJ, Mackenbach JP (2005) Quantitative health impact assessment: current practice and future directions. J Epidemiol Community Health 59:361–370
18. Jacobson E, DeCoursey WJ, Rosenberg N (2011) The Health-Impact Assessment (HIA): a useful tool. Published as a supplement to Healthy Communities: a resource guide for Delaware municipalities, 2011. http://www.ipa.udel.edu/healthydetoolkit/docs/HIA_Web.pdf. Accessed 6 June 2013
19. Human Impact Organization FAQ. http://www.humanimpact.org/faq#howmuch. Accessed 6 June 2013
20. Scott-Samuel A, Birley M, Ardern K (2001) The Merseyside guidelines for Health Impact Assessment, 2nd edn. IHIA Consortium, Liverpool. http://www.liv.ac.uk/ihia/IMPACT%20Reports/2001_merseyside_guidelines_31.pdf. Accessed 6 June 2013

21. Brodin H, Hodge S (2008) A guide to quantitative methods in Health Impact Assessment. Swedish National Institute of Public Health. http://www†.fhi.se/PageFiles†/6057/R2008-41-Quantitative-Methods-in-HIA.pdf. Accessed 7 June 2013
22. Bhatia R (2010) A guide for Health Impact Assessment. CDPH 10:40–41. http://www.cdph.ca.gov/pubsforms/Guidelines/Documents/HIA%20Guide%20FINAL%2010-19-10.pdf. Accessed 5 June 2013
23. United States Environmental Protection Agency–USEPA–(2000) Guidelines for preparing economic analyses. http://www.dof.ca.gov/research/economic_research_unit/documents/Section%202001%20ISOR%205%20EPA%20Guidelines%20for%20Preparing%20Economic%20Analysis%20EE-0228C-07.pdf. Accessed 5 June 2013
24. O'Connell E, Hurley F (2009) A review of the strengths and weaknesses of quantitative methods used in health impact assessment. Public Health 123(4):306–310
25. Health Canada. EA within a Canadian context. In: Canadian handbook on health impact assessment. Ottawa: Health Canada, 1999:4-1–4-4. Available at: http://publications.gc.ca/collections/Collection/H46-2-99-235E-1.pd
26. Stockholm County Council, Landstingsforbundet (2004). Examples of how to start up and implement health impact assessments (HIA). Stockholm County Council, Southwestern Health District. www.lf.svekom.se/artikel.asp%3FC=900%26A=1327. Accessed 9 June 2013
27. Fehr R (1999) Environmental health impact assessmentevaluation of a ten-step model. Epidemiology 10:618–625
28. Environmental Health Council (2000) Health Impact Assessment Implementation Guidelines, Consultation Draft 2000, Department for Health and Aged Care, Commonwealth of Australia, Canberra. http://www.health.gov.au/pubhlth/strateg/envhlth/hia/. Accessed 7 June 2013
29. Kjellstrom T, Hill S (2002) New Zealand evidence for health impacts of transport. A background paper prepared for the Public Health Advisory Committee. New Zealand National Advisory Committee on Health and Disability. http://nhc.health.govt.nz/system/files/documents/publications/health-impact-transport-phac.pdf. Accessed 7 June 2013
30. Acheson D (1998) Independent inquiry into inequalities in health report. Department of Health, England Stationery Office, London
31. Dannenberg AL, Bhatia R, Cole BL, Heaton SK, Feldman JD, Rutt CD (2008) Use of health impact assessment in the U.S.: 27 case studies, 1999–2007. Am J Prev Med 34(3):241–256
32. Health Impact Assessment Clearinghouse Learning and Information Center (2010). Completed HIAs. University of California, Los Angeles. http://www†.hiaguide.org/hias. Accessed 8 June 2013
33. The Robert Wood Johnson Foundation and The Pew Charitable Trusts (2011) Health Impact Project 2011. http://www.healthimpactproject.org/. Accessed 8 June 2013
34. Harris-Roxas B, Harris E (2011) Differing forms, differing purposes: a typology of health impact assessment. Environ Impact Assess Rev 31(4):396–403.
35. San Francisco Department of Public Health (2009) A health impact assessment of the healthy families act of 2009. Human Impact Partners, Oakland
36. City of Pittsburg (2008) Railroad Avenue Specific Plan HIA. Human Impact Partners, 2008. http://www.hiaguide.org/sites/default/files/PittsburgRRAve.pdf. Accessed 9 June 2013

Chapter 16
Health in All Policies

Agnese Lazzari, Chiara de Waure and Natasha Azzopardi-Muscat

Nowadays, looking at its current state of art, it may be strongly stated that Health in All Policies (HiAP) represents one of the key principles of the European Union (EU) Health Strategy and is recognized as an integral part of all policies at the European level as well as at the global level. As a horizontal, policy-related strategy, HiAP has a high potential for contributing to improved population health but the implementing challenge may find several barriers once into practice. The institutionalization of HiAP within the governmental process, for instance, implies a strong leadership of the health sector in order to make population health a priority of the highest level of government. Evidences from case studies have been reported below to show how various mechanisms can be included and potentially adopted for pursuing the defined strategy for health protection and social gradient improvement. Final key recommendations have been provided for supporting policy makers in effectively implementing HiAP.

A. Lazzari (✉) · C. de Waure
Institute of Public Health, Università Cattolica del Sacro Cuore,
L.go F. Vito 1, 00168 Rome, Italy
e-mail: agneselazzari@gmail.com

C. de Waure
e-mail: chiara.dewaure@rm.unicatt.it

N. Azzopardi-Muscat
Department of Health Services Management, Faculty of Health Sciences,
University of Malta, Msida, Malta
e-mail: natasha.muscat@gov.mt

Department of International Health, CAPHRI School for Public Health
and Primary Care, Maastricht University, Maastricht, The Netherlands

S. Boccia et al. (eds.), *A Systematic Review of Key Issues in Public Health*,
DOI 10.1007/978-3-319-13620-2_16

Definitions of HiAP

HiAP is a policy-related strategy addressing determinants of health which are controlled by policies belonging to different sectors [1]. The HiAP approach relies on the fact that the population health is a product of both health sector activities and social, environmental, and economic factors. The latter may be influenced by policies and actions beyond the health sector which are put in place at all levels of governance, including European, national, regional, and local ones. The goal of HiAP is to improve evidence-based policy making in order to promote the health and well-being of countries. In particular, HiAP is directed to improve the accountability of policy makers for health impacts across all decisions, emphasizing the consequences of public policies on health determinants, and to contribute to sustainable development [2].

Because of its application to policy development and implementation, a possible barrier to HiAP is represented by political factors preventing long-term and shared strategies. The promotion of a "trans-sectoral" approach to policy making as well as the development of strategies and tools to collect and systematically analyze the impact of HiAP actions could be useful to overcome potential barriers and resistances [3].

Current Status

HiAP is by now recognized as a necessary approach at both the European and global level [4].

In Europe, HiAP was formally legitimated as an EU approach in 2006 with the Finnish EU presidency [5, 6] even though the topic of HiAP was tackled by several EU presidencies such as the Portuguese, the German, the British, and the Dutch ones [1]. Furthermore, the need for the integration of health protection in community policies was pointed out in several resolutions of the European Council in the 1990s [7–9]. Nevertheless, the European Commission, which is the only institution able to make initiatives, did not act on the matter so far despite the Council recommendations [6]. Nowadays, HiAP represents one of the key principles of the EU Health Strategy and is recognized as an integral part of all policies at the EU level [1]. Furthermore, HiAP is required by the EU treaties as an approach to be followed in the development of EU policies. Health protection in all policies was signed as a European priority in 1992 first with the Maastricht Treaty which stated that "health protection requirements should form a constituent part of the Community's other policies" [10]. Later on, this statement was strengthened in the Amsterdam Treaty, in particular, article 152 incorporated a strong public health statement, requiring the EU to protect and promote the health of all European citizens. The guarantee of high level of health protection in all policies was also maintained in the Lisbon Treaty which included HiAP in article 168 using similar wording to article 152 of the Amsterdam Treaty [11, 12].

The incorporation of health into EU policy areas with respect to social policy, taxation, environment, education, and research was promoted also by the Directorate of Health and Consumer Protection through project funding.

As suggested by the European Observatory [13], there are several tools useful in order to implement HiAP. They address organizational structures — such as establishing committees, networks, or dedicated organizations/unions; processes—in that planning and setting priority, policy formulation, and joined-up evaluation; finance mechanisms and regulation—such as laws and agreement protocols. The promotion and the strengthening of the use of these tools have received recognition by European governments.

The institutionalization of HiAP within the governmental process implies a strong leadership of the health sector in order to make population health a priority of the highest level of the government.

Furthermore, a formal commitment is envisaged within countries. The implementation of HiAP in governmental processes should depend upon and, at the same time, encourage the interaction between the different sectors of public administration promoting a horizontal management approach [14].

In brief, key findings from literature reviews, qualitative interviews, and institutional recommendations [15] suggest the following top tips for implementing HiAP and ensuring that it functions better than has traditionally been the case: (a) a transparent and clear mandate for HiAP guarantees effectively joined-up government to coordinate policy-making processes; (b) the presence of systematic processes supports the evaluation of all possible interactions across sectors; (c) different interests need to be mediated; (d) mechanisms of transparency, responsibility, and accountability, alongside with engagement into the process have to be developed and maintained; (e) partnerships and trust can be better built through practical integrative initiatives across sectors; and (f) stakeholders outside of government are required to be involved [16].

With reference to this last point, experience with stakeholder engagement has taught that barriers and limits to HiAP are usually heterogeneous and that such engagement may present several strengths and opportunities. Key stakeholder commitment is considered essential for intersectoral action and social participation aimed at positively affecting the social determinants of health, although this approach does not necessary ensure equity to be achieved. A strong awareness of the influence of social determinants of health across all sectors must to be sustained in order to also guarantee equity.

In addition, tight coordination between national–regional–local levels is required and intersectoral action needs a structure to support it, with a specific budget and human resources dedicated to spend time and pay due attention to the project.

On the other hand, strengths can be identified once a legal framework (i.e., a New Public Health Act) is enacted and there is a potential to effect the necessary capacity building on HiAP. Intersectoral work is also taken into account during the planning phase in order to better perform HiAP. The external context, therefore, can contribute to undermine the health protection initiatives with the pressure of the current financial crisis (i.e., budget shortcuts; aggravation of social determinants of health) and the lack of thorough methodology and know-how. On the other hand, the international agenda is increasingly recognizing the importance of social determinants of health, promoting and supporting institutional commitment, as well as other sectors have begun to include health in their intersectoral work. The role of synergies with key tools such as health impact assessment is also to be considered fundamental in encouraging a new model towards social determinants of health approach [15].

In this context, England, Finland, New Zealand, Norway, Sweden, and Québec are leading examples because of the establishment of a cross-departmental collaboration at the highest level of government [13].

At the worldwide level, HiAP was recognized in the World Health Organization (WHO) Adelaide Statement which introduced a strategic approach for governments to take in planning and setting policies, as part of a broader strategy across WHO regional and national members [16].

The awareness of the relevance of a global and strategic approach to health has gradually developed. In 1978, the Alma Ata declaration defined health as a "social goal whose realization requires the action of many other social and economic sectors in addition to the health sector." Later on, the Ottawa Charter on Health Promotion called for health-promoting public policy and supportive environments and underlined the importance of health promoters' action across sectors. The 1997 WHO Conference on Intersectoral Action for Health strived health authorities to establish partnership with other sectors and in 2005 the WHO Commission on Social Determinants of Health encouraged health-promoting policies in education, industrial affairs, taxation, and welfare [17].

From a literature search run until July 2013 on PubMed with the keywords "Health in all policies" OR "HiAP," several case studies or initiatives aimed at promoting HiAP were identified.

In Spain, Franco et al. used the HiAP approach in order to point out a series of policies aimed to prevent and control childhood obesity epidemics [18]. For their relevance and their role with respect to socioeconomic status, gender differences and the work–life balance, authors identified advertising, transportation, built environment, education, and food environment as the main areas to be studied. The authors discussed several actions helpful in order to control obesity such as advertising regulation policies, the building of track for bicycling and walking as well as of recreational areas, the adjustment of school curriculum, the adaption of school cafeteria menus, and the development of policies aimed at making healthy food available at reasonable prices. Also, Israel's National Program to Promote Active, Healthy Lifestyle addressed obesity through an inter-sectoral, interministerial approach which encompassed joint planning, integration in the policy agendas, and budget sharing [19].

In Finland, the need to influence health determinants through sectors beyond the health sector became evident since the early 1970s [20]. In particular, in the 1970s, Finland launched several inter-sectoral actions to change national diets in order to reduce mortality associated with cardiovascular diseases [21]. In 1972, following a report delivered by the Economic Council emphasizing the need for measures outside the health sector, the North Karelia Project was launched. The project led to innovative partnerships with industry in product development and relied on the work of an inter-sectoral advisory board set up by the Ministry of Agriculture and Forestry.

With the political consensus, the government set up a committee—the Coronary Heart Disease Committee—entrusted to make proposals on the practical implementation of recommendations. The Committee had representatives of the Ministries of Social Affairs and Health, of Finance and of Agriculture and Forestry, as well as administrative sectors of the Ministries of Trade and Industry and of Education. The Committee worked on the reduction in consumption of animal-based fat through several actions including tax policies, switching in priority for agricultural production, educational campaigns, and product labeling [20].

In The Netherlands, municipal organizations are entrusted to develop and implement HiAP [22, 23]. Notwithstanding, the level of implementation of HiAP is quite heterogeneous. Most of the municipalities recognize the importance of HiAP and describe it in policy documents but few are carrying out concrete collaboration agreements and structural consultations or are sharing HiAP vision [24]. The regional Public Health Service of South Limburg together with the National Institute on Health Promotion and Disease Prevention developed a coaching program for nine municipals in order to improve HiAP, using obesity as an example. Several initiatives were launched at the strategic, tactical, and operational level. With respect to the first, three regional conferences were held for municipal councilors with a public health portfolio. At the tactical level, managers were informed by the municipal councilors and civil servants about the coaching program, the need for HiAP, and organizational transition in order to facilitate inter-sectoral collaboration. Finally, at the operational level the active learning was stimulated and a masterclass for regional civil servants and Public Health Service professionals was organized with the aim of stimulating inter-sectoral collaboration. At the end of the day, concrete outcomes in terms of HiAP proposals were observed in six out of nine coached municipalities [25].

Another experience carried out in The Netherlands was about the reduction of health inequalities [24]. The National Institute for Public Health and the Environment was committed to analyze opportunities to address health inequalities through the HiAP strategy. On the basis of data derived from the document analysis, 38 out of 153 policy resolutions were identified to have a potential impact on determinants of health inequalities. Resolutions often consisted of a combination of policy measures, projects, and programs and were mostly released by the Ministry of Housing, Communities, and Integration and by the Ministry of the Education, Culture, and Science. Fifteen resolutions were on the enhancement of socioeconomic position; 4 on striving participation of people with health problems; 19 on improving living and working environment and lifestyle; and 4 on accessibility and quality of care. Interestingly, only 11 were inter-sectoral collaboration between the Ministry of Health and other ministries. This aspect allows us to conclude that even though HiAP is officially recognized as a strategic approach to be followed in setting policies and programs, further efforts are needed at European and global levels in order to implement in a practical manner.

Identification of Best Practices

The essence of a healthy population lies in tackling and reducing health and social inequalities. Good health equates with good quality of life, enhances workforce productivity and education, strengthens social relations and safety within the community, promotes behavioral and environmental sustainability, and reduces poverty and social exclusion.

The adoption of the HiAP approach has been offered to governments by WHO as a framework to develop healthy populations, this being a desirable policy achievement for highly developed societies. Stronger coordinated action has been increasingly demanded by key stakeholders and this has reached the top of political agenda at the international level. Yet, key factors such as the financial crisis and the increasingly costs of an infinite demand for health and social care are placing unsustainable burdens on national and local resources. This threatens to undermine further enhancement of the HiAP multifaceted policy approach [16]. Further obstacles derive from the ill-defined boundaries of the many complex interdependencies.

A cooperative mechanism, aimed at promoting a new policy paradigm and innovative solutions beyond sectional and organizational silos, is strongly required to address social gradient improvements avoiding duplication and fragmented actions [16]. Such a complex HiAP policy-making process aimed at health protection, prevention, and promotion has been piloted, challenged, and applied across several countries at different levels (local–national–international). It is undoubtedly supportive to decision makers and leaders providing integrative suggestions and consultations on health, well-being, and equity while defining, applying, and assessing policies and public services [16].

The English experience in tackling health and social inequalities is worth a mention as an interesting example in terms of cross-sectoral methods. This country in fact has been characterized for the broad range of policy initiatives and programs addressing health inequalities, especially since the advent of the Labour Government in 1997. "Reducing health inequalities: an action report" represents the first example of formal recognition of the consistent influence of social policies on the reduction of health inequalities, with measures addressing living standards improvement, the reduction of road traffic accidents, as well as a safe walking environment and the cycling routes diffusion. Additionally, the joint interplay of policy-making processes across different departments has been enhanced under the pressure of the "cross-cutting review" operated by Her Majesty's Treasury. Thus, the resulting health outcomes have been strongly related to diverse sectors and their coordinated actions, gaining more "out-health" outcomes rather than just "in-health" outcomes. Multi-sectoral plans and future priorities for health protection and equity have to be sustained by HiAP and government initiatives have to consider how health inequalities track the social gradient and pursue cross-sectoral work in all areas to promote progress [1].

In this sense, a remarkable experience has been tested by Wales where the government is currently leading a national consultation on whether and how to introduce the HiAP principles to tackle inequalities and better the health of the nation. According to the proposed "mass strategy" approach, healthier public policy would be made statutory and certain public health duties should be made compulsory for public bodies across all sectors (education, social care, housing and working places, transport, environmental and urban planning, etc.). If this plan succeeds, Wales would be the first country to establish a legal obligation for improving health across all non-health sectors; this HiAP duty would be a pioneering and radical action in response to WHO's inputs and definitely a leading best practice that would challenge policy makers all over countries [26, 27].

Such a strategy, indeed, lays on the previous South Australian (SA) Government experiences of the HiAP through the "health lens analysis" approach. This method, used for a set of different areas (i.e., water security, digital technology access), is a key tool that includes also health impact assessment considerations (see *Health Impact Assessment Chapter for further reading*) and provides evaluation results to sustain continuous improvement of policy models, ongoing processes and future policy directions. According to this approach, South Australia has included health in its national strategic plan (so-called SASP) and, above all, it has called for a new outlook of shared governance where public health is an essential element for strategic policy adjustments across all sectors. This implies a mutual contribution, benefiting well-being and health through the other sectors influence and, conversely, using health inputs to gain achievements in other sectors achievements.

An outstanding experience, in this sense, has been recorded with reference to regional migrant settlement in SA, run in 2008 by the Department of Trade and Economic Development in partnership with Multicultural SA and SA Health. A multiple stakeholders commitment was developed, involving participants from different departments (Department of Education and Children's Services; Department of Premier and Cabinet and Department of Further Education, Employment, Science and Technology) in order to promote population growth in regional areas of South Australia through overseas migration programs. The health lens application to settlement services and the reported assessment brought about new and more complete understandings of migrant settlement dynamics (conceptual learning). The interaction between the socioeconomic and health factors impacting on migrant settlement emerged and led the involved stakeholders to a better understanding and redefinition of their top agenda priorities (social learning). All participants' positive attitude toward HiAP, favored by an initial engagement process and an early establishment of partnership processes, resulted in a unified vision and shared language, key elements for driving and supporting further intersectoral work, model, and policy processes [28, 29].

Key Elements for Decisions Makers

HiAP is a collaborative approach that has been used internationally to address multi-factorial health and social inequalities. The implementing challenge of HiAP, as described above, has shown how various mechanisms can be included and potentially adopted for pursuing the defined strategy for health protection and social gradient improvement (i.e., health impact assessments, advocacy promotion and preventive campaigns, key stakeholders commitment in policy consultations up to the publication of national policy reports and bills) [6]. In particular, the policy-making processes have witnessed to be effectively supported by different tools, each of them better fitting a different stage of their cycles: establishment of interministerial and interdepartmental committees; use of community consultations; team working action across different sectors; activation of partnership platforms; definition of integrated budgets and accounting; cross-cutting information and evaluation systems; "health lens" analysis assessments and health impact assessments; and set-up of joined-up workforces and definition of legislative frameworks [16]. Anyway, no matter what the tools, as highlighted by evidences review and qualitative interviews [15], policy makers' willingness to implement HiAP is likely to be more successful once they consider the following key areas:

- The *leadership role:* HiAP has to be clearly supported by governments and at the top level of decisional processes. Call and advocacy for HiAP approach has to be exercised by health systems and departments, with an explicit political commitment capable of facing the current reluctance due to the economic crisis.
- *Joined-up governance and clear strategy* to endorse the HiAP approach is suggested. Action plans and an overarching strategy help to better mediate once potential contrasting goals between sectors would raise, define shared achievements across government and finalize the use of resources for specific projects.
- Stakeholders' commitment as well as working with key partners are considered essential for intersectoral action and social participation. Particular attention has to be paid to *partnership promotion* and *stakeholder engagement* that can, indeed, include potential reluctance among different parts to cooperate and team working at the national level and sometimes also integration among private and community services.
- Moreover, there is an evident need to encourage *capacity building* and *technical skills* for managing and implementing HiAP both within and external to the health sector. Softer skills related to conflict resolutions, team working, and integrated communication, in addition to core abilities (i.e., data analysis and interpretation), are capable of supporting the common awareness of health equity.
- *Health equity* remains an elusive concept that needs further data and investigations. Both national and local levels have to be able to appropriately distinguish among health equality and health equity and evidence should better focus on providing good equity examples of HiAP.
- Additionally, a precise *tactic* is a useful technique for a successful implementation of HiAP. A truly cooperative approach would be, then, possible through the

use of "win–win" policies with mutual benefits for health and other areas clearly stated and shared ("Health for All Policies" as well as "Health in All Policies").

- *Culture* and *values* of the implementing context is a key factor, too often not properly considered in the literature and by policy makers. Public health history and tradition can, in fact, strongly affect the way interventionists accept and play the HiAP approach [15].
- Finally, it is clear that there is a need for *research* to strengthen HiAP investigations as well as for policy makers to advocate for it. Multidisciplinary capacities in policy analysis and methods have to be developed and different perspectives taken into account to guarantee a reasonable success of implementation. Furthermore, HiAP has to move from rhetoric to action and reports and follow-up on the concrete outcomes of implementing HiAP are ultimately required [30].

References

1. Ståhl T, Wismar M, Ollila E, Lahtinen E, Leppo K (eds) (2006) Health in all policies. Prospects and potentials. Ministry of Social Affairs and Health, Helsinki. http://ec.europa.eu/health/archive/ph_information/documents/health_in_all_policies.pdf. Accessed 30 Nov 2013
2. WHO (2013) Working definition prepared for the 8th global conference on health promotion. Helsinki. http://www.healthpromotion2013.org/health-promotion/health-in-all-policies. Accessed 30 Nov 2013
3. Greaves LJ, Bialystok LR (2011) Health in all policies—all talk and little action? Can J Public Health 102(6):407–409
4. European Portal for Action on Health Inequalities. Health in All Policies (HiAP): EuroHealthNet. http://www.health-inequalities.eu/HEALTHEQUITY/EN/policies/health_in_all_policies/. Accessed 30 Nov 2013
5. Employment Social Policy Health and Consumer Affairs Council of the European Union [EPSCO] Council conclusions on Health in All Policies (HiAP). Brussels, 30 November and 1 December 2006
6. Koivusalo M (2010) The state of health in all policies (HiAP). The European Union: potential and pitfalls. J Epidemiol Community Health 64:500–503
7. European Council (1995) Council resolution of 20 December on the integration of health protection requirements in Community policies, Brussels
8. European Council (1996) Council resolution of 12 November on the integration of health protection requirements in Community policies, Brussels
9. European Council (1998) Council conclusion of 30 April on the integration of health protection requirements in Community policies, Brussels
10. European Commission (1992) Treaty on European Union (Maastricht text). Article 129. Public Health. Official Journal of the European Union C 191/1
11. European Commission (1997) Treaty of Amsterdam amending the Treaty on European Union, the Treaties Establishing the European Communities and Related Acts. Article 152. Public Health. Official Journal of the European Union C 340/1
12. European Commission (2009) Treaty of Lisbon: amending the Treaty on European Union and the Treaty Establishing the European Community. Official Journal of the European Union C 306/1
13. St-Pierre L, Hamel G, Lapointe G, McQueen D, Wismar M (2009) Governance tools and framework for health in all policies: European Observatory on health systems and policies

14. Bekker M (2007) The politics of healthy policies. Redesigning health impact assessment to integrate health in public policy. Eburon, Delft
15. Howard R, Gunther S (2012) Health in all policies: an EU literature review 2006–2011 and interview with key stakeholders. Equity Action.
16. WHO (2010) Adelaide statement on health in all policies. Moving towards a shared governance for health and well-being. Government of South Australia, Adelaide. http://www.who.int/social_determinants/hiap_statement_who_sa_final.pdf. Accessed 30 Nov 2013
17. Kickbusch I (2010) Health in all policies: the evolution of the concept of horizontal health governance. In: Kickbusch I, Buckett DK (eds) Implementing health in all policies. Government of South Australia, Adelaide
18. Franco M, Sanz B, Otero L, Domínguez-Vila A, Caballero B (2010) Prevention of childhood obesity in Spain: a focus on policies outside the health sector. SESPAS Report 2010. Gac Sanit 24(1):49–55
19. Kranzler Y, Davidovich N, Fleischman Y, Grotto I, Moran DS, Weinstein R (2013) A health in all policies approach to promote active, healthy lifestyle in Israel. Isr J Health Policy Res 2(1):16
20. Melkas T (2013) Health in all policies as a priority in Finnish health policy: a case study on national health policy development. Scand J Public Health 41(11):3–28
21. Puska P, Ståhl T (2010) Health in all policies-the Finnish initiative: background, principles, and current issues. Annu Rev Public Health 31:315–328
22. The Council for Public Health and Health Care (RVZ), Council of Public Administration (Rob), Netherlands, Education Council of the Netherlands (2009) Off the beaten track. Advice on cross-sectoral policy. The Hague
23. The Netherlands Ministry of Health. Welfare and sports. Being healthy and staying healthy: a vision of health and prevention (2007). The Hague
24. Storm I, Harting J, Stronks K, Schuit AJ (2013) Measuring stages of health in all policies on a local level: The applicability of a maturity model Health Policy Jun 10
25. Steenbakkers M, Jansen M, Maarse H, de Vries N (2012) Challenging health in all policies, an action research study in Dutch municipalities. Health Policy 105(2–3):288–295
26. Rose G (1981) Strategy of prevention: lessons from cardiovascular disease Br Med J 282:1847–1851
27. Fletcher A (2013) Working towards "health in all policies" at a national level. Wales as a world leader? BMJ 346:1-2
28. Government of South Australia (2010) Final report of the regional migration health lens, Adelaide. www.sahealth.sa.gov.au/healthinallpolicies. Accessed 30 Nov 2013
29. Hurley C, Lawless A (2010) Applying a health lens analysis to regional migrant settlement. Government of South Australia, Adelaide
30. Storm I, Aarts MJ, Harting J, Schuit AJ (2011) Opportunities to reduce health inequalities by 'Health in All Policies' in the Netherlands: an explorative study on the national level. Health Policy 103(2–3):130–140

Index

A

Active ageing, 130, 131, 135, 146, 235
Aged, 24, 26, 37, 47, 59, 81, 91, 98, 100, 101, 110, 114, 116, 131, 132, 137
Anxiety disorders, 206, 207, 209, 210
Asthma, 28, 93, 109–113, 119, 237

B

Best buys, 27, 34, 49, 57, 58
Best practices, 19, 28, 34, 51, 59, 76–83, 97, 105, 112, 113, 117, 135, 178, 234, 282
Breast cancer, 23, 28, 71, 73, 79, 252
Burden of disease, 2, 5, 10, 14, 16, 38, 42–44, 46, 101, 116, 120, 163, 205, 228

C

Capacity building, 279, 284
Cardiovascular diseases (CVD), 5, 19, 20, 30, 33, 35–37, 48, 51, 57, 93, 101, 118, 133, 138, 139, 145, 174, 193, 238
Child accident, 184, 185
Chronic obstructive pulmonary disease (COPD), 20, 27, 114–118, 122
City planning *See* Urban planning, 155
Colorectal cancers, 23, 25, 44, 69, 75, 80
Communicable diseases, 5, 154, 162, 229, 240
Communication, 8, 16, 50, 157, 163, 197, 198, 216, 240, 241, 243, 268, 284
Cost of injuries, 125, 140
Cost-effectiveness, 3, 12, 27, 34, 48, 51, 53–55, 57–59, 81, 113, 122, 135, 234
Culture, 3, 8, 130, 172, 180, 181, 190, 192, 240, 241, 285

D

Dementias, 206, 210, 212, 214
Depressive disorders, 206
Diabetes, 5, 19, 20, 23–26, 28, 33, 37, 43, 45, 46, 91, 98–105
Diarrhoeal diseases, 6, 16
Disease prevention, 25, 51, 154–158, 250, 253
Disparities, 66, 158, 228, 232, 271
Diversity, 105, 130, 195, 197, 198, 200

E

Economic burden, 19, 26, 30, 39, 40, 101, 112
Environmental health, 1, 259, 269
Epidemiologic transition, 133
Epidemiology, 66, 91, 92, 99, 110, 114, 169
Equity, 196, 197, 264
Ethics, 158
Ethnicity, 189, 190

F

Fatalities, 176, 181, 184, 232

G

Genetic tests, 253, 254, 258, 259
Genomic medicine, 250
Genomic profiling, 251
Genomic tests, 251, 255
Global Initiative for Asthma (GINA), 112
Global initiative for chronic Obstructive Lung Disease (GOLD), 114, 117

H

Health equity, 284
Health equity *See also* Equity, 227
Health inequalities, 2, 190, 192, 227, 264, 270, 281, 282

S. Boccia et al. (eds.), *A Systematic Review of Key Issues in Public Health*,
DOI 10.1007/978-3-319-13620-2

Health policy, 2, 3, 49, 59, 93, 101, 200
Health promotion, 51, 55, 146, 154, 155, 158, 239, 258
Health trends, 20
Healthy ageing, 130, 134–136, 138, 142, 145
Healthy cities, 224, 242, 243
Heart disease, 2, 21, 25, 33–35, 37, 42, 139, 251
High-risk prevention, 48
HIV/AIDS, 5, 8, 39, 229
Human Genome Project, 249, 251

I
Indoor air pollution, 119, 122–124, 237
Inequalities *See* Health inequalities, 2
Infectious diseases, 2, 5, 21, 34, 39, 122, 142, 143, 146, 157, 228, 243, 256, 257, 259, 269
Influenza, 13–15, 38, 142, 242
Injuries prevention, 169–172, 176, 180, 184–186, 237
Intervention programs, 93, 141

J
Justice, 154, 155, 165, 166, 212

L
Leadership role, 284
Life expectancy, 2, 29, 34, 120, 130–132, 136, 139, 144, 227, 228, 243
Liver cancer, 23, 28, 66, 72, 73, 81, 82
Longevity, 21, 133, 145, 238
Lung cancer, 23, 24, 43, 68, 69, 72, 75, 76, 79, 109, 118, 119, 122–124, 232

M
Malaria, 6, 15, 16, 39, 256, 258
Monitoring, 2, 8, 49, 95, 96, 102, 113, 119, 154, 172, 174, 257, 264
Morbidity, 2, 5, 19, 22, 38, 53, 59, 112, 118, 119, 133, 137, 138, 145, 156, 157, 207, 226, 243, 254
Mortality, 2, 5, 7, 9, 19, 20, 22, 24, 25, 29, 33, 36–39, 43, 45, 46, 53, 81, 112, 175, 280

N
Non-communicable diseases (NCD), 2, 19, 20, 34, 37, 99, 105, 190, 195, 228, 230, 243

O
Obesity, 70, 89–92, 138
Obstructive sleep apnea syndrome (OSAS), 109, 124, 125
Oldest old, 129, 131, 145, 213, 235, 243
Outdoor air pollution, 119–121, 124, 232, 243
Overweight, 25, 33, 34, 44–46, 49, 53, 54, 70, 80, 89–92

P
Partnership promotion, 284
Personalized medicine, 250
Policy making, 270, 279, 282, 284
Population-wide prevention, 48, 49, 53
Prevalence, 37
Prevention, 49–51, 79–83, 181–185
Prostate cancer, 71, 73, 75, 80, 258
Public health, 158, 159, 165, 256
Public Health Genomics (PHG), 250, 252, 256, 258, 259

R
Research, 200, 253
Respiratory allergies, 20, 110, 113
Respiratory diseases, 19, 20, 92, 109, 110, 120, 229
Responsibility, 142, 154–157, 159–162, 251, 279
Risk assessment, 46
Risk factors, 8, 20, 22–24, 27, 28, 30, 33, 40, 47, 56, 66, 99, 113, 172, 263

S
Safety promotion, 170, 174
Schizophrenia, 206, 210–212
Secondary prevention, 34, 48, 50–52, 56–58, 74, 76, 77, 252
Stakeholder engagement, 284
Stomach cancer, 25, 72, 81
Stroke, 20, 21, 24, 25, 33–35, 37–40, 42, 44, 193
Sustainable ecosystem, 243

T
Technical skills, 284
Tobacco smoke, 27, 49, 109, 111, 113, 118, 122, 124
Translational research, 253
Tuberculosis (TB), 6, 10, 39, 109, 118, 123, 227, 229, 256, 258

U
Urban dwellers, 223, 226, 232
Urban health, 223, 224, 229, 231, 233, 234, 238, 243
Urban planning, 230, 236, 239, 240, 243, 283
Urban population, 196, 224, 226, 227, 242
Urbanization, 100, 224, 226, 230, 234, 242
Uterine cervix cancer, 68, 80

V
Vaccinations, 34, 159, 160, 162
Vaccinomics, 257, 258
Victims, 7, 176, 232

Printed in the United States
By Bookmasters